Clinical Leadership in Nursing and Healthcare

Clinical Leadership in Nursing and Healthcare

Third Edition

Edited by David Stanley

The University of New England
Armidale
NSW, Australia

Clare L. Bennett and Alison H. James

Cardiff University
Cardiff, Wales, UK

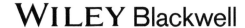

Registered Offices
John Wiley & Sons, Inc., 111 River Street, Hoboken, NJ 07030, USA
John Wiley & Sons Ltd, The Atrium, Southern Gate, Chichester, West Sussex, PO19 8SQ, UK

Editorial Office
9600 Garsington Road, Oxford, OX4 2DQ, UK

For details of our global editorial offices, customer services, and more information about Wiley products visit us at www.wiley.com.

Wiley also publishes its books in a variety of electronic formats and by print-on-demand. Some content that appears in standard print versions of this book may not be available in other formats.

Library of Congress Cataloging-in-Publication Data
Names: Stanley, David, 1960- author. | Bennett, Clare L., author. | James,
   Alison H., author.
Title: Clinical leadership in nursing and healthcare / David Stanley, Clare L.
   Bennett, and Alison H. James.
Description: Third edition. | Hoboken, NJ : Wiley-Blackwell, 2023. |
   Includes bibliographical references and index.
Identifiers: LCCN 2022026724 (print) | LCCN 2022026725 (ebook) | ISBN
   9781119869344 (paperback) | ISBN 9781119869351 (Adobe PDF) | ISBN
   9781119869368 (epub)
Subjects: MESH: Leadership | Nurses–organization & administration | Health
   Services Administration | Nursing–organization & administration
Classification: LCC RA971.35 (print) | LCC RA971.35 (ebook) | NLM WY 105
   | DDC 610.69068/3–dc23/eng/20220727
LC record available at https://lccn.loc.gov/2022026724
LC ebook record available at https://lccn.loc.gov/2022026725

Cover design by Wiley
Cover images: © Govindanmarudhai/Getty Images

Set in 9.5/12.5pt STIXTwoText by Straive, Chennai, India
Printed and bound by CPI Group (UK) Ltd, Croydon, CR0 4YY

C9781119869344_280923

Contents

Notes on Contributors

Dr Judith Anderson - RN, BN, MHSM, MN, PhD.
Judith is a healthcare manager with extensive experience in management, including high-level roles overseeing aged-care services, clinical teams and rural health services. This work has given her skills in people management, change management, education and quality improvement. Judith is a highly motivated and committed academic having achieved over $290 000 in research grant funding. In addition to her national academic profile as an expert in rural nursing, including multi-purpose health services, Judith has assumed several leadership roles in the School of Nursing, Midwifery and Indigenous Health (SNMIH), including Course Director, in which she has overseen the implementation of substantial organisational change within the school; and the accreditation of the Bachelor of Nursing and Master of Clinical Nursing (Nurse Practitioner) Courses. Judith was awarded a Fellowship from the Australian College of Nursing for her contributions to the profession in 2010.

Dr Clare L. Bennett - D.Nurs, SFHEA, PGCE, MSc, BSc (Hons), Dip.N, RGN.
Clare is a Registered Nurse with a background in Immunology, HIV, Infectious Diseases and Sexual Health. She is a Doctor of Nursing and is currently a Senior Lecturer at Cardiff University. She teaches Leadership, Quality Improvement and Patient Safety on undergraduate and postgraduate programmes for nurses and allied health professionals and has conducted realist evaluations of leadership programmes for the Royal College of Nursing, Health Education England and a number of National Health Services (NHS) Trusts in England. Clare is also an honorary lecturer at the University of Freiburg, Germany, where she teaches leadership and research methods. She is an active researcher, teaches research methods and supervises doctoral students. Clare also conducts systematic reviews and teaches and coaches in the field of evidence implementation.

Dr Denise Blanchard - RN PhD.
Associate Professor Denise Blanchard is the Head of Discipline Nursing at the School of Nursing and Midwifery at the University of Newcastle. As the Head of Discipline Nursing, she is accountable for the effective leadership of nursing and provides strategic leadership to the broader university and undertakes a strong engagement role nationally and internationally for nursing. Associate Professor Blanchard combines her extensive experience in

education and leadership with more recent research and policy development to make a research contribution to issues related to aged care and aged-care nursing, self-care for long-term conditions and evidence-based practice. She is recognised for her work with evidence-based healthcare and teaching and learning in the tertiary sector.

Sally Carvalho - FHEA, PG Cert HE, MSc, BSc (Hons), RNT, RGN.

Sally is a Registered Nurse with a practice and leadership background within Emergency Department nursing, NHS nurse-led Walk-in Centre services and General Practitioner Out of Hours care provision. She is a Senior Lecturer at the Three Counties School of Nursing and Midwifery, University of Worcester. Sally has a diverse teaching skillset, but mainly focuses upon teaching pre-registration student nurses, specifically concentrating in the areas of leadership and management in nursing, law, ethics and professional issues.

Dr Tracey Coventry – RN, MW, BSc(Nursing), MNEd, PhD.

Tracey is the Program Coordinator/Senior Lecturer for the University of Notre Dame Australia, Fremantle, School of Medicine Health Leadership programs and a senior leader in mental health, working as a Policy Analyst in an acute Mental Health Service. As previous Postgraduate Coordinator for the School of Nursing and Midwifery, Tracey coordinated postgraduate work integrated learning programs in clinical, mental health and perioperative nursing and on campus programs in nursing. She has many years of experience in the hospital acute care sector in healthcare policy development, student placement and general and paediatric education roles. Tracey completed her PhD on the clinical nurse educator and the influence of the role and leadership specifically related to the graduate nurse. As an active researcher, Tracey is currently engaged in research in health professional education and leadership and supervises PhD and Masters (Research) students.

Dr Sarah Dineen-Griffin - PhD MPharm, GradCertPharmPrac, BBSci, AACPA, MPS.

Sarah has significant experience in clinical roles as a community, hospital, and medicines review pharmacist. She is a Lecturer in Health Management and Leadership at Charles Sturt University in Australia. She completed her PhD in pharmacy practice focusing on consumer self-care and the co-design, evaluation, and implementation of pharmacy services (2020). Dr. Dineen-Griffin has been an investigator on national and international research projects. At an international level, she was elected to the Community Pharmacy Section Executive Committee of the International Pharmaceutical Federation (2021–2025) and is Vice Chair of the International Pharmaceutical Federation New Generation of Pharmaceutical Scientists Group (2019–2022). Sarah is an editorial board member for Research in Social and Administrative Pharmacy and *Pharmacy Practice* journal and has published in international journals. At a national level, she is vice president of the Pharmaceutical Society of Australia NSW Branch (2021–2023), chair of the Early Career Pharmacist Group for the Pharmaceutical Society of Australia NSW Branch (2020–2021) and a member of the National Self-Care Policy Advisory group (2020). Sarah was named the Pharmaceutical Society of Australia NSW Young Pharmacist of the Year (2021). She was recently appointed to the Expert Advisory Committee (the Committee) to lead the Review of the National Medicines Policy by Federal Health Minister Greg Hunt (2021).

Dr Alison H. James - DAHP, SFHEA, PGCE, MA, BA (Hons), Dip Critical Care, RGN.
Alison is a Registered Nurse and Doctor of Advanced Healthcare Practice with a background in Neurosciences, Critical Care, Osteoporosis and Knowledge Transfer consultancy in health and social care. She is a Senior Lecturer at the School of Healthcare Sciences at Cardiff University and teaches Leadership and Quality Improvement on programmes across the nursing and allied health programmes at undergraduate and postgraduate level and is a coach and mentor for student leadership in the UK. Alison's developing research interests lie in the preparation of students for values-based leadership, experiential pedagogies and social justice.

Dr Julie Reis - PhD, BN (Hons), RN.
Julie is a Senior Lecturer in the School of Nursing, Paramedicine and Healthcare Sciences at Charles Sturt University. Julie is passionate about issues relating to health, education, and community. Julie believes strong, healthy, and sustainable communities are critical for quality of life with health and education fundamental to life outcomes. Her beliefs about health and education stem from Primary Health Care philosophy, underpinned by principles of social justice and equity. Julie's professional career includes experience in the health and tertiary education sectors as a clinician, clinical facilitator, and academic. She is a Senior Fellow with the Higher Education Academy in the UK. Julie has also been an elected local government member.

Dr Kylie Russell – PhD, RN
Kylie is the Head of Program Development, Quality and Assessment in the School of Medicine at the University of Notre Dame, Australia. Kylie has held several roles in the School of Nursing and Midwifery, including Postgraduate Coordinator, Associate Dean and Clinical Placement Coordinator. Kylie has over 20 years' experience in Western Australian government health in various roles including Clinical Nurse Manager, Staff Development Educator, Clinical Nurse Consultant, HR Manager, and various project officer roles. Kylie completed her PhD on the impact of belongingness and workplace culture on student clinical learning. Kylie is actively engaged in research, supervises research students, and sits on a number of external research committees and trusts. Kylie is a long-standing mentor to nurse leaders and board member of an NFP residential care provider.

Dr David Stanley, RN, RM, Gerontic Cert, Grad Cert HPE, Dip HE (Nursing),
BN, MSc (Health Sciences), TF, NursD.
David began his nursing career at the Whyalla and District Hospital, South Australia in 1980. These were the final days of PTS (preliminary training school) training and capping ceremonies, and he entered nursing without much thought about its history or future. He completed his training as a Registered Nurse and Midwife in South Australia and worked through his formative career in a number of hospitals and clinical environments. In 1993, he completed a Bachelor of Nursing at Flinders University, Adelaide (for which he was awarded the University Medal) and worked for a short time on Thursday Island before volunteering to teach midwifery for several years in Africa. Following this wonderful experience, he moved to the UK and worked as the Coordinator of Children's Services in York

and as a Nurse Practitioner in the Midlands. He completed a Master of Health Science degree at Birmingham University, and after a short return to Australia, where he worked in Central Australia for Remote Health Services in Alice Springs, he returned to the UK in 2001 to complete his Nursing Doctorate at Nottingham University. There he undertook research in the area of clinical leadership. While he studied, he worked as a Senior Lecturer at University College Worcester (now Worcester University). Returning to Australia in 2006, he worked at several universities in Perth and then Charles Sturt University, NSW, before moving to the University of New England, where he was a Professor in Nursing.

David's career has taken him to several countries (Thailand, China, Singapore, Tanzania, Zimbabwe and the UK), where he has worked in a range of different roles. His professional interests have focused on leadership and management, aged care, the experience of transition to university for first-year nursing students, physical assessment, the experience of men in nursing and the impact the media has had on the nursing profession. He has also retained a long interest in international nursing issues and supports the benefits of nurses and midwives learning more by exploring other parts of the world with clinically focused practice opportunities. David has arranged or been part of several international clinical practice opportunities to the Philippines, Tanzania and Thailand and has supported other international trips in a number of roles associated with international coordination. He is currently an Adjunct Professor in Nursing at Charles Sturt University and Research advisor for the Fiji National University.

Preface

In the first edition of this book, Janelle Boston, an experienced clinician and educator in Perth, Western Australia, offered the following paragraph as part of her contribution:

> In today's rapidly changing clinical environment and ever-increasing junior work-force, it is essential to develop and maintain strong nursing leaders who will be able to foster our future nurses for generations to come. As a Clinical Liaison Support Practitioner working with undergraduate nursing students, I believe it is important to lead by example striving for the best possible outcomes in clinical excellence by providing ongoing opportunities for professional growth in learning and develop-ment. For me outstanding clinical leaders are experts in their field, who share their passion and knowledge, who motivate and support their team members and provide positive direction no matter how challenging the situation.

We include this again here because although this book has developed to become increas-ingly focused on the wider healthcare team, we are sure Janelle is on to something and feel that it is important to lead by example and support the clinical leaders who are experts in their field, and who share their passion. This book is for them.

The third edition of this book is the culmination of a considerable effort to understand clinical leadership (and followership) and reflects the authors' professional interest in this topic. The book is primarily based on several extensive research projects that considered who clinical leaders are, why they are seen as clinical leaders, what the characteristics of clinical leadership might be and the experience of being a clinical leader. It is also based on our years of involvement in clinical leadership, as senior clinicians, academics, researchers and educators, dealing with the issue of clinical leadership from a practical, applied posi-tion or as an educator and researcher. Collectively, our aim has been to try to understand and share our understandings with clinically focused health professionals from a range of disciplines.

David's interest is also firmly based on his own experience of being a nurse and midwife. He recalls rejoicing in the pleasure of working with effective, wonderful and inspiring clin-ical healthcare leaders. A number of names come easily to mind: Sister Johnson and Paul Fennell, both of whom I had the joy of working with when I was a student and then a registered nurse at the Whyalla and District Hospital in South Australia; Sister Barbra, Sister Helen, Doctor Mike and Doctor Monica, from my days as a volunteer in Zimbabwe at the Murambinda Mission Hospital; and Christina Schwerdt and Penny Rackham from my short stay as an educator on Thursday Island. There are many, many others; but I also recall the depths of facing shift after shift with 'leaders' who were never at the bedside, always at meetings or only showed up on the ward to criticise and ridicule (I won't name any, but sadly their names come quite crisply to mind too). Likewise, Clare can recall the joy of working in clinical teams where values-based leadership led to shared understandings and a shared passion for improvement, meaning that patient care was of the highest standard. However, like David, she can also readily recall the damaging effect of poor leadership that rewarded those who maintained the status quo and punished those who wished to innovate, with deleterious effects on staff morale and, importantly, patient outcomes. Alison's interest in leadership has developed through her clinical nursing career and her time working with health and social care teams, and her awareness of how leadership impacts the dynamics of teams and cultures in practice. She has continued to focus on leadership in her research and is particularly interested in how students are prepared for leadership, and how experiencing both positive and negative styles of leadership can influence others in practice.

Collectively, we were drawn to investigate this topic because of our long association with the nursing profession and other healthcare disciplines. We have held a long and passionate interest in clinical leadership, particularly from the perspective of promoting better healthcare. We have sought to understand and promote greater clinical leadership and healthcare empowerment and support the development of insight into clinical leadership that can have positive impacts on the quality of care provided to patients and clients in a plethora of healthcare environments.

Clinical Leadership in Nursing and Healthcare was written for healthcare professionals who act principally in direct client/patient care. It will also be useful for students studying health-related courses at undergraduate and postgraduate levels, and for nurses and other healthcare professionals in roles of increasing autonomy, such as nurse practitioners and specialist health providers, health professionals studying leadership (or management) and anyone who wants to maximise their contribution to healthcare.

The purpose of the text is to motivate and inspire, as well as to offer guidance and support for clinical leaders (or aspiring clinical leaders) to take change and innovation forward and to initiate greater quality in care or therapies and treatments by basing these on their professional values. There are many books about management (and leadership) for nurse managers or healthcare managers, and, while their contribution to the health service is great, this book was not necessarily written with these professionals in mind. If you are a manager of some sort and you have this book in your hand now, by all means read on, as we are sure there are lessons and messages in the text for any health professional. However, our hope when we sat to write *Clinical Leadership in Nursing and Healthcare* was to generate an understanding of leadership for clinical leaders: leaders at the bedside or who remain 'hands on' in their interaction with clients or patients; leaders who might not have the badge, or the title, or the confidence, or the realisation, but who are leaders in the health service, nonetheless. These are leaders in the eyes of the people who follow them (their junior colleagues, their senior colleagues, patients or clients, other professionals, students and learners, qualified practitioners or yet-to-be-qualified practitioners), although they might not realise it themselves. These are the key leaders who can and will have a vast impact on the provision of quality healthcare, innovation and change within the health service.

The book presents the information in three parts. First it addresses the topic of clinical leadership and leadership in general. Much of what healthcare professionals know about leadership is based on insights and writings from the management paradigm. The first section redresses this by outlining why clinical leadership and quality or innovation are linked. It also discusses what leadership means by describing the theories that underpin what we know about leadership. As well, it describes the difference between leadership and management; looks at the attributes and value of followers; offers a description of the characteristics of clinical leaders; and sets out a number of theories of leadership that point to a values-based approach to leadership, including a new theory: congruent leadership. This theory, developed from research specifically undertaken with a range of health professionals, is directly relevant for bedside, clinical leaders to gain an understanding about what leadership means.

The second part of the book deals with the 'tools' for developing effective clinical leadership skills and insights. Chapters in this part offer information about organisational culture, managing change, decision making, team working, reflection, creativity, motivation and inspiration, networking, delegation, how to deal effectively with conflict, the relevance of quality initiatives and project management for clinical leaders and the use of evidence-based practice. These topics are all provided so that clinical leaders can orchestrate successful change and innovation and focus on their values or lead effective quality initiatives.

The final part of the book addresses issues that put clinical leadership into context. The topics relate to gender, generational groups, power, politics, empowerment, oppression, leading in challenging times or during times of crisis and how clinical leaders can (using a *congruent leadership* or a *values-based* style) have positive impacts on the quality of healthcare and lead their patients or clients, colleagues, team mates, co-workers, organisation and the heath service in general towards a better tomorrow.

Within most chapters there are 'Clinical Leader Stories' – these offer an example of clinical leadership in practice from the view of a clinician. Most were provided by students undertaking clinical leadership courses or as part of the undergraduate degrees. Thank you to the many students who gave their permission to use these stories. Also, at the end of each chapter, you will find a short biography of a different leader. When we set out on the journey to explore clinical leadership, we realised that there were few (if any) texts that addressed clinical leadership and few texts addressed leadership without reference to management (this is discussed further in Chapter 2). The second realisation was that the examples of leaders presented in the past published texts were, with few exceptions (e.g. Florence Nightingale, Boudica or Queen Elizabeth the 1st), all men and all from positions traditionally associated with leadership or management. This edition has expanded the profile of the leaders considered to include leaders and people who are often under-represented or fail to be recognised in terms of leadership. Leaders are indeed present at any level of an organisation, in the health service or across the spectrum of society, and the examples given show that leaders can be anyone who leads with their values to the fore. We make no apologies for focusing on underrepresented leaders in this book or for using many examples of women leaders. However, it does pose a dilemma because the lack of male leaders in the health service (particularly in nursing) means that in redressing one imbalance we are creating another. There are many significant men we know who have led in the health service, even in nursing (e.g. Walt Whitman, Phil Della, Luke Yokota and others), but the aim of this text is to make clear the part of many under-represented leaders who have contributed and led in a variety of fields. We hope you enjoy reading about their significant contributions.

David Stanley
Clare L. Bennett
Alison H. James

Acknowledgements

We should like to thank all the students who have taken part in the clinical leadership courses and subjects we have each been involved with in the UK, Australia, Singapore, Tanzania, Europe, and other parts of the world. Your enthusiasm and commitment to learning and improving care and clinical services have been an inspiration. We also thank all the health professionals and colleagues who have contributed to our understanding of clinical leadership by willingly contributing to our research or teaching resources with their insights and knowledge. We should also like to thank our education-based colleagues who (over many years) have supported each of us and contributed their ideas, time and talents to the delivery of clinical leadership education: They are too numerous to mention.

A special thank-you is extended to Stephen Stanley for contributing the wonderful cartoons and illustrations used throughout the book. In Australia, Stephen is a nationally recognised cartoonist, and it was a delight that he agreed to support this book with his talents and time.

The third edition of this book rests on the support and encouragement of Magenta Styles, Associate Editorial Director at Wiley, who provided excellent review feedback and encouraged David to seek additional UK based co-authors. Thanks too to the reviewers and to Wiley for making recommendations for developing the text further. This led to the initiation of an excellent collaboration and wonderful collaborative working relationship, and we are truly grateful for this wider author profile.

We are also deeply indebted to the book production and procurement department at Wiley for their faith in us and their support. In addition, Anne Hunt and Chris Sabooni and other editorial team members must be thanked for their wonderful and ongoing editorial support. Particularly Chris Sabooni, who undertook the final and most detailed edit to really bring polish to the text.

We should also like to thank the chapter contributors: Judith Anderson, Sarah Dineen-Griffin, Julie Reis Tracey Coventry, Kylie Russell, and Denise Blanchard from Australia, and Sally Carvalho from the UK. Each provided their respective chapters on time and with due care over the content. We could not have completed the book on time without their support, hard work and able great contributions.

In the first edition, *Clinical Leadership: Innovation into Action* (2011), David neglected to acknowledge the wonderful input from his doctoral supervisors, Karen Cox and Linda Ellison (both from Nottingham University in England), and he hopes they will forgive this oversight. Karen Cox was an inspirational supervisor who prompted him to look beyond the end of his doctoral studies and keep asking the 'so what?' question, and Linda offered sound doctoral advice from an educational perspective that David found invaluable.

There are many others who have in many ways added to the completion of this project. Colleagues have offered support and encouragement, and undergraduate and postgraduate students have kept us keenly interested in the topic of clinical leadership. They have all fueled our desire to do our best for them and remind us always that at the core of our learning is the client, patient, healthcare consumer – or person. Thank you all.

It is not only giants that do great things.

November 2021

David Stanley
Clare L. Bennett
Alison H. James

Part I

Clinical Leaders: Role Models for Values-Based Leadership

Nothing in life is to be feared. It is only to be understood.
Marie Curie, Polish-born French physicist and chemist,
famous for her work on radioactivity, first recipient of two Nobel prizes,
the first female professor, University of Paris

Clinical Leadership in Nursing and Healthcare suggests that clinically focused leadership or clinical leadership and administration-based or managerial leadership are not the same thing. The case for this view is set out in this first part of the book. To support this statement, the book outlines a number of principles, frameworks, tools and topics describing how nurses and other health professionals can develop, lead and deliver effective clinical care – as clinical leaders, not as managers or as administrative leaders in the academic, political or managerial sphere. It also outlines a new theory of values-based leadership – congruent leadership, which has been developed from a number of research studies exploring the nature and characteristics of clinical leadership from a wide range of different health professional disciplines, in the UK and Australia.

Congruent leadership theory suggests that leaders demonstrate a match (congruence) between the leader's values and beliefs and their actions. As such, clinically focused health professionals have moved decisively and clearly in the direction of their values and beliefs and can be seen expressing congruent leadership. They may simply have stood by their values, working not because they wanted to change the world but because they knew that what they were doing was the right thing to do and that their actions were making a difference, if only in the life of one person.

It is timely that clinical leadership is being re-evaluated and frameworks developed that support it (Stanton et al. 2010; Martin and Learmonth 2012; Mannix et al. 2013; Storey and Holti 2013; Scully 2014; McLellan 2015; Rose 2015; West et al. 2015; Bender 2016; Swanwick and McKimm 2017; James et al. 2021), because it is clear that in attempting to climb the career ladder, many health professionals have faced the dilemma of having to move further

Clinical Leadership in Nursing and Healthcare, Third Edition.
Edited by David Stanley, Clare L. Bennett and Alison H. James.
© 2023 John Wiley & Sons Ltd. Published 2023 by John Wiley & Sons Ltd.

away from the core reason they first became health professionals, resulting in role confusion and blurring of values (Stanley 2006c; Copeland 2014; Stanley 2019). Many have had to move into management or administrative positions or academic roles and leave their clinical roles further behind with each promotion. However, if leadership happens at all levels (Cook 2001; Stanley 2006a, b, 2008, 2011; Higgins et al. 2014; Swanwick and McKimm 2017; Stanley 2019), identifying who the clinical leaders are and attempting to gain an understanding of what clinical leadership means becomes vital.

The first part of this book comprises five chapters. Chapter 1 deals with an exploration of the concept of clinical leadership. It explores the attributes of effective clinical leaders and outlines the rationale behind these attributes, then discusses why an understanding of clinical leadership matters now. The chapter considers what clinical leadership is and who clinical leaders are. Could a therapy team leader, who is busy telephoning staffing agencies in order to find staff to fill vacancies for a busy clinic, be the clinical leader? Could it be a nurse consultant, paramedic lead or nurse practitioner who is in the process of initiating a reform of clinically based practice on a recent research project? Could a healthcare assistant or physiotherapy aid who, day in and day out, has cared for sick and frail medical patients on a busy orthopaedic rehabilitation ward be the clinical leader? Could the bright-eyed, newly qualified occupational therapist who approaches work with enthusiasm and the hope that they are making a difference to people's lives on a busy rehabilitation day-case unit be the clinical leader? Could it be the junior registered nurse who remains focused on essential bedside care and refuses to become drawn into the ward management issues? Or is the manager the clinical leader, as they keep staff focused on issues of quality, cleanliness and care?

Reflection Point

There are 'Reflection Points' throughout this book. These are to encourage you to pause and reflect on the topic or issues being discussed.

Start the book by pausing to reflect on who you think the clinical leaders are in your clinical area or practice location. Imagine that a relative or friend is ill and requires care in the clinical area you work in. Who are the people you would point to as clinical leaders? Who would confidently care for and lead the care for your relative or friend? What are your thoughts? Could it be any or all of the people described earlier?

Chapter 2 offers an introduction to the various definitions, styles and theories of leadership. A spectrum of perspectives are presented to help health professionals come to grips with the concept of leadership. It is suggested that there are a wide range of views, beliefs and ideas about what leadership means, what types of leadership there are and how the types of leadership might be employed to build relationships, communicate more effectively, promote vision or values and bring about change or innovation. Chapter 3 offers an insight into values-based leadership, what it means and the theories that support it. One of these is congruent leadership theory (Stanley 2006a, b, 2008, 2011, 2014, 2019). This theory of leadership was developed specifically from research exploring clinically focused leadership as it relates to health professionals. Congruent leadership is promoted in this book as a valuable way to gain an understanding of how clinical leaders lead and why clinical leaders are seen as leaders. Examples of clinical leadership applied to congruent leadership are offered, as is a discussion about the strengths and limitations of the theory. Moreover, the relationship of congruent leadership to change, innovation, power and quality is considered. Chapter 4 offers an insight into the important and often overlooked concept of followership. The concept of followership is defined, and followers' responsibilities and the attributes of effective and not so effective followers are explored. Chapter 5 offers a discussion of the difference between management and leadership, suggesting that managers and leaders are driven and governed by a different set of values and beliefs, goals and objectives. The differences between management and leadership outlined here make it clear that while a manager may be an effective leader and a leader may be an effective manager, their diverse drives, motivators and objectives may in fact make it very difficult for one professional to hold both sets of responsibilities successfully. Most significantly, the differences may be most evident in relation to the values that drive clinically focused health professionals, therefore attempting to combine these different roles may lead to internal conflict and ineffective care (Stanley 2006c, 2011, 2019).

Part I aims to explore clinical leadership, leadership theory, followership, values-based leadership and the difference between leadership and management. It will outline the characteristics, qualities and attributes of clinically focused leaders and help identify what they are, as well as what a health professional might look for to become a clinical leader.

References

Bender, M. (2016). Conceptualizing clinical nurse leader practice: an interpretive synthesis. *Journal of Nursing Management* 24: 23–31. http://dx.doi.org/10.1111/jonm.12285.

Cook, M. (2001). The attributes of effective clinical nurse leaders. *Nursing Standard* 15 (35): 33–36.

Copeland, M.K. (2014). 'The emerging significance of values-based leadership: a literature review', Business faculty Publications, St. John Fisher College. Fisher Digital Publications. *International Journal of Leadership Studies* 8 (2): 105–135.

Higgins, A., Begley, C., Lalor, J. et al. (2014). Factors influencing advancing practitioners' ability to enact leadership: a case study within Irish healthcare. *Journal of Nursing Management* 22: 894–905.

James, A.H., Bennett, C.L., Blanchard, D., and Stanley, D. (2021). 'Nursing and values-based leadership: a literature review. *Journal of Nurse Management* 29 (5): 916–930.

Mannix, J., Wilkes, L., and Daly, J. (2013). Attributes of clinical leadership in contemporary nursing: an integrative review. *Contemporary Nurse* 45 (1): 10–21.

Martin, G.P. and Learmonth, M. (2012). A critical account of the rise and spread of "leadership": the case of UK healthcare. *Social Science & Medicine* 74 (3): 281–288.

McLellan, A. (ed.) (2015). Ending the crisis in NHS leadership: A plan for renewal. *Health Service Journal*, special edition, 1–11.

Rose, Lord (2015). Better Leadership for Tomorrow: NHS Leadership Review. London: Department of Health. http://thelarreysociety.org/wpcontent/uploads/2015/08/Lord_Rose_NHS_Report_acc.pdf (accessed 1 May 2016).

Scully, N.J. (2014). Leadership in nursing: the importance of recognising values and attributes to secure a positive future for the profession. *Collegian* 22 (4): 439–444.

Stanley, D. (2006a). In command of care: clinical nurse leadership explored. *Journal of Research in Nursing* 2 (1): 20–39.

Stanley, D. (2006b). In command of care: towards the theory of congruent leadership. *Journal of Research in Nursing* 2 (2): 134–144.

Stanley, D. (2006c). Role conflict: leaders and managers. *Nursing Management* 13 (5): 31–37.

Stanley, D. (2008). Congruent leadership: values in action. *Journal of Nursing Management* 16: 519–524.

Stanley, D. (2011). *Clinical Leadership: Innovation into Action*. South Yarra, VIC: Palgrave Macmillan.

Stanley, D. (2014). Clinical leadership characteristics confirmed. *Journal of Research in Nursing* 19 (2): 118–128.

Stanley, D. (2019). *Values-Based Leadership in Healthcare: Congruent Leadership Explored*. London: SAGE.

Stanton, E., Lemer, C., and Mountford, J. (2010). *Clinical Leadership: Bridging the Divide*. London: Quay Books.

Storey, J. and Holti, R. (2013). Towards a New Model of Leadership for the NHS, Leeds: NHS Leadership Academy. http://www.leadershipacademy.nhs.uk/wp-content/uploads/2013/05/Towards-a-New-Model-of-Leadership-2013.pdf (accessed 1 July 2016).

Swanwick, T. and McKimm, J. (2017). *ABC of Clinical Leadership*, 2e. Oxford: Wiley Blackwell.

West, M., Loewenthal, L., Eckert, R., West, T. and Lee, A. (2015). Leadership and Leadership Development in Healthcare: The Evidence Base, London: Faculty of Medical Leadership and Management/Center for Creative Leadership/The King's Fund, https://www.fmlm.ac.uk/resources/leadership-andleadership-development-in-health-care-the-evidence-base (accessed 1 July 2016).

1

Clinical Leadership Explored

David Stanley

> *Find people who share your values, and you'll conquer the world together.*
> John Ratzenberger, author of *We've Got It Made in America*

Introduction

Jesse Jackson, the American political and civil rights leader, has said: 'Change isn't about processes or structure. It is about courageous people who are prepared to act.' This book is about people in the health service who are courageously driven by their values and prepared to act on them. These people may apply courage: suggesting the best available evidence in the face of luddite behaviour; care when time is pressing; clinical competence; commitment; compassion or any of the foundational and traditional values evident and relevant in modern health care. For me, these are **clinical leaders**: women and men, across the spectrum of the health service, who explore the boundaries of their practice and who press for continual improvements in quality care, increased innovation and productive changes in practice. They are leaders because they put their values (about care, compassion, competence, commitment, courage, etc.) into action. Others see these values in practice and follow, because they hold, aspire to or believe in the same values and beliefs.

While nursing leadership and healthcare leadership are terms that have been evident in the nursing and health industry literature for many decades, clinical leadership is a relatively new term. However, what do we know about the concept of clinical leadership and what does the term mean? This chapter sets out to explore definitions of clinical leadership, the attributes of effective clinical leaders, and attributes less likely to be associated with clinical leadership. It will also consider who clinical leaders might be, and will outline the implications for health organisations when understanding and recognising clinical leaders. It suggests that if an organisation – or indeed the health service as a whole – is to adapt and develop, there is an urgent need to identify who the clinical leaders are and to understand how they see themselves or are recognised by others (Mountford and Webb 2009; Jeon 2011; Storey and Holti 2013a; Bender 2016).

Clinical Leadership in Nursing and Healthcare, Third Edition.
Edited by David Stanley, Clare L. Bennett and Alison H. James.
© 2023 John Wiley & Sons Ltd. Published 2023 by John Wiley & Sons Ltd.

Clinical Leadership: What Do We Know?

Attempts to define clinical leadership, like insights into the concept, are relatively new (Stanley and Stanley 2017). There were early contributions from Peach (1995) and Lett (2002), both from an Australian perspective, and US authors Dean-Barr (1998), McCormack and Hopkins (1995), and Rocchiccioli and Tilbury (1998) added to the dialogue. Berwick (1994) and Wyatt (1995) from a medical perspective, Forest et al. (2013) from a dentistry perspective and Schneider (1999) from a pharmacological standpoint have also added to the discussion. Most recently and also from a medical perspective, Stanton et al. (2010), Swanwick and McKimm (2017), and Storey and Holti (2013a) have offered a summary of what clinical leadership may mean. However, and in spite of this growing body of literature, a clear definition remains elusive (Mannix et al. 2013; Jeon et al. 2014). Fortunately, more literature is evident each year that addresses Malby's (1997) suggestion that there has been limited agreement on a definition of clinical leadership.

Harper (1995) offered one of the earliest definitions, suggesting that a clinical leader possesses clinical expertise in a specialist practice area and uses interpersonal skills to enable nurses and other healthcare providers to deliver quality patient care. McCormack and Hopkins (1995), Cook (2001b), and Lett (2002) support Harper's view, suggesting that clinical leadership can be described as the work of clinicians who practise at an expert level and who have or hold a leadership position.

Rocchiccioli and Tilbury (1998), writing from a nursing perspective, also cite excellence in clinical practice, but add that it also involves an environment where staff are empowered and where there is a vision for the future. Lett (2002) and Swanwick and McKimm (2017) suggest that a clinical leader is a clinical expert who leads their followers to better healthcare by providing a vision to those followers and so empowering them. Expert practice and a positive impact on quality patient care again feature, but each also links clinical leadership with vision, and this is at odds with the research results that support this book (Stanley 2006a, b, 2008, 2011, 2014; Stanley et al. 2012, 2014, 2015; Stanley and Stanley 2019). These publications suggest that clinical leadership and vision are seldom directly linked. Instead, clinical leaders are more likely to be followed because they match their values and beliefs with their actions in clinical practice; a perspective elaborated on in Chapter 4. This perspective aligns clinical leadership with approaches to leadership driven or based on a values-based leadership style; James et al. (2021).

Stanton et al. (2010, p. 5) offer the view that anyone who is in a clinical role and who exercises leadership is a clinical leader, before suggesting that a clinical leader's role is to 'empower clinicians to have the confidence and capability to continually improve health care on both the small and the large scale'. The UK Department of Health's (2007) definition *(and I feel it is still one of the best)* is that the role of a clinical leader is:

> To motivate, to inspire, to promote the values of the NHS, to empower and create a consistent focus on the needs of patients being served. Leadership is necessary not just to maintain high standards of care, but to transform services to achieve even higher levels of excellence.
>
> (DoH 2007, p. 49)

Bender (2016) recently attempted to develop a theoretical understanding of clinical nurse leader practice and suggested that the core attributes of clinical nurse leaders rest on links to clinical practice, effective communication, effective interprofessional relationships, team working and supporting other staff.

Clark (2008) and Cook (2001a) suggest that clinical leaders are in non-hierarchical positions, with Cook adding that clinical nurse leaders are directly involved in providing clinical care that continually improves care through influencing others, with Cook and Holt (2000) supporting this perspective. Clinical nurse leaders also have a relationship with quality patient care and are able to influence others, implying perhaps that they may not need to be in positions of power or those that are hierarchically significant to lead in the clinical arena. The research that supports this book bolsters such views. These authors also imply that clinical leaders must be good communicators, and that they need effective team-building skills and respect for others.

The *McKinsey Quarterly* definition of clinical leadership; another that I particularly like (cited in Stanton et al. 2010) is that:

> Clinical leadership is putting the clinician at the heart of shaping and running clinical services, so as to deliver excellent outcomes for patients and population, not as a one-off task or project, but as a core part of clinicians' professional identity.

In addition, the literature points to a number of key elements in the recognition of clinical leadership (Stavrianopoulos 2012; Chavez and Yoder 2014; Stanley and Stanley 2017):

- **Clinical expertise** (Berwick 1994; Harper 1995; Rocchiccioli and Tilbury 1998; Schneider 1999; Lett 2002; Stanley 2006a, b, 2008, 2011, 2014; Stanton et al. 2010; Swanwick and McKimm 2017; Stanley et al. 2012, 2014, 2015; Won 2015; Bender 2016; Stanley and Stanley 2019).
- **Effective communication and interpersonal skills** (Harper 1995; Cook and Holt 2000; Cook 2001b; Stanley 2006a, b, 2008, 2011, 2014; Swanwick and McKimm 2017; Stanley et al. 2012, 2014, 2015; Jeon et al. 2014; Won 2015; Bender 2016).
- **Empowerment and respect for others** (Rocchiccioli and Tilbury 1998; Cook and Holt 2000; Lett 2002; Stanley 2006a, b, 2008, 2011, 2014; Stanton et al. 2010; Stanley et al. 2012, 2014, 2015; Bender 2016; Boamah 2018; Stanley and Stanley 2019).
- **Team working or team building** (Rocchiccioli and Tilbury 1998; Cook and Holt 2000; Lett 2002; Stanley 2006a, b, 2008, 2011, 2014; Stanton et al. 2010; Stanley et al. 2012, 2014, 2015; Bender 2016).
- **Driving change, making care better and providing quality care** (Berwick 1994; Harper 1995; Schneider 1999; Cook 2001b; Lett 2002; Stanley 2006a, b, 2008, 2011, 2014; Ferguson et al. 2007; Clark 2008; Stanton et al. 2010; Swanwick and McKimm 2017; Stanley et al. 2012, 2014; Byers 2015; Demeh and Rosengren 2015; Stanley et al. 2015; Stanley and Stanley 2019).
- **Vision** (Rocchiccioli and Tilbury 1998; Cook and Holt 2000; Lett 2002; Clark 2008; Swanwick and McKimm 2017).

However, it is my contention that there is much more to understanding clinical leadership than these definitions and views.

> **Reflection Point**
>
> Look around the area where you work. Who would you identify as a clinical leader? Why would you select this person or people? How does your choice of clinical leader fit with the definitions already offered in this chapter?

Attributes *Less* Likely to Be Seen in Clinical Leaders

Clinical Leaders Are Not Seen as Controlling

Being viewed as 'controlling' was consistently seen as less likely to be associated with the qualities of a clinical leader, a view supported by Coventry and Russell (2021), who explored the clinical leadership attributes of clinical nurse educators. Table 1.1 indicates emphatically that in the six research studies that support this book, being 'controlling' was always the attribute identified as least likely to be linked to clinical leadership (for more on these see Chapter 4). Moreover, the percentages are remarkably similar across a range of professional disciplines, cementing a disassociation between being controlling and clinical leadership. In the sixth study with rural and remote area nurses' clinical leaders who 'did not listen, gave poor feedback, were not focused on staff, did not connect or engage with the team or were dishonest, aggressive or inflexible,' were seen as poor clinical leader (Stanley and Stanley 2019, p. 6).

Clinical Leaders Are Not Seen as Visionary

'Being visionary' was also poorly associated with clinical leadership. As with Cook's (2001a) study, having a vision or articulating a vision appeared to be unrelated and unrecognisable as a dominant feature of the qualities and characteristics for which clinical leaders were recognised.

Table 1.1 'Being controlling': The characteristic least commonly associated with clinical leaders.

	Study 1	Study 2	Study 3	Study 4	Study 5	Study 6
	Nurses	Paramedics	Residential care staff	Volunteer ambulance officers	Allied health professionals	Rural and remote area nurses
Percentage of respondents who identified *controlling* as the attribute least likely to be linked to clinical leadership	78%	84%	80%	84%	83%	Being controlling was mentioned by 32 of the 56 (57%) participants as an attribute least likely to be associated with a clinical leader

In Study 1 the term 'visionary' was identified by 72.3% of respondents as affiliated with clinical leadership, although even with this percentage it was ranked 27th on a list of 42 words to describe the qualities and characteristics most associated with clinical leadership. In each of the six studies, being visionary or having a vision failed to be rated highly in terms of a percentage factor, or as an attribute of clinical leadership. Table 1.2 offers data from all six studies to support this view. Interestingly, the percentages seemed to drop as the studies progressed in time (from 72% with nurses in 2005 to 34.2% with allied health professionals in 2015). The sixth study was based on interviews and did not gather percentage responses, although it was rarely discussed by participants.

These results question the significance of 'vision' or 'being visionary' as a quality or characteristic sought or seen in clinical leaders. In each of the studies, respondents were invited to list their own attributes of clinical leaders and, as such, many additional attributes were offered. However, very few related to 'vision', 'being visionary' or 'being forward thinking' (Stanley 2006a, b, 2008, 2011, 2014; Stanley et al. 2012, 2014, 2015; Stanley and Stanley 2019). The lack of characteristics centred around clinical leaders being visionary was borne out by the results of the interviews or free-text comments, where 'vision' was hardly mentioned as an attribute looked for in clinical leaders, and rarely described as the motivation behind being a clinical leader. One person in the sixth study said, 'Sometimes as leader you might have a vision' (Stanley and Stanley 2019), but this was the closest comment and one of only two that even mentioned vision in the context of clinical leadership in this study. Some respondents discussed goals or objective setting, but these were commonly focused on work tasks or professional development aspirations and only loosely related to vision.

This may be because respondents were drawn to or identify with clinical leaders who can lead them through the 'here and now' issues of busy and chaotic clinical work – who can cope with the demands of each day as it comes, rather than postulate and pontificate about how things could or should be. Clinical leaders were seen and selected if they had their values on show and stood on a solid foundation of care and compassion that governed and drove their practice standards. Clinical leadership is therefore defined in action, as clinical leaders mobilise their values and beliefs to guide and direct what they do when faced with challenges and critical problems in the clinical area (Clark 2008;

Table 1.2 'Being visionary' as associated with clinical leadership.

	Study 1	Study 2	Study 3	Study 4	Study 5	Study 6
	Nurses	Paramedics	Residential care staff	Volunteer ambulance officers	Allied health professionals	Rural and remote area nurses
Percentage of respondents who identified *visionary* as an attribute likely to be linked to clinical leadership	72% Ranking 27th out of 42 attributes	51% Ranking 37th out of 54 attributes	20% Ranking 33rd out of 54 attributes	40.9% Ranking 38th out of 54 attributes	34.2% Ranking 36th out of 54 attributes	Being visionary was mentioned by only 2 of the 56 (3.5%) participants as an attribute of a clinical leader

Stanley 2006a, b, 2008, 2011, 2014; Edmondstone 2009; Stanley et al. 2012; Forest et al. 2013; Stanley et al. 2014; Scully 2014; McLellan 2015; Stanley et al. 2015; Stanley and Stanley 2019).

Clinical Leaders Are Not Seen as 'Shapers'

Cook (2001a) saw clinical leaders as 'creative', identifying the typology of 'shapers' to describe them (see later in this chapter). In each of the six research studies that influence this book, creativity was rarely identified as a defining characteristic of a clinical leader. As indicated in Table 1.3, being 'creative/innovative' or 'artistic' was seldom ranked highly on the clinical leader attribute list.

Artistic was ranked second only to 'controlling' as the characteristic least associated with clinical leadership in the first study among nurses and was continually ranked near the end of the order in all the other studies. Higher percentages of respondents did still consider being 'creative/innovative' a feature of clinical leadership. However, this failed to be as strongly associated with clinical leadership as other attributes, and in interviews with clinical leaders or in other data sources, creativity and innovation were seldom expressed as an attribute worthy of note (Stanley 2006a, b, 2008, 2011, 2014; Stanley et al. 2012, 2014, 2015; Stanley and Stanley 2019).

I have struggled with this aspect of the results since my initial publications. Rolfe (2006), who wrote a commentary on the 2006 article (Stanley 2006b), was likewise unsure of the validity of the results, given that creativity was ranked so low. However, this feature of the results has been confirmed again and again with each subsequent study (see Table 1.3). I am sure that some clinical leaders are creative and that being creative is a substantial skill

Table 1.3 'Creative/innovative' and 'artistic' as associated with clinical leadership.

	Study 1	Study 2	Study 3	Study 4	Study 5	Study 6
	Nurses	Paramedics	Residential care staff	Volunteer ambulance officers	Allied health professionals	Rural and remote area nurses
Percentage of respondents who identified *creative/innovative* as an attribute likely to be linked to clinical leadership	76.5% Ranking 25th out of 42 attributes	51% Ranking 32nd out of 54 attributes	60% Ranking 27th out of 54 attributes	59.0% Ranking 27th out of 54 attributes	56% Ranking 22nd out of 54 attributes	Being innovative was identified by only 3 of the 56 (5.3%) participants in this study.
Percentage of respondents who identified *artistic* as an attribute likely to be linked to clinical leadership	13% Ranking 41st out of 42 attributes	24% Ranking 50th out of 54 attributes	0% Ranking 54th out of 54 attributes	42.5% Ranking 48th out of 54 attributes	8.5% Ranking 50th out of 54 attributes	This was not identified by any of the participants in this study.

for clinical leaders to employ, but I am now sure that being creative is not something that others look for in their clinical leaders. Creativity does remain a key attribute that clinical leaders should aspire to, and it is of particular relevance if clinical leaders are to influence innovation or change or to find new ways to bring their values into practice. Chapter 9 elaborates on the issue of creativity and identifies a number of strategies that clinical leaders can employ to bolster their creative capacity.

Attributes *More* Likely to Be Seen in Clinical Leaders

While the previous section has focused on the attributes less likely to be recognised in clinical leaders (control, vision and creativity), this section addresses the attributes that the six research studies, and others, have identified as being directly linked to clinical leaders.

Cook attempted to identify the attributes of effective clinical leaders by focusing not on nurses at the 'hierarchical apex of the organisation . . . but on those nurses that directly deliver nursing care' (2001a, p. 33). His study focused on nurses who were not deemed to be in conventional nursing leadership positions but who displayed many of the attributes of highly effective leaders. Following his data analysis, he produced a table that set out the clinical leaders' attributes – described as 'typologies' – with associated constraining and facilitating factors related to each attribute.

Cook (2001a) recognised clinical leaders or 'discoverers', who had a desire to improve the care they provided, and 'valuers', who valued both themselves and those around them and were able to empathise with their colleagues and patients. 'Enablers' encouraged others to see what needed to be done and assisted them to do it; 'shapers' possessed the 'creativity' to generate new ways of working and were able to help others make decisions; and 'modifiers' supported and helped others with the process of change. Cook indicates that his 'research identified aspects of leadership that are unique to clinical nursing' (2001a, p. 36), but suggested that further research was required to identify these with confidence.

Many clinical leadership attributes were identified in the six research studies (Table 1.4), although 10 were most prominent. Many are also interrelated and interdependent, so it would be unusual if a clinical leader who was considered clinically competent and clinically knowledgeable was not also seen as a role model in their clinical area. However, each of these attributes has been singled out and will be explored separately as a way of establishing a complete map of a clinical leader's attributes.

Clinical Competence/Clinical Knowledge

One of the key elements of clinical leadership relates to the clinical leader's ability to remain credible and competent in the provision of clinical care. High numbers of participants in all six studies, as well as information from Jonas et al. (2017), Mannix et al. (2013), McDonnell et al. (2015), Won (2015), Bender (2016), Stanley and Stanley (2017), and Coventry and Russell (2021) supported this perspective. Clinical leadership appears to be firmly embedded in the domain of clinical activity. Clinical competence was clearly linked to clinical experience and the confidence that others saw in the clinical leader's ability. It meant being able to show or to do – as well as to know or to teach others about – clinical

Table 1.4 Attributes most likely to be associated with clinical leadership.

Attributes	Study 1 Nurses	Study 2 Paramedics	Study 3 Residential care staff	Study 4 Volunteer ambulance officers	Study 5 Allied health professionals	Study 6 Nurses in rural and remote areas
Clinical competence	95.2%	96.2%	100%	90.1%	83.7%	98.2%
Approachable	97.3%	96.2%	100%	90.1%	83.1%	83.9%
Empowered, motivated/ motivator	94.1%	86.5%	80%	77.0%	72.6%	64.2%
Supportive	94.1%	91.3%	100%	77.0%	75.2%	64.2%
Inspires confidence	93.0%	85.6%	40%	85.2%	52.1%	53.5%
Has integrity/is honest	87.2%	93.3%	100%	78.6%	83.1%	53.5%
Role model for others	Not covered in this study	93.3%	80%	88.5%	79.8%	78.5%
An effective communicator	Not covered in this study	89.4%	100%	86.8%	88.3%	82.1%
Visible in practice	85.6%	85.6%	100%	65.6%	55.0%	78.5%
Copes well with change	90.9%	79.8%	100%	73.7%	76.9%	33.9%

issues. Interestingly, being an 'expert' in their clinical field was not specifically mentioned, although this was a central feature of the characteristics identified by Cook (2001a) and by Berwick (1994), Stanton et al. (2010), and Schneider (1999) in relation to clinical leadership from a medical, pharmacological and nursing perspective, respectively.

Clinical leaders were identified as clinically competent – that is, as credible in their clinical field and working in a 'hands-on' capacity (Stanley 2006a, b, 2008, 2011, 2014; Stanley et al. 2012, 2014, 2015; Stanley and Stanley 2019) – and were therefore recognisable because they possessed a set of knowledge that was specific to their clinical field. In the sixth clinical leadership study with rural and remote area nurses. the main attribute sought from effective clinical leaders was that of 'good clinical skills' (Stanley and Stanley 2019). While this knowledge base may extend into a broad range of topics or areas, clinical leaders were often identified because they knew, and could do well, the 'stuff' central to their clinical area and practice.

One nurse said, 'You've got to be knowledgeable, but you've also got to have knowledge that's applicable to the area that you work in.' Others said that 'being good clinically' was important, and another added that clinical leaders needed to be 'knowledgeable in their area of practice.' Effective clinical leadership rested on sound clinical knowledge that extended into having knowledge not just about clinical issues, but knowing how teams worked, how individuals worked and about relationships between people. One study respondent said that it was about being 'aware of people's limitations . . . aware of who works well together, who needs a lot of support and who doesn't. Who needs time effectively on their own and who doesn't and who needs continual prompting and back up.'

Approachability

Approachability was rated very highly as a clinical leader attribute, a view also supported by Coventry and Russell (2021) in their exploration of clinical leadership with clinical nurse educators. This was exemplified by an allied health professional who described a clinical leader as one who is 'supportive, fair, reasonable, willing to change, understanding and approachable'. In the study with rural and remote area nurses, clinical leaders were sought who were 'approachable, valued respect for others, were trustworthy, calm, caring and compassionate', all attributes described or identified in the previous studies (Stanley and Stanley 2019). Ineffective clinical leaders were described as being 'basically dictators', while effective clinical leaders had a more relaxed approach and saw staff as 'equal in their own right'. Poor clinical leaders were described as being 'bossy, they try to control things, they make changes without talking to people and they don't listen', while many respondents reacted well when a clinical leader 'valued' them, or made 'staff feel they were there for them', or when clinical leaders were 'approachable, friendly and understanding'. These views were supported by Cook (2001a), Clark (2008), Edmondstone (2009), Mannix et al. (2013), Won (2015), and Bender (2016).

Empowered/Motivator or Motivated

Clinical leaders and front-line professionals were identified because they were confident, a view supported by Van Dyk et al. (2016), or because of their enthusiasm and their ability to make others feel confident. Clinical leaders were motivated and able to motivate others because they showed

> belief in what you're doing . . . because I know people who are higher, you know a higher level than me are not necessarily good leaders . . . they're not . . . they don't necessarily have any belief in what they're doing.

Clinical leadership was seen to be about empowering people to perform better, deal with quality care (Jonas et al. 2017) and sow the seeds to let others take the lead. One participant in the rural and remote area study said a clinical leader is 'approachable, very organized, know the ward, inside out have very good clinical skills and they are good enough to stand up to management and tell them no' (Stanley and Stanley 2018).

Supportive

Being supportive was linked to being approachable, with a high number of respondents suggesting that effective clinical leaders needed to support others in their team. This view was again evident in the results of Coventry and Russell (2021) study and was also identified as important by Mannix et al. (2013) and Bender (2016), who saw support as a central role of building and sustaining effective teams. In the study with rural and remote area nurses, one said,

> It's about the way they treat the patients and family members, the way they stay positive with all staff, they are fair with all staff, congratulating the team for a job well done, providing positive feedback (Stanley and Stanley 2018).

Inspires Confidence

Linked to being motivational, inspiring confidence was suggested by a large number of respondents as central to the attributes of clinical leaders. This view was significant in areas of rural and remote practice where staff were more isolated and needed to be more self-reliant (Stanley and Stanley 2019). In support of this view, an allied health professional suggested that a clinical leader is one whom 'others view as the best example of excellent performance and that motivates others to grow and succeed' (Stanley et al. 2015). Coventry and Russell (2021) suggested that inspiring confidence was linked to role modelling and implementing change.

Integrity/Honesty

Being honest and having integrity are linked to attributes of approachability and being supportive. Being seen as honest was consistently rated highly as a clinical leader attribute (Coventry and Russell 2021). Edmondstone (2009) added that clinical leaders needed to enjoy the trust and respect of their colleagues to be successful. One allied health professional described an ideal clinical leader by saying 'they should not be a bully and have clear understanding of people's roles and responsibilities', they should have 'integrity, be honest and be transparent' (Stanley et al. 2015). Rural and remote area nurses also looked for clinical leaders who were 'open and honest' (Stanley and Stanley 2019).

Role Model

In addition to clinical competence and clinical knowledge, clinical leaders were also identifiable because – unlike managers and, to a lesser extent, leaders – in general – respondents viewed them as role models (Watson 2008; Coventry and Russell 2021). Clinical leaders had their standards of practice on show and others indicated that it was the ability of a health professional to care effectively for their patients or clients that made them stand out as a clinical leader. One respondent indicated that being a good clinical leader meant 'being a good role model, making sure that your practice is evidence-based, that you pick up on poor standards of care and you pick up on problems and identify them'. Another added, 'a good manager may not lead by example, whereas a good clinical leader would'. Clinical leaders were seen as 'someone you would look up to', 'people that have been inspirational or people you've thought, "oh that's what I really want to be like"'. These views were supported by Cook (2001a), Watson (2008), Mannix et al. (2013), Bender (2016), and Coventry and Russell (2021).

Effective Communicator

High numbers of study respondents and information from Cook (2001a), Clark (2008), Edmondstone (2009), Jonas et al. (2017), Mannix et al. (2013), and Bender (2016) indicate that a central attribute of clinical leadership is effective communication. This meant that clinical leaders needed to be 'extremely good at explaining things at the right level that you understand', as one study respondent said. Clinical leaders were also respected if they listened and effective communication was fundamental if clinical leaders – who were not managers or titled leaders – were to influence their colleagues. One respondent indicated that 'the ward manager has got the title and therefore they manage and are seen to be leaders because of the title, but there are other people that lead by virtue of their opinion'.

Visible in Practice

Although this was less evident than some of the other attributes, in order to be approachable, supportive and an effective role model, clinical leaders needed to be visible, available and present. The maxim, **'you can't be what you can't see'** applies here. One respondent indicated:

> If you want information, or if you want the best way to do something on the ward at that moment you're not going to get, or you don't have time to go looking for matron or phoning the nurse consultant, who's maybe in the middle of a clinic and can't come up until . . .
> *Because they're not around?*
> . . . because they're not around. I want somebody right there on the ward.
> *So, is being a clinical leader about being visible and present?*
> I think it does help to have leadership on the ward, that is visible . . . I think you need clinical leaders on the ward where they can be utilised and their knowledge shared and lead from the front.

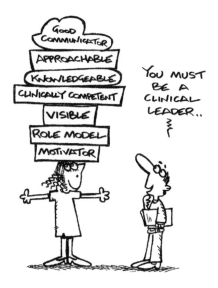

Another respondent supported this view: 'to lead it is very, very difficult, very time-consuming and exhausting and I think you have to . . . give of yourself, and that's why you have to be visible'. Clark (2008) agrees and adds that visibility means that clinical leaders were present in the clinical area: not just that they were there, but that they were engaged and involved. When another respondent said of a colleague that she was 'an ideal clinical leader' because 'she is very visible', it captured all the characteristics and attributes discussed here. Visibility implied clinical competence, clinical knowledge, effective communication, support, empowerment and motivation, being open and approachable and acting as a role model. Not being visible, or being unable to be involved in patient/client care activity, was seen by some respondents to place the person in a difficult position, or one that weakened their clinical leadership potential or clinical credibility.

Copes Well with Change

Finally, clinical leaders were also identified as being able to cope well with change, a view supported by Mannix et al. (2013) and also evident in Coventry and Russell's (2021) study, with clinical nurse educators being seen as change agents who were the go-to people if something needed to be changed or implemented (Coventry and Russell 2021). Dealing well with change is recognised as a key attribute in the modern health service and is one that is valued in clinical leaders.

Other Attributes

Over the years I have shared my views on clinical nurse leadership attributes and found considerable support for the characteristics I offered. However, I have always been keen to explore further attributes. After many discussions to solicit further views and based on my own and others' research, the following attributes are also worthy of consideration:

- courage
- ability to make decisions
- ability to offer direction
- sense of humour
- persistence and determination
- dynamism/energy
- calm under pressure
- positivity
- empathy
- compassion (critical for the application of compassionate leadership) (West 2021)
- change facilitation
- passion

These additional characteristics enhance an understanding of clinical leadership and can be seen to add a further perspective to the characteristics and attributes required to grasp what makes an effective clinical leader.

Values: The Glue that Binds

Values can be described as deeply held views that act as guiding principles for individuals and organisations (Pendleton and King 2002; Clark 2008; Gentile 2010). When they are stated and made explicit – or even if they are inferred from observable behaviour, then followed – they form the basis of trust in any relationship; and if values are stated or shown and not followed, then trust can be harmed. Values also relate to where individuals or organisations stand on a range of issues and point towards actions or statements that reflect what is important to that person or organisation. In the study with rural and remote area nurses one participant said,

> my view is that it's about people putting their values and beliefs into action. . . if my mother gets sick that's the nurse I want to have look after my mother, because she puts into practice what I think is the important values of nursing. That's what I think clinical leadership is all about (P50) (Stanley and Stanley 2019).

Antrobus and Kitson (1999, p. 750) identified 'understanding self and having a clear understanding of values, purpose and personal meaning' as part of the skills repertoire that they identified for effective nurse leaders. Cook (2001a) also saw clinical nurse leaders as 'valuers' who empathised with others and who tried to gauge their own and others' feelings. However, in the data from the research for this book, clinical leaders described themselves as being driven by their values and 'passion' for high-quality patient care. Coventry and Russell (2021) found in their study with clinical nurse educators that clinical leaders were seen as sharing their values, encouraging a positive culture and being guided by concern and compassion most of the time. Ultimately, holding and demonstrating values and beliefs emerged as a strong attribute of clinically focused leaders, with clinical leaders being identified if they were seen to demonstrate their values or had their values on show. Therefore, they were followed not because they had control, or for their vision and creativity (although they may have had these attributes), but because their values and beliefs were the driving force behind their ability to engage in critical problems and face the challenges of clinical care.

Being creative and having a vision remain central to the successful application of transformational leadership (Frankel 2008; Marriner-Tomey 2009), although they appeared not to be features for which clinical leaders are recognised (Stanley 2006a, b, 2008, 2011, 2014; Stanley et al. 2012; Scully 2014; Stanley et al. 2014; McLellan 2015; Stanley et al. 2015; Coventry and Russell 2021). There is a view that values are inextricable from vision, although Pendleton and King (2002) declare that it may be even more important to know where you stand (a values-centred position) rather than where you are going (pertaining to vision). This implies that values are rooted in understanding an individual's and organisation's principles, while vision is about being able to drive through or respond to changes in the future.

Clinical leaders are identifiable because of where they stand and how they behave when dealing with patients and colleagues. When facing challenges in the clinical arena, they are recognisable because they display their principles about the quality of care and they deal with patients in a 'hands-on' fashion, living out their values in the actions of clinical care. They stand apart from novice clinicians, poor decision makers, staff who are 'hidebound', managers who are tied up with other functions and those who are less visible in the clinical environment. They may be experts in their clinical field, but they are recognised not necessarily because of their expert practice, but because when faced with challenges and critical problems their actions are directed, and their leadership is defined by the values and beliefs that they hold about care, healthcare and respect for others.

Who Are the Clinical Leaders?

In the past, leadership studies were very much focused on leadership at the high end of the organisational hierarchy, shining a light on the academic, political and management domains (Antrobus and Kitson 1999). The proliferation of these studies and literature has to some extent overshadowed leadership by others, at other levels of the health service, although this trend has slowed and been redressed in recent years. Indeed, as a nurse practitioner in the late 1990s, it was the lack of appropriate literature or studies about clinical-level leadership that spurred me on to my own research journey in the topic of clinical leadership. It is now clear that leadership is everyone's business (Ogawa and Bossert 1995; Cook 2001a; Higgins et al. 2014; Jonas et al. 2017;). Because clinical-level leaders are central to the provision of healthcare, they have found themselves more and more the focus of leadership studies and the recipients of leadership education. Burns (2001) supports these views and believes that in a chaotic healthcare environment, front-line leaders are not only required at all levels, they may understand the environment's complexities even more than executive leaders removed from direct operations.

The success and appeal of television programmes like *Undercover Boss* support this view, and demonstrate the value of understanding the workplace from a front-line staff perspective, what Mintzberg (1983) calls the 'operating core' of a healthcare organisation. However, clinical leadership has historically been less valued than senior management and, as such, health service management has dominated the leadership debate in health to the detriment of clinical, bedside or front-line leadership. Clark (2008, p. 30) suggests that organisations should be tapping into 'the leadership skills and potential of all front line staff to deliver high-quality, safe and effective care to patients and service users'.

Indeed, when I began my clinical leadership research journey as a student at Nottingham University, doctors and nurse consultants were identified as the clinical leaders. Allied health professionals were not even considered in the mix, and to a large extent leadership training or education was the domain of those in identified hierarchical management positions. Coventry and Russell (2021) sought to explore if clinical nurse educators were seen as clinical leaders. They found that they were, and indeed had much in common with the attributes and characteristics identified in the clinical leader studies that underpin this text.

The six studies that support this book confirmed that clinical leaders exist in vast quantities and at all levels within all clinical areas. The 188 questionnaire respondents in the initial study nominated 326 people as clinical leaders, and in the 4 clinical areas of the focused interviews, the 42 nurses interviewed nominated 130 people as clinical leaders, most of whom (although not all) were middle-level nurses or lower. Clark (2008, p. 30) also suggested that 'some nurses may not think of themselves as leaders because they equate leadership with authority or with specific job titles rather than as a way of thinking or behaving'. Coventry and Russell (2021) found that in spite of the informal nature of the clinical nurse educators' role, clinical nurse educators encouraged, promoted, supported and engaged in advancing the nursing profession and promoting excellence in nursing care. As the study results show, health professionals see clearly that their clinical colleagues are leaders – and rightly so.

The initial study and the four that followed demonstrated that clinical leaders were to be seen at all levels, with nominations offered for doctors, other health professionals, area managers, directors of nursing, clinical nurses, registered nurses and even healthcare assistants; although again, mid-level health professionals who were focused on clinical activities received the most recognition as clinical leaders. No direction was given on the questionnaires about whom to nominate and only 8.8% of all nominations in the initial study were for medical staff – a figure that might stun Stanton et al. (2010) or Swanwick and McKimm (2017), or others who write about the pivotal place of medical professionals as clinical leaders.

Medical professionals may be clinical leaders, but it is equally the case that any health professional, at any level, who has the attributes identified in this chapter and who is followed because they have their values and beliefs on show and match these to their actions, may be seen as a clinical leader.

From a nursing perspective, the mid-level registered nurse was the candidate most likely to be viewed as a clinical leader by their colleagues, both senior and junior. The results (Stanley 2006a, b) also showed that differences exist between specialist units and general wards; in the latter, lower-level registered nurses followed mid-level registered nurses in being commonly nominated as clinical leaders. In specialist clinical units, as well as mid-level registered nurses, more senior registered nurses or clinically based specialist nurses were common candidates for selection. Moreover, significantly fewer clinical leaders were identified in non-specialist clinical areas. It was worryingly noted that clinical areas that commonly took new graduates and neophyte practitioners into their first experiences of healthcare had fewer clinical leaders in place to support them. However, the attributes that identified clinical leaders were the same, regardless of the clinical area in which they worked.

There was little support for managers to be seen as clinical leaders. If a manager had an element of 'control' built into their role, or if they had minimal clinical engagement, they were seldom identified as a clinical leader. This view was supported in the results of Coventry and Russell's (2021) study with clinical nurse educators.

This is not a new point, and publications for some time have drawn attention to the tension between clinical leadership responsibilities and management functions (Rafferty 1993; Christian and Norman 1998; Antrobus and Kitson 1999; Stanley 2000; Firth 2002; McCormack and Garbett 2003; Thyer 2003; Stanley 2006c). The main focus of the conflict was between the clinician's desire to remain clinically focused and the need to be able to maintain the management and resource capabilities of their clinical area. For many allied health professionals, this was a common feature of their clinical leadership/management dichotomy. A research transcription extract demonstrates this point:

> The main one I think is really the issue from the [organisation's] point of view . . . the [organisations] want to implement schemes or whatever which I don't feel are in the best interests of the patients or staff . . . for example the [organisations] are trying to

have [middle-level nurses] carry a hospital bleep, now I disagree with that because I feel my role should be ward-based, clinically based and I don't want to see my role as managing the hospital.

This highlights the observation that clinical leaders are selected because they have their values on show. As such, when health professionals are promoted away from the clinical area or lose direct client contact, many face a crisis of conscience as they struggle to remain rooted to their core professional values while being directed and drawn into areas of management and administration that are often either removed from or in conflict with their values and beliefs about patient/client care (Stanley 2006c). Even if this is not the case and a crisis of conscience is avoided, others may recognise the 'controlling' elements in their role, and this may diminish their identification or effectiveness as a clinical leader.

Clinical leaders, therefore, are not identified because of their position, job title, role in the health service or badge. They can be in any clinical area and involved in any aspect of patient care or clinical service. They are rarely found in offices, removed from clinical contact or interaction with clients or patients, and they are generally experienced health professionals focused on their desire or 'passion' for developing a high standard of care and best-quality service.

Clinical leaders are recognised for having their values and beliefs sit behind their actions and interventions. They are not recognised for their vision or creativity (although some are creative and visionary). They are found across the spectrum of health organisations, often at the highest level for clinical interaction, but not commonly at the highest management level in a ward or unit team, and they are seen in all clinical environments.

Clinical Leader Stories: 1 Leading by Example

While I was a second-year physio student, I was fortunate enough to work alongside someone who I believe was the epitome of clinical leadership in healthcare. When I reflect on the type of physio I want to be I always think about my interactions with this instructor. This physio clinical supervisor was professional, approachable and open. She was an effective communicator and clinically competent. I observed many physios gravitating to her on the ward as she was so knowledgeable and always happy to help. She empowered other physios to engage professionally with other members of the healthcare team and actively sought out students to practice or observe clinical skills and practices that were uncommon on the ward. I really appreciated this encouragement, as I was new to the ward environment and lacked the confidence to really engage with senior staff members or seek out learning opportunities on my own. I feel this was an extremely positive experience for me as it has increased my awareness of the difference you can make to a student's transition to practice by empowering them and encouraging them to speak up. I feel she offered a good example of Congruent Leadership and Transformational Leadership. The physio clinical supervisor's values were evident in their practice and the clinical leadership displayed by her has inspired me to want to lead others by setting a positive example myself. I know that in the future I'll be a positive role model by putting what I learnt into action and leading by the example that was shown to me. *Lisa: Physiotherapy Student.*

Reflection Point

Do you need to have a title or hierarchical role to be an effective clinical leader? Why might this matter? Discuss this with a senior colleague. What are their views on this question?

Clinical Leadership Defined

The definition offered in this book is that:

> **clinical leaders are clinical experts in their field and are followed because they match their actions with their values and beliefs about quality patient care.**

In addition, it is suggested that the attributes of effective clinical leaders are those of clinical competence, clinical knowledge and effective communication, and that they are empowered motivators, role models, visible in practice, supportive, have integrity, are inspirational, cope well with change and are open and approachable.

It is suggested that clinical leaders can be found in all areas of care and that they are seldom managers or even the most senior health professional. Instead, clinical leaders are identified in large numbers and represent the clinician who is visible in practice with their values and beliefs about care on display (Coventry and Russell 2021).

Reflection Point

When in your career have you undertaken leadership training? Was it at an undergraduate or postgraduate level? Or has your employer, recognising the value of having clinical-level leaders who understand the value of leadership instruction, sent you on or supported you to undertake further training? Speak with your clinical colleagues. What leadership instruction have they received?

Why Clinical Leadership Now?

Why should we consider clinical leadership at this time and in this context? When I was a student nurse in the 1980s, no one mentioned 'leadership', let alone 'clinical leadership'. Indeed, I recall a strong element of subservience running as an undercurrent through the profile of our nursing curriculum and within our training, suggesting that doctors were nurses' leaders and their betters, and that we did not need to make decisions or think too much. I can recall, too, the beginnings of a quiet rebellion as nurses abandoned their nurses' cap and moved to competency-based assessment, university-based education, new roles, new dress codes and new titles. Yet the subservience was evident, nonetheless.

So why has clinical leadership become an issue for current and future health professional students and practitioners?

A New Agenda

Leadership development is being seen as central to the development and modification of the health agenda (Stanton et al. 2010; Mannix et al. 2013; Phillips and Byrne 2013; Rose 2015; Townsend et al. 2015; West et al. 2015; Bender 2016; Swanwick and McKimm 2017; West 2021). The UK Department of Health said as long ago as 1999 that it required staff who can establish direction and purpose, inspire, motivate and empower teams around common goals, in order to help produce improvements in quality, clinical practice and service (DoH 1999), and nothing has changed to modify this requirement. Similar calls to action are evident in other parts of the world where leadership development is seen as central to the development of the healthcare agenda. Leadership is needed at all levels (DoH WA 2004) and it is suggested that clinical leadership needs to be increased, that clinical networks for change need to be initiated and that growing change management and leadership skills are essential for all health professionals (DoH WA 2004; Martin and Learmouth 2012; Storey and Holti 2013b; Scully 2014; Byers 2015; McLellan 2015; Rose 2015; West et al. 2015; West 2021).

Changing Care Contexts

It is recognised that the context of healthcare is changing. Care provision is no longer (and has really never been) solely in the domain of the acute hospital. Therefore, as new healthcare environments are developed, new ways of working with new roles and staff mean that new approaches to care and greater innovation are required. The development of nurse practitioners, for example, and wider skill sets for allied health professionals and paramedics offer examples of how the healthcare environment is developing. Patients can now be treated and cared for in a range of clinical areas (and indeed, remotely via telehealth) and environments by experienced and skilled health professionals, who can deliver and prescribe care and implement clinical decisions based on their critical thinking.

Change Equates to More Leadership

There is also a recognition that the health service needs more staff with greater leadership (as opposed to management) skills and insights (Stanton et al. 2010; Byers 2015; McLellan 2015; Swanwick and McKimm 2017). This is partly in response to the realisation that the more change there is, the greater is the need for leaders (Kotter 1990). It is also an acknowledgement that until quite recently there has been under-investment in leadership training and leadership development and even a lack of discussion about clinical leadership within healthcare (Rafferty 1993; Hurst 1997; Lett 2002; Stanley 2008; Martin and Learmouth 2012; Storey and Holti 2013a; Scully 2014; Byers 2015; McLellan 2015; Rose 2015; West et al. 2015; West 2021). I would suggest that the core reason for a surge in leadership, and clinical leadership in particular, is the realisation that change, innovation, the development of quality care and the links between values and care, compassion and quality are all based on effective leadership (West 2021). While management is essential, the development of grassroots, front-line leaders opens up genuine opportunities for a positive impact on innovation, creativity and change (James et al. 2020).

More Emphasis on Quality

As Francis (2013) shows, there is a pressing need to do better, often with limited resources (Storey and Holti 2013a; Scully 2014; McLellan 2015; Byers 2015; Rose 2015; West et al. 2015; West 2021). The drive to improve quality and support the integration of quality improvement sits at the heart of a need to generate more effective clinical leadership. In the UK, initiatives such as the 'Payment by Results' scheme mean that care providers are rewarded for the volume of work they do and are assessed against an ever-stricter quality reporting mechanism (Stanton et al. 2010). An emphasis on quality supported by the adoption of clinical governance strategies also places more pressure on clinicians to continuously improve the quality of care.

Clinicians are best placed to address quality initiatives, change and innovation in clinical practice. Linking all of these is the realisation that if care is to improve and develop, then change and innovation in practice are required. It is often the clinician, working with clients, other colleagues, relatives and patients, who is best placed to identify inefficiencies, bottlenecks and problems, and who can identify the most appropriate solutions for these issues. Clinicians are indeed the 'operational core' of the health service (Mintzberg 1983).

Therefore, if the health service is to grow, support innovation and initiate change, it needs leaders with skills and talents to take their ideas and projects forward. As well, if the health service is to retain a focus on the core values that underpin the provision of quality health care then an exploration of values-based leadership approaches is vital (James et al. 2020; West 2021). In the clinical arena, it is clinical leaders who are in an ideal position to fulfil this role and who are ideally situated to support other clinicians to develop the health service. Clinical leaders, however, need the skills, attributes, tools and techniques to initiate and manage change effectively and the personal will and abilities to recognise themselves as 'change agents' and as a force for positive growth in the health service.

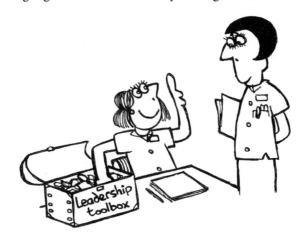

Case Study 1.1   Vivian Bullwinkel

Vivian Bullwinkel is rightly regarded as a clinical leader. Read about her and consider how holding on to her values during her struggle in difficult conditions was central to her survival and shaped her ensuring career as a health professional leader.

Vivian was born in 1915 and began her education in Broken Hill, New South Wales before training as a nurse and midwife in 1934. At the outbreak of World War II she travelled to Melbourne with a view to join the war effort. Enlisting took time, and while she waited for an opportunity to contribute she worked as a nurse at the Jessie MacPherson Hospital in Melbourne.

In May 1941, Vivian volunteered for the Australian Army Nursing Service (AANS) and was posted to Singapore, the bastion of the British Empire in the Far East. She served at the 2/13th Australian General Hospital, and with other Australian nurses she cared for wounded Allied soldiers, often under difficult conditions as the war reached closer. By early February 1942, the Japanese army was on the brink of taking Singapore. Vivian boarded the SS *Vyner Brooke* with 65 other nurses fleeing the Japanese advance, but the ship was struck by Japanese aircraft a few days later and sank. A large number of passengers, including Vivian and many of the nurses, made it to shore on the island of Banka (now part of Indonesia). The nurses surrendered to the occupying Japanese army; however, the following day they were ordered to walk out to sea, where they were machine gunned. Vivian was shot and injured, but survived by feigning death until the Japanese had moved off. Twenty-one nurses were murdered.

Following the massacre, Vivian dragged herself back to the beach, the sole survivor of the atrocity. In the jungle just off the shore she discovered a wounded British soldier and for several weeks they both hid in the jungle, scavenging food and managing their wounds as best they could. However, their deteriorating condition forced them to surrender. The British soldier died shortly afterwards. Vivian and other Australian nurses spent a further three and a half years in captivity, being starved, tortured, refused medical care or treatment, and moved from one jungle camp to another. Death was a constant threat, but Vivian's determination to survive and willingness to offer others compassion and companionship saw her survive to be released at the war's end.

Following World War II, 'Sister Bullwinkel' served with the Australian army in Japan in 1946 and 1947 before resigning from the military at the rank of captain. In 1955 she joined the Citizen Military Forces and served until 1970, reaching the rank of lieutenant colonel. In addition, she spent 16 years as matron and 7 years as Director of Nursing at Melbourne's Fairfield Hospital. She retired in 1977, married Colonel F.W. Statham and moved to Perth, Western Australia, where she died in 2000.

Vivian was awarded the Royal Red Cross Medal in 1947 for services to the veteran and ex-prisoner of war communities, to nursing, to the Red Cross Society and to the wider community. She was appointed a Member of the Order of the British Empire (MBE) in 1973, was awarded the Order of Australia (AO) in 1993, and was also a recipient of the Florence Nightingale Medal.

In 1993 she returned to Banka Island to unveil a shrine to the nurses who were murdered there. She survived multiple difficulties and challenges during her years of

---

(Continued)

captivity, and if persistence and determination are invincible, Vivian Bullwinkel is surely the personification of this tenet.

Challenge: Can you recognise any of the attributes of a clinical leader in Vivian's story? How might these attributes have contributed to her survival as a Japanese prisoner and her ongoing career success?

Summary

- Change and quality in the health service are not all about processes and structure; they are also about courageous people who are prepared to act.
- The main attributes of clinical leaders are approachability; empowerment and motivation; being visible in practice; clinically competent and clinically knowledgeable; having values and beliefs on show; having effective communication skills; coping well with change; having integrity; and is supportive, inspires confidence and is a positive clinical role model.
- Clinical leaders are not identified because of their position, job title, role in the health service or badge.
- Clinical leaders can be found in any clinical area and are involved in any aspect of patient care or clinical service.
- Clinical leaders are generally experienced, clinically focused health professionals driven by their desire or 'passion' for developing a high standard of care/service.
- Clinical leaders are the people at the 'coal face' (operating core) and are in the best position to identify change initiatives and to drive change or quality in clinical practice.
- Six research projects that explored who clinical leaders are, why clinical leaders are seen as such and what the experiences of clinical leaders are sit at the heart of this book and the theory presented here.
- Clinical leadership and the clinical leader's time has come. There is a new agenda in the health service focusing on innovation, change, a drive for quality and leaders who use values-based leadership approaches. Care practices and the context of care provision are changing. There is a recognition that greater change needs stronger leadership and that leaders can come from any stratum of the health industry. Indeed, effective change, quality improvements and innovation may be more successful if they are initiated and developed by clinicians who are empowered to lead and apply their values about compassion, care, competence, communication, and other values held within healthcare.

Mind Press-Ups

Exercise 1.1

If you can, approach a person who you feel is a clinical leader. Explain to them that you see them as a clinical leader and ask them how they feel. Were they shocked, surprised, delighted? How did they respond to your announcement?

Exercise 1.2

What are your experiences of leadership development from your undergraduate or formative healthcare education? Do you feel well prepared and instructed in leadership theories and techniques? Ask some colleagues how they learnt about leadership and what they understand leadership to be.

Exercise 1.3

Draw a 'mind map' with the word 'leadership' in the centre. You could start the map here and build or add to it as you progress through the book or over the trajectory of your studies.

Exercise 1.4

Who are your leaders? Who might you direct an alien or stranger to if they asked you to take them to your leader? Would these be the same people if you were asked to take them to your 'clinical leader'?

References

Antrobus, S. and Kitson, A. (1999). Nursing leadership: influencing and shaping health policy and nursing practice. *Journal of Advanced Nursing* 29 (3): 746–753.

Bender, M. (2016). Conceptualizing clinical nurse leader practice: an interpretive synthesis. *Journal of Nursing Management* 24: 23–31. https://doi.org/10.1111/jonm.12285.

Berwick, D. (1994). Eleven worthy aims for clinical leadership of health care reform. *Journal of the American Medical Association* 272 (10): 797.

Boamah, S. (2018). Linking nurses' clinical leadership to patient care quality: the role of transformational leadership and workplace empowerment. *Canadian Journal of Nursing Research* 50 (1): 9–19.

Burns, J.P. (2001). Complexity science and leadership in healthcare. *Journal of Nursing Administration* 3 (10): 474–482.

Byers, V. (2015). The challenges of leading change in health-care delivery from the frontline. *Journal of Nursing Management* 25: early view. https://doi.org/10.1111/jonm.12342.

Chavez, E.C. and Yoder, L.H. (2014). Staff nurse clinical leadership: a concept analysis. *Nursing Forum* 50 (2): 90–100.

Christian, S.L. and Norman, I.J. (1998). Clinical leadership in nursing development units. *Journal of Advanced Nursing* 27: 108–116.

Clark, L. (2008). Clinical leadership values, beliefs and vision. *Nursing Management* 15 (7): 30–35.

Cook, M. (2001a). The attributes of effective clinical nurse leaders. *Nursing Standard* 15 (35): 33–36.

Cook, M. (2001b). Clinical leadership that works. *Nursing Management* 7 (10): 24–28.

Cook, A. and Holt, L. (2000). Clinical leadership and supervision. In: *Accident and Emergency Theory into Practice* (ed. B. Dolan and L. Holt), 497–503. London: Baillière Tindall.

Coventry, T.H. and Russell, K.P. (2021). The clinical nurse educator as a congruent leader: a mixed method study. *Journal of Nursing Education and Practice* 11 (1): 8–18.

Dean-Barr, S. (1998). Translating clinical leadership into organizational leadership. *Rehabilitation Nursing* 23 (3): 118.

Demeh, W. and Rosengren, K. (2015). The visualisation of clinical leadership in the context of nursing education: a qualitative study of nursing students' experiences. *Nurse Education Today* 35: 888–893.

Department of Health (1999). *Making a Difference.* London: Stationery Office.

Department of Health (2007). *Our NHS: Our Future.* NHS Next Stage Review Interim Report. London: HM Stationery Office.

Department of Health, Western Australia (2004). *Strategic Intent 2005–2010.* Perth: Department of Health http://www.health.wa.gov.au/hrit/docs/publications/clinicalframework.pdf (accessed 1 May 2016).

Edmondstone, J. (2009). Clinical leadership: the elephant in the room. *International Journal of Health Planning and Management* 24: 290–305.

Ferguson, L., Calvert, J., Davie, M. et al. (2007). Clinical leadership: using observations of care to focus on risk management and quality improvement activities in the clinical setting. *Contemporary Nurse* 24: 212–224.

Firth, K. (2002). Ward leadership: balancing the clinical and managerial roles. *Professional Nurse* 17 (8): 486–489.

Forest, A.E., Taichman, R.S., and Inglehart, M.R. (2013). Dentists' leadership-related perceptions, values, experiences and behaviour: results of a national survey. *Journal of the American Dental Association* 144 (12): 1397–1405.

Francis, R. (2013). *Report of the Mid Staffordshire NHS Foundation Trust Public Inquiry.* London: HM Stationery Office.

Frankel, A. (2008). What leadership styles should senior nurses develop? *Nursing Times* 104 (35): 23–24.

Gentile, M.C. (2010). *Giving Voice to Values.* London: Yale University Press.

Harper, J. (1995). Clinical leadership: bridging theory and practice. *Nurse Educator* 20 (3): 11–12.

Higgins, A., Begley, C., Lalor, J. et al. (2014). Factors influencing advancing practitioners' ability to enact leadership: a case study within Irish healthcare. *Journal of Nursing Management* 22: 894–905.

Hurst, K. (1997). *A Review of the Nursing Leadership Literature.* Leeds: Nuffield Institute, University of Leeds.

James, A., Bennett, C., and Stanley, D. (2020). How to maintain enthusiasm and demonstrate values-driven leadership in challenging times. *Nursing Managmemnt* https://rcni.com/nursing-management/opinion/comment/how-to-maintain-enthusiasm-and-demonstrate-values-driven-leadership-challenging-times-167876.

James, A.H., Bennett, C.L., Blanchard, D., and Stanley, D. (2021). 'Nursing and values-based leadership: a literature review. *Journal of Nurse Management* 29 (5): 916–930.

Jeon, Y.-H. (2011). Clinical leadership: the key to optimising the aged care workforce. *Connections* 14 (4): 18–19.

Jeon, Y.-H., Conway, J., Chenweth, L. et al. (2014). Validation of a clinical leadership qualities framework for managers in aged care: a Delphi study. *Journal of Clinical Nursing* 24 (7–8): 999–1010. https://doi.org/10.1111/jocn.12682.

Jonas, S., McCay, L., and Keogh, B. (2017). The importance of clinical leadership. In: *ABC of Clinical Leadership*, 2e (ed. T. Swanwick and J. McKimm), 1–3. Oxford: Wiley-Blackwell/ BMJ Books.

Kotter, J.P. (1990). What leaders really do. In: *Harvard Business Review: On Leadership* (ed. M.A. Boston), 37–60. Harvard Business School Press.

Lett, M. (2002). The concept of clinical leadership. *Contemporary Nurse* 12 (1): 16–20.

Malby, R. (1997). Developing the future leaders of nursing in the UK. *European Nurse* 2 (1): 27–36.

Mannix, J., Wilkes, L., and Daly, J. (2013). Attributes of clinical leadership in contemporary nursing: an integrative review. *Contemporary Nurse* 45 (1): 10–21.

Marriner-Tomey, A. (2009). *Guide to Nursing Management and Leadership*, 8e. St Louis: Elsevier.

Martin, G.P. and Learmouth, M. (2012). A critical account of the rise and spread of "leadership": the case of UK healthcare. *Social Science & Medicine* 74 (3): 281–288.

McCormack, B. and Garbett, R. (2003). The characteristics and skills of practice developers. *Journal of Clinical Nursing* 12 (3): 317–325.

McCormack, B. and Hopkins, E. (1995). The development of clinical leadership through supported reflective practice. *Journal of Clinical Nursing* 4 (3): 161–168.

McDonnell, A., Goodwin, E., Kennedy, F. et al. (2015). An evaluation of the implementation of advanced nurse practitioner (ANP) roles in an acute hospital setting. *Journal of Advanced Nursing* 71 (4): 789–799. https://doi.org/10.1111/jan.12558.

McLellan, A. (2015). Ending the crisis in NHS leadership: a plan for renewal. *Health Service Journal*, Special ed. 1–11.

Mintzberg, H. (1983). *Structure in 5 s: Designing Effective Organisations*. Upper Saddle River, NJ: Prentice-Hall.

Mountford, J. and Webb, C. (2009). When clinicians lead. McKinsey Quarterly. http://www. mckinsey.com/industries/healthcare-systems-and-services/our-insights/when-clinicians-lead (accessed 1 May 2016).

Ogawa, R.T. and Bossert, S.T. (1995). Leadership as an organisational quality. *Educational Administration Quarterly* 31 (2): 224–243.

Peach, M. (1995). Reflection on clinical leadership behaviours. *Contemporary Nurse* 4 (1): 33–37.

Pendleton, D. and King, J. (2002). Values and leadership: education and debate. *British Medical Journal* 325: 1352–1355.

Phillips, N. and Byrne, G. (2013). Enhancing frontline clinical leadership in an acute hospital trust. *Journal of Clinical Nursing* 17 (18): 2625–2635.

Rafferty, A.M. (1993). *Leading Questions: A Discussion Paper on the Issues of Nurse Leadership*. London: King's Fund.

Rocchiccioli, J.T. and Tilbury, M.S. (1998). *Clinical Leadership in Nursing*. Philadelphia, PA: W. B. Saunders.

Rolfe, G. (2006). In command of care: towards a theory of congruent leadership. *Journal of Research in Nursing* 2 (2): 145–146.

Rose, L. (2015). *Better Leadership for Tomorrow: NHS Leadership Review*. London: Department of Health http://thelarreysociety.org/wp-content/uploads/2015/08/Lord_Rose_NHS_Report_acc.pdf (accessed 1 May 2016).

Schneider, P. (1999). Five worthy aims for pharmacy's clinical leadership to pursue in improving medication use. *American Journal of Health-System Pharmacy* 56 (24): 2549–2552.

Scully, N.J. (2014). Leadership in nursing: the importance of recognising values and attributes to secure a positive future for the profession. *Collegian* 22 (4): 439–444.

Stanley, D. (2000). *In the trenches*. Unpublished MSc thesis, University of Birmingham.

Stanley, D. (2006a). In command of care: clinical nurse leadership explored. *Journal of Research in Nursing* 11 (1): 20–39.

Stanley, D. (2006b). In command of care: towards the theory of congruent leadership. *Journal of Research in Nursing* 11 (2): 134–144.

Stanley, D. (2006c). Role conflict: leaders and managers. *Nursing Management* 13 (5): 31–37.

Stanley, D. (2008). Congruent leadership: values in action. *Journal of Nursing Management* 16: 519–524.

Stanley, D. (2011). *Clinical Leadership: Innovation into Action*. South Yarra, VIC: Palgrave Macmillan.

Stanley, D. (2014). Clinical leadership characteristics confirmed. *Journal of Research in Nursing* 19 (2): 118–128.

Stanley, D. and Stanley, K. (2017). 'Clinical leadership and nursing explored: a literature search. *Journal of Clinical Nursing* 27: 1730–1743.

Stanley, D. and Stanley, K. (2018). *Report: there where the 'bullets can fly': Clinical leadership in rural and remote North-Western New South Wales*. Research Report. 2018 UNE Print.

Stanley, D. and Stanley, K. (2019). 'Clinical leadership and rural and remote practice: a qualitative study. *Journal of Nursing Management* 27 (6): 1314–1324.

Stanley, D., Cuthbertson, J., and Latimer, K. (2012). Perceptions of clinical leadership in the St. John Ambulance Service in WA. *Response* 39 (1): 31–37.

Stanley, D., Latimer, K., and Atkinson, J. (2014). Perceptions of clinical leadership in an aged care residential facility in Perth, Western Australia. *Health Care: Current Reviews* 2 (2): http://www.esciencecentral.org/journals/perceptions-of-clinical-leadership-in-an-aged-care-residential-facility-in-perth-western-australia.hccr.1000122.php?aid=24341 (accessed 1 May 2016).

Stanley, D., Hutton, M., and McDonald, A. (2015). *Western Australian Allied Health Professionals' Perceptions of Clinical Leadership: A Research Report*. Bathurst: CSU Print.

Stanton, E., Lemer, C., and Mountford, J. (2010). *Clinical Leadership: Bridging the Divide*. London: Quay Books.

Stavrianopoulos, T. (2012). 'The clinical nurse leader. *Health Science Journal* 6 (3): 392–401.

Storey, J. and Holti, R. (2013a). *Possibilities and Pitfalls for Clinical Leadership in Improving Service Quality, Innovation and Productivity*, Final Report, NIHR Service Delivery and Organisation Programme. London: HM Stationery Office.

Storey, J. and Holti, R. (2013b). *Towards a New Model of Leadership for the NHS*. Leeds: NHS Leadership Academy http://www.leadershipacademy.nhs.uk/wp-content/uploads/2013/05/Towards-a-New-Model-of-Leadership-2013.pdf (accessed 1 July 2016).

Swanwick, T. and McKimm, J. (2017). *ABC of Clinical Leadership*, 2e. Oxford: Wiley-Blackwell.

Thyer, G. (2003). Dare to be different: transformational leadership may hold the key to reducing the nursing shortage. *Journal of Nursing Management* 11: 73–79.

Townsend, K., Wilkinson, A., and Kellner, A. (2015). Opening the black box in nursing work and management practice: the role of ward managers. *Journal of Nursing Management* 23 (2): 211–220.

Van Dyk, J., Siedlecki, S.L., and Fitzpatrick, J.J. (2016). Frontline nurse managers' confidence and self-efficacy. *Journal of Nursing Management* 24 (4): 533–539. https://doi.org/10.1111/jonm.12355.

Watson, C. (2008). Assessing leadership in nurse practitioner candidates. *Australian Journal of Advanced Nursing* 26 (1): 67–76.

West, M. (2021). *Compassionate Leadership: Sustaining Wisdom, Humanity and Presence in Health and Social*. Swirling Leaf Press.

West, M., Loewenthal, L., Eckert, R. et al. (2015). *Leadership and Leadership Development in Healthcare the Evidence Base*. London: Faculty of Medical Leadership and Management/Center for Creative Leadership/The King's Fund www.fmlm.ac.uk/resources/leadership-and-leadership-development-in-health-care-the-evidence-base (accessed 23 Sept. 2021).

Won, H. (2015). Clinical leadership of staff nurse: a phenomenological study. *Indian Journal of Science and Technology* 8 (1): 1–4.

Wyatt, J. (1995). Hospital information management: the need for clinical leadership. *British Medical Journal* 311 (6998): 175–178.

2

Leadership Theories and Styles

David Stanley

The brain can be hired. The heart and soul have to be earned.
John Christensen, ChartHouse Learning

If I have seen further it is by standing on the shoulders of giants.
Sir Isaac Newton, letter to Robert Hooke, circa 1675

Introduction: Leadership – What Does It All Mean?

Leadership has long been a feature of educational, business, industry, military and medical or health service debate. A plethora of books, journal articles, web pages and papers has resulted, offering a wide variety of theories, definitions and perspectives about how to recognise effective leadership, develop better leaders, promote change or innovation and promote more effective organisations. Although the focus of this book is clinical leadership and leadership related to healthcare professionals, it will draw on concepts, definitions and theories of leadership from business, industry, educational and military perspectives. In addition, it will explore leadership related to healthcare and care in the clinical setting to support a better understanding of clinically focused leadership.

This chapter attempts to define leadership. Leadership can be a vexed and convoluted concept, and it is commonly seen as linked to theories of management and associated with elevated hierarchical positions and power. This book is not specifically directed at titled leaders, people in authority, managers or senior managers. Indeed, leadership and leaders are considered to be different from management and managers (Zaleznik 1977; Kotter 1990; Stanley 2006, 2011). While it is acknowledged that they are related, for the purposes of this book concepts of management are not explored or considered, although the differences between management and leadership are discussed in Chapter 5.

Many people from a range of different groups have been interested in discovering more about leadership, and for a long time the nature of leadership has been extensively

Clinical Leadership in Nursing and Healthcare, Third Edition.
Edited by David Stanley, Clare L. Bennett and Alison H. James.
© 2023 John Wiley & Sons Ltd. Published 2023 by John Wiley & Sons Ltd.

researched (Swanwick and McKimm 2017). Chinese and Indian scholars have studied and written about leadership. It is referred to in the Old Testament, and numerous mythical stories from civilisations across the globe address the act of leadership. Confucius wrote about leadership, and Plato, who lived between 427 and 347 BCE, wrote in *The Republic* about the value of developing leadership characteristics by describing the attributes required to navigate and command a sea vessel (Adair 2002a). In almost any field of endeavour, from leading large corporations or massive armies to leading the editorial committee of a monthly newsletter, a clinical area or the local junior football club, leadership and the experience of being a leader are common themes.

Theories and definitions of leadership abound. Stogdill (1974, p. 7) believes that 'there are almost as many different definitions of leadership as there are people who have attempted to define the concept'. Northouse (2007, p. 2) also indicates that as soon as 'we try to define leadership, we immediately discover that leadership has many different meanings', while Bennis and Nanus (1985, p. 4) feel that in relation to leadership, 'never have so many laboured so long to say so little'.

Here is a smattering of quotations about leadership to help enhance your insight:

> Leadership is the capacity to translate vision into reality.
> *(Warren G. Bennis, President, University of Cincinnati,*
> *University of Maryland Symposium, 21 January 1988)*

> The key to successful leadership today is influence, not authority.
> *(Kenneth Schatz, Managing by Influence, Prentice-Hall, 1986)*

> A leader is a dealer in hope.
> *(Napoleon Bonaparte, 1769–1821, Emperor of France,*
> *Maxims of Napoleon)*

> I am certainly not one of those who needs to be prodded. In fact, if anything, I am a prod.
> *(Winston Churchill, 1874–1965, UK Prime Minister, writer and Lord of*
> *the Admiralty, speech in Parliament, 11 November 1942)*

> Charisma becomes the undoing of leaders. It makes them inflexible, convinced of their own infallibility, unable to change.
> *(Peter F. Drucker, management consultant and writer,*
> *Wall Street Journal, 6 January 1988)*

> Leadership is practiced not so much in words as in attitude and in actions.
> *(Harold Geneen, CEO of ITT, Managing, Doubleday, 1984)*

> The reward of the general is not a bigger tent, but command.
> *(Oliver Wendell Holmes, Jr, 1841–1935, US Supreme Court Justice, 1917)*

The rotting fish begins to stink at the head. (Italian proverb)
When the best leader's work is done the people say, 'We did it ourselves'.
(Lao-Tzu, 604–531 BCE, Chinese philosopher and founder of Taoism,
Tao Te Ching)

If the blind lead the blind, both shall fall into the ditch.
(New Testament, Matthew 15:14)

More than knowledge, leaders need character. Values and ethics are vitally important.
(Oscar Arias, former president of Costa Rica, humanitarian, June 2001)

Leadership Defined: The Blind Man's Elephant

An understanding of leadership is central to understanding the experience of leading in any environment, which also applies to the clinical environment (Kibbe 2019). As such, it is useful to begin with an exploration of the terms 'leadership' and 'leader'. As the quotations show, defining leadership can be like the parable of the blind men and the elephant, and in many respects the definition offered depends on which part is grasped (Box 2.1).

There are a wide variety of beliefs, definitions and perspectives of leadership, with many complex dimensions (Northouse 2007; Jones and Bennett 2018). Because of this, a number of definitions are explored here to elaborate on the concept of leadership and offer a prelude to understanding clinical leadership. These are taken from a wide range of fields and perspectives and support considerable breadth in the definition of leadership.

Fiedler (1967), who primarily studied military and managerial leadership, felt that the leader has long been considered to be the individual in the group with the task of directing and coordinating the group's activities. Others view leadership from a personality perspective, a power relationship perspective, as an instrument of goal achievement (Bass 1990) or as the process of influencing people to accomplish goals (Northouse 2007; Grossman and Valiga 2021).

Box 2.1   The Parable of the Blind Men and the Elephant

Three blind men were asked to lead an elephant and, in the process, to describe what the elephant might be like by touch alone. The first grasped the trunk and declared that an elephant must be like a giant snake; the second felt the rough hide and said that the elephant must be like a giant warthog; and the third grasped the tusk and said that an elephant must be like an enormous walrus.

The point of the parable is that taking only a part of an elephant cannot lead to a complete understanding of the beast. I have always wondered, though, how these three blind men knew what a snake, a warthog and a walrus felt like in the first place. I guess you can only take a parable so far.

Leadership can also be described as achieving things with the support of others (Leigh and Maynard 1995), and Wedderburn-Tate, writing from a nursing perspective, feels that the leader's function is to get others to 'perform at consistently high levels, voluntarily' (1999, p. 107). This is in keeping with U.S. President Eisenhower's view that leadership is the art of getting someone else to do something you want done because he wants to do it (Stanton et al. 2010, p. 3). These definitions imply that influence is a factor.

Fiedler (1967) and Dublin (1968) suggest that leadership is more than influence and propose that it is the exercise of authority and the making of decisions. They see the leader as the person who has formal authority (power) and functional capacity over a group. Maxwell (2002), however, supporting Leigh and Maynard (1995) and Wedderburn-Tate (1999), feels that this is going too far, and that leadership is influence – nothing more, nothing less. Stogdill (1950) also considers that leadership and influence are related but believes that there may be more than just this. He proposes another view, that leadership is the process of influencing people or the activities of a group to accomplish goals. This perspective brings in the concept of influence and acknowledges that people without formal power can exercise leadership. Leadership is also seen as 'a talent that each of us has and that can be learned, developed and nurtured. Most importantly it is not necessarily tied to a position of authority in an organisation' (Grossman and Valiga 2021, p. 18).

As well as goal setting and influence, leadership is an important element in effecting change (Stogdill 1950). Kotter (1990, p. 40) supports this, indicating that 'leadership is all about coping with change'. However, Bennis and Nanus describe a leader as 'one who commits people to action, who converts followers into leaders and who converts leaders into agents of change' (1985, p. 3). Lipman, from a business/management perspective, defines leadership as 'the initiation of a new structure or procedure for accomplishing an organisation's goals and objectives' (1964, p. 122).

These views appear to suggest that change is central to leadership and they rest on the assumption that leaders function within an organisation where change, rather than stability, is the goal. Pedler et al. (2004), also from a management perspective, indicate that while leadership includes elements of the leader's character and the context within which the leadership takes place, it focuses on the critical tasks that the leader must perform, the problems and challenges that leaders face. Again, defining leadership by the leader's ability to change or respond to challenges, Figure 2.1 demonstrates these ideas.

Leadership has also been viewed as attending to the meanings and values of the group, rather than just the authority, function, challenges and traits of the leader (James et al. 2021). Covey (1992) describes what he calls 'principle-centred leadership', and Pondy (1978) similarly proposes that the ability to make activities meaningful and not necessarily to change behaviour, but to give others a sense of understanding of what they are doing, is at the core of leadership. Therefore, the act of leading is about making the meaning of an activity explicit:

> Unlike the supposed individualistic leadership of the past, now leadership is influenced by the impact of the immediate and surrounding context . . . the contention put forward is that [the] organisational context provides the parameters within which current leadership is contained.
>
> *(Kakabadse and Kakabadse 1999, p. 2)*

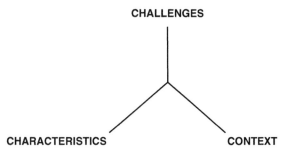

Figure 2.1 The three domains of leadership. **Challenges** are the critical tasks, problems and issues requiring action. **Characteristics** are the qualities, competencies and skills that enable us to contribute to the practice of leadership in challenging situations. **Context** is the 'on-site' conditions found in the challenging situation. Source: Pedler et al. 2004, with permission of The McGraw Hill Companies.

From this perspective it can be argued that the task of the leader is to interpret and clarify the context and thus provide a platform for communicating meaning within the activity.

As a result, leadership becomes more about selecting, synthesising and articulating an appropriate vision for the follower (Bennis et al. 1995). Greenfield takes this concept of vision further by implying that rather than just clarifying meaning or making the activity meaningful, leadership is about setting meaning, describing leadership as

> a willful act where one person attempts to construct the social world for others . . . leaders will try to commit others to the values that they themselves believe are good and that organisations are built on the unification of people around values.
> *(Greenfield 1986, p. 166)*

Similarly, Bell and Ritchie (1999) and Day et al. (2000), from an education perspective, commonly refer to the 'head teacher' as the person within a school who is responsible for 'establishing core characteristics' (Bell and Ritchie 1999, p. 24), for committing others to their values and for setting the overall aims for the school.

However, no one definition can be considered wholly right or wrong and there are a multitude of others that have not been outlined here. Therefore, adding to the already numerous definitions may seem irresponsible, although I offer a definition nonetheless, as a way of identifying how leadership is understood within the context of this book:

> Leadership is unifying people around values and then constructing the social world for others around those values and helping people get through change.

Like the blind men describing an elephant, there is considerable overlap and blurring at the edges of these varied perspectives, and perhaps an eclectic view of leadership may prove most beneficial, with Duke suggesting that 'leadership seems to be a gestalt phenomenon; greater than the sum of its parts' (1986, p. 10).

No One Way

Leadership has been studied in many fields of endeavour and by many scholars and individuals for a very long time. Rather than this resulting in a clear and unequivocal understanding, many different and sometimes opposing definitions have evolved and still exist (Rigolosi 2013; Swanwick and McKimm 2017; Jones and Bennett 2018). These varied definitions could easily lead to confusion or unsettle our concept of leadership. Instead, I feel that they function like the dishes at a banquet, each individual dish adding to the glory of the collective whole and each offering something that helps explain what leadership is and how leadership can be understood.

However, definitions alone offer only a taste of the meaning of leadership. As with the blind men in their understanding of the elephant, a wider view may be more helpful. To this end, this chapter now explores the theoretical perspectives of leadership and brings a greater array of dishes to the banquet.

Reflection Point

Throughout my teaching career I have asked students to identify who they see as great leaders. Most of those identified were men (Nelson, Churchill, Lincoln, Mandela, etc.) and often I have had to prompt students to consider female leaders. Think about great leaders from history, politics, the arts, education, sports or any field of endeavour. List two people for each category you choose and try to describe what it was that made them stand out as a great leader for you. As well, make another two lists. One of male and one of female leaders that stand out to you. Are the attributes of the people on each list different? Is gender an issue that defines or divides leaders?

Leadership Theories and Styles

In order to clarify information about leadership and leaders, it is prudent to consider the theories of leadership that are prominent in the literature and important to explore the concepts, theories and styles of leadership that have previously been developed and described. They are not proposed as a linear progression, although the later theories have grown from, or are at least a reaction to, or are influenced by earlier ones. The following pages offer only an introduction to leadership theories, but it is hoped that they set the stage for a consideration of congruent leadership in Chapter 4 and for clinical leadership in the overall context of this book.

The Great Man Theory: Born to Lead?

The 'great man theory' (Galton 1869) is one of the earliest theories of leadership (Khan et al. 2016). It suggests that leadership is a matter of birth, with the characteristics of leadership being inherited or, as Man (2010) suggests, assigned by divine decree. Bennis and Nanus explain this theory by saying that 'those of the right breed could lead; all others must be led' (1985, p. 5).

Therefore, individuals born into 'great' families were considered to be infused with the skills and characteristics of a leader, and indeed some individuals born into the 'right' family did accomplish great things and changed the course of human history. However, the idea that leaders are born and not made lost credibility after a number of significant changes in the fabric of western society (Grossman and Valiga 2021). The French and Russian Revolutions and World War I are examples of the types of changes that led people to see that leaders could come from any stratum of society. As such, the great man theory, dominated by an old leadership culture, literally died out as those who supported it were replaced by a new breed of self-styled leaders.

The Heroic Leader: Great People Lead

To some extent this theory is aligned with the 'great man' theory. Heroic leadership (sometimes called 'charismatic' leadership) (Khan et al. 2016) is based on four principles – self-awareness, ingenuity, love and heroism (Lowney 2003). However, heroic leaders make use of their power or position to make decisions unilaterally. The heroic leader is often described as a charismatic, goal-scoring superstar who doesn't mind carrying the team on his back. The role of heroic leadership is to set expectations for everyone to commit to and follow. These can be values but are most commonly seen as a set of courageous actions. Accountability starts with the leader's actions, and followers align themselves because the leader models the behaviours and actions others see as courageous or heroic. The leader leads by virtue of their heroic stance or heroic actions.

The Big Bang Theory: From Great Events, Great People Come

The 'big bang theory' proposes that calamitous circumstances provide the elements essential for the creation of leaders. Leaders, it suggests, are created by the great events that affect their lives (Grossman and Valiga 2021). Again, the revolutions of the nineteenth and twentieth centuries and World War I are cited as examples of major calamitous circumstances, but this type of event could as easily be a local disaster (such as the floods in Yorkshire in 2015 and fires in the state of Victoria in 2009, 2015, and 2019/2020), a family crisis or a personal catastrophe. Bennis and Nanus explain this by saying that 'great events made leaders of otherwise ordinary people' (1985, p. 5), suggesting that it is the situation and the followers that combine to create the leader. The lives of a number of great political and military leaders might be used to substantiate this theory of leadership, with the life and presidency of Abraham Lincoln offering a sound example of a poor person's rise to prominence during the dramatic events of mid-eighteenth-century America (McPherson 1988; Carwardine 2003; Gallagher et al. 2003). The rise to power of Napoleon Bonaparte following the after-effects of the French Revolution is another. The theory that otherwise ordinary people become great leaders because of great events may be true for some leaders, but, as with Lincoln and Bonaparte, much of the leader's success may be attributable to their hard work and knowledge in preparation for the great events that are common features of many people's lives.

From an Australian standpoint the notorious career of the bushranger Ned Kelly could be viewed from the perspective of the big bang theory. A series of calamitous personal and family events during Ned's early life resulted in his decision to take up a life of crime, and ultimately he led a small group of outlaws who committed a series of robberies and murders across the countryside of northern Victoria. The theory argues that without the events that sparked Ned's behaviour and reactions, he is unlikely to have risen to prominence in his chosen field and become Australia's most notorious bushranger.

Trait Theory: The Man, Not the Game

The 'trait theory' of leadership rests on the assumption that the individual is more important than the situation. Therefore, it is proposed that identifying distinguishing characteristics of successful leaders will give clues about leadership (Khan et al. 2016; Swanwick and McKimm 2017; Grossman and Valiga 2021). Rafferty (1993) and Jones and Bennett (2018) refer to this as the constitutional approach, where part of the assumption is that if great leaders cannot be trained or taught, they can at least be selected, linking this with attributes of the great man theory.

A large number of studies in the early part of the twentieth century (Northouse 2007; Yoder-Wise 2015) were initiated to consider the traits of great leaders. However, as Bass (1990) indicates, while a number of traits did seem to correspond with leadership, no qualities were found that were universal to all leaders. Stogdill (1948), who undertook a major review of universal leadership traits between 1904 and 1947, concluded that no consistent set of traits differentiated leaders from non-leaders in a range of work environments and situations. The traits that he identified in 1948 and again in 1974, as well as others identified by Mann (1959), Kirkpatrick and Locke (1991), Smith (1999), and Grossman and Valiga (2021) are listed in Table 2.1.

The descriptive words on these lists indicate that trait theories have evolved and changed with time, but all remain unable to capture any great degree of consistency between the traits identified. Stogdill found in 1948 and again in 1974 that the traits that lead to success may differ according to the situation the leader is in, as well as the personality of the leader. Therefore, the traits themselves could be seen as misleading, although it has been proposed that the leader's characteristics play a critical part in effective leadership (Northouse 2007). It is also suggested that possession of all the traits is an impossible ideal and that there are a considerable number of cases where people who possess a few, or even none, of the principal traits achieve notable success as leaders (Stogdill 1974).

The disadvantage of trait theory is that it does not lead to a comprehensive theory of leadership and it neglects both the impact of the situational context within which the leader operates (Stogdill 1948; Northouse 2007) and the impact of the leader's personality (Mann 1959). Rafferty (1993) also points out that trait theory ignores or underestimates the

Table 2.1 Leadership traits.

Stogdill 1948 (cited in Northouse 2007, p. 18)

Intelligence	Alertness
Insight	Responsibility
Initiative	Persistence
Self-control	Sociability

Stogdill 1974 (cited in Northouse 2007, p. 18)

Achievement	Persistence
Insight	Initiative
Self-confidence	Responsibility
Cooperativeness	Tolerance
Influence	Sociability

Smith (1999, p. 6)

Early loss of a parent
Escape from squalor
First-born child
Tall
High energy levels
Work long hours
Can manage with little sleep
Introverted and psychologically on edge
Outsiders coming from beyond the group
they lead
Enormous self-belief

Mann (1959, p. 253)

Intelligence	Masculinity
Adjustment	Dominance
Extroversion	Conservatism

Kirkpatrick and Locke (1991, p. 52)

Drive	Motivation
Integrity	Confidence
Cognitive ability	Task knowledge

Grossman and Valiga (2021, p. 5)

Abundant reserve of energy
Ability to maintain a high level of activity, better education
Superior judgement
Decisiveness
Breadth of general knowledge
High degree of verbal facility
Good interpersonal skills
Self-confidence
Creativity
Above average height and weight

degree to which the leader's role could be structured by issues of class, gender or racial inequalities and that it assumes a passive role for the followers.

Trait theory developed as an elaboration of the great man theory and remains central to what Grint (2000) describes as 'the arts of leadership'. However, the investigation and establishment of trait theory developed in line with business and management development in the early twentieth century (Northouse 2007), where it was hoped that once the appropriate qualities and traits were identified, a potential leader could be hired who demonstrated these traits, or who could be supported in acquiring them through study and experience (Bernhard and Walsh 1990). Then, if the appropriate conditions prevailed or could be predicted, appropriate people (who showed the relevant traits) could be selected or trained for the leadership situation.

While it is possible to acquire some (but not all) of the traits, this theory remains divorced from the notion that leadership (in isolation from the traits) could be learnt and, as such, it found limited purchase with the liberated and increasingly educated masses of the Western world. Therefore, as community values altered and research about leadership increased, other perspectives of leadership developed (Lett 2002).

Style Theory: It's How You Play the Game

Studies of leadership and management and their relationship to productivity and group behaviour resulted in what are generally called style theories (Adair 1998; Handy 1999; Northouse 2007). Style theories explore how leaders behave, what they do, how they act, as well as how groups respond, with leaders being described as either democratic, paternalistic, laissez-faire, authoritarian and/or dictatorial (Handy 1999; Lett 2002; Northouse 2007; see Table 2.2). As these words were found to have an 'emotive connotation', aspects of style theory are also described as 'structuring and supportive styles' (Handy 1999, p. 101), and much of the literature related to style theory emphasises the benefits or drawbacks of one or another approach to motivating a group (usually of subordinates to the leader).

Early investigations of style theory were undertaken by the Ohio State University, where a Leader Behaviour Description Questionnaire (LBDQ) was developed and tested in educational, military and industrial settings. Leaders, they concluded, exhibited either *structuring* behaviour, which defined the work context and role responsibilities of subordinates, or *consideration* behaviour, which focused on building relationships such as trust and respect with subordinates. These studies were elaborated on by the University of Michigan with an approach more focused on the leader's behaviours in relation to the performance of small groups (Northouse 2007). By the 1960s, Blake and Mouton (1964) had developed the 'managerial grid' (now called the leadership grid) as a model to support organisational leadership and management training, by exploring how leaders (managers) could help organisations reach their potential through developing either support for production or concern for people.

The management/leadership grid (Blake and Mouton 1964; Blake and McCanse 1991) can be used to explain how leaders or managers within an organisation function by focusing on the relationship between two factors: concern for people and concern for production or results.

Table 2.2 Management/leadership styles.

Autocratic: characterised by being highly directive, viewed as having a right to manage.

Good points: clear objective, single-minded, based on orders, no thinking required.	**Negative points:** diminished autonomy, problem if the vision is false or off, power vacuum if the leader leaves, no debate, no opportunity to experience power before promotion.

Paternalistic: characterised by a caring but overprotective, interfering manager. Manager knows best, may consult, but always decides. High degree of support but no corresponding responsibility or autonomy.

Good points: followers/ employees may feel 'cared for', may foster a sense that they belong or have a team or esprit de corps.	**Negative points:** stifles autonomy. High reliance on the manager/organisation, even for basic human needs (like some 1970s Japanese companies – when some employees were off sick they felt so lost without their work they were encouraged to come in and spend their time, even if ill, with their colleagues and co-workers).

Democratic: characterised by discussion, debate and shared vision.

Good points: promotes a shared vision, ownership of outcomes and problems, involvement of the whole team, flatter structure employed.	**Negative points:** can allow the more vocal or more outspoken to dominate; mob may rule and may be wrong. Can lead to ineffective decision making.

Laissez-faire: characterised by an easygoing, non-directive and non-hierarchical approach.

Good points: promotes autonomy, self-survival, self-direction, individuality, freedom, and self-expression.	**Negative points:** assumes everyone is willing or capable of leadership, or that people are happy to be left to their own devices. This approach can lead to chaos or anarchy.

Based on Handy 1999; Lett 2002; Northouse 2007.

Concern for people deals with how a manager or leader supports people within an organisation as they try to work towards their goals. This can be achieved by focusing on issues of trust and commitment, motivation, working conditions, fair play and the promotion of strong social support structures (Blake and Mouton 1964). *Concern for results* addresses how the manager/leader achieves various tasks and can include factors such as policies, sales figures, quality targets and other activities and processes concerned with production or the organisation's goals. The original grid was developed as a nine-point scale on which one represents minimum concern and nine represents maximum concern. By plotting the scores from the vertical and horizontal axes, various leadership/management styles could be identified.

The style theory approach to leadership is not designed to instruct leaders in how to behave, but it is useful in supporting leaders (managers) in identifying the major components of their behaviour. However, the theory failed to elaborate on why some leaders were successful in certain situations and not in others.

Different organisations require different styles of management or leadership at different times, depending on their approach, their goals and their stage of development. Many authors use different terms (democratic = participative), but often they end up describing the same thing. It was Kurt Lewin who in 1948 set out the three basic leadership/management styles of autocratic, democratic and laissez-faire. Since then, other terms have been used and other views expressed. Here are some of them:

- **Supporting:** where leaders pass day-to-day decisions to the follower. The leader facilitates and takes part in decisions, but control is with the follower.
- **Delegating:** leaders are still involved in decisions and problem solving, but control is with the follower. The follower decides when and how the leader will be involved.
- **Directing:** leaders define the roles and tasks of the follower and supervise them closely. Decisions are made by the leader and announced, so communication is largely one way.
- **Coaching:** leaders still define roles and tasks but seek ideas and suggestions from followers. Decisions remain the leader's prerogative, but communication is much more two-way.

The leadership style that individuals use will be based on a combination of their beliefs, values and preferences, as well as the organisational culture and norms, which encourage some styles and discourage others. Examples of these styles are:

- charismatic leadership
- participatory leadership
- situational leadership
- transactional leadership
- transformational leadership
- the quiet leader

Clearly some of these relate to leadership theories, and this is where the matter of styles and theories become intertwined. Tannenbaum and Schmidt (1958) suggest that there are seven leadership styles; Tayeb (1996) claims that there are four styles; and Morgan (1986) proposes six styles of leadership (and management). Confused yet? I'd be surprised if you weren't. Goleman et al. (2002) consider that there are six styles – coaching, visionary, affiliative, democratic, pace-setting and commanding – although as you will see from any internet search for 'leadership styles', there are many more.

Situational or Contingency Theory: It's about Relationships

To address the failure of style theory and to elaborate on why some leaders are successful in certain situations and not in others, Fiedler (1967) proposed the 'situational' or 'contingency theory' of leadership (Wedderburn-Tate 1999), which was popularised by Hersey and Blanchard in 1988 (Swanwick and McKimm 2017). Here, Fiedler (1967) and others (Tannenbaum and Schmidt 1958; Vroom and Yetton 1973; House and Mitchell 1974; Hersey and Blanchard 1988) believed that leadership effectiveness depends on the relationship between the leader's task at hand, the leader's interpersonal skills and the favourableness of the work situation. Fiedler (1967) found – after what has more recently been criticised as limited research (Handy 1999) – that leaders were more effective if the situation within which they were trying to function was more favourable to them or even, surprisingly, less favourable. The three factors (Handy 1999, pp. 103–5) relate to:

- the degree of trust and respect that the followers have for the leader
- the clarity of the objectives to be achieved
- the degree of power in terms of whether the leader could reward or punish the followers or if the leader had clear organisational backing

From Fiedler's perspective, the key to understanding leadership is to be able to adapt the leadership approach to complement the issue being faced or to determine the appropriate action based on the people involved and the prevailing situation (Adair 1998). Adair also offers an example of how situational leadership might be applied by describing the actions of a group of survivors following a shipwreck:

> The soldier in the party might take command if natives attacked them, the builder might organise the work of erecting houses and the farmer might direct the labour of growing food . . . leadership would pass from member to member according to the situation. (1998, p. 15)

Central to Fiedler's (1967) work was the ability to analyse how the leader could use power and influence without losing respect and credibility with the subordinate group. Tannenbaum and Schmidt (1958) felt that organisations could help more by structuring the task, improving the formal power of the leader or changing the composition of the follower group to give the leaders a more favourable climate within which to work. Vroom and Yetton's (1973) decision tree model (Box 2.2) also recognises the relationship among the leader, the followers and the task at hand, and proposes that there are five types of leadership style to choose from, decided by answering a series of questions.

Criticism of both Vroom and Yetton's decision tree model and Fiedler's situational–contingency model includes that leadership is more complicated than a series of questions and broader than the extent of the relationship between three central factors (Adair 1998). Handy (1999) also feels that even the pleasingly rational decision tree is not complicated enough to fully describe and address the convoluted nature of leadership decision making.

Blanchard et al. (1994) suggest that the development of situational leadership has been in support of the activity of management: that it is used as a 'practical approach to managing and motivating people' and that it has been 'taught to managers at all levels of most of the Fortune 500 companies as well as to managers in fast-growing entrepreneurial organisations' (p. 8). As a result, theories of leadership and management remained closely intertwined and, although Zaleznik (1977) and Kotter (1990) make it clear that management and leadership are different, many of the perspectives and theories that developed to explore and explain leadership grew from a desire to understand human resource management, improve employee and workforce production and support the development of managers.

Box 2.2   Vroom and Yetton's Decision Tree Model

The leader has five styles to choose from. These are:

AI You solve the problem or make the decision yourself, using information available to you at the time.

AII You obtain the necessary information from your subordinate(s) then decide on the solution to the problem yourself.

CI You share the problem with relevant subordinates individually, getting their ideas and suggestions. Then you make the decision.

CII You share the problem with your subordinates in a group, then you make the decision.

GII You share the problem with your subordinates as a group, then together you make the decision.

The seven questions, which could be set out like a decision tree, are:

1) Is one decision likely to be better than another? (if not, go to AI)
2) Does the leader know enough to take it on her or his own? (if not, avoid AI)
3) Is the problem clear and structured? (if not, go to CII or GII)
4) Must the subordinates accept the decision? (if not, then AI and AII are possible)
5) Would they accept your decision? (if not, then GII is preferable)
6) Do subordinates share your goals for the organisation? (if not, then GII is risky)
7) Are subordinates likely to conflict with each other? (if yes, then CII is better)

Source: Handy 1999, pp. 103–7.

Reflection Point

Think about any outstanding leaders from your experience as a clinician/student. Reflect on their influence on you and write a short commentary about what it was about these people that made them stand out as leaders. Also reflect on the great leaders in your discipline. There may be some obvious ones that come to mind, and some you may know personally. Make a list of three great leaders in your discipline from across the globe. You should find an abundance of them! Finally, after considering the information here (and after reading Chapter 4), if given the opportunity to publish the definitive definition of leadership, what would you write?

Transformational Theory: Making Change Happen

In an attempt to understand the distinction between leadership and management – and to address the question of why some leaders are able to inspire their followers even when the situation is less than ideal – the theory of 'transformational leadership' was developed (Northouse 2007). The term was coined by Downton (1973) and later adopted and developed by House (1976) and Burns (1978), who really secured its distinctiveness by firmly linking leaders' and the followers' motives. It was Bass (1985), while seeking to identify the distinctions between leadership and management, who later refined the theory and felt that transformational leadership motivated followers to do more than was expected by providing an idealised influence, inspirational motivation and vision. Transformational leadership is also strongly associated with the qualitative studies of Bennis and Nanus (1985) and, more recently, of Fuda (2014). These scholars also sought to tease out the differentiation between management and leadership, with transformational leadership seen as connected to a process of attending to the needs of followers, so that interaction between them raised the motivation and energy of both. Transformational leadership is therefore about challenging the status quo, creating a vision and sharing that vision, with successful transformational leaders being able to establish and gain support for their vision, while being consistently and persistently driven towards maintaining momentum and empowering others (Kakabadse and Kakabadse 1999; Swanwick and McKimm 2017).

Bennis and Nanus (1985), expanding on Burns' (1978) theory, identified four themes that they felt were pivotal to effective transformational leadership:

- **Vision**, or the ability to have a dream and actually deliver on it.
- **Communication**, or the ability to articulate the vision so that it steals into the imagination and minds of followers.
- **Trust**, or the ability of followers to feel that their leader is consistent, has integrity and can be relied on.
- **Self-knowledge (self-knowing)**, or what Bennis and Nanus describe as the ability to 'know their worth . . . trust themselves without letting their ego or image get in the way' (1985, p. 57).

In effect, 'self-knowing' is about looking for the fit between who the leaders are and who they need to be to fulfil the task. Handy (1999, p. 117) aligns 'self-knowing' with 'emotional wisdom' and Goleman (1996) and Goleman et al. (2002) elaborate on this aspect of leadership, connecting it to the concept of 'emotional intelligence' where a person is able to motivate themselves, be creative and perform at their peak, sensing what others are feeling and handling relationships effectively. The transformational leader need not be associated with status or power and is seen as being appropriate at all levels of an organisation. The leader's role is to communicate a vision that gives meaning to the work of others. Crucially, the role of the transformational leader is reconstruction of the context in which people work, removing the old and replacing it with the new.

The interdependence of followers and leaders within this theory has meant that transformational leadership has found favour in care-related and teaching fields (Day et al. 2000) and, according to Welford, 'transformational leadership is arguably the most favourable leadership theory for clinical nursing in the general medical or surgical ward setting' (2002, p. 9). Thyer also feels that it is 'ideologically suited to nurses' (2003, p. 73), and Goertz Koerner (2010) identifies Florence Nightingale as an ideal example of a transformational leader. Sofarelli and Brown (1998), Freshwater et al. (2009), Weberg (2010), Marshall (2011), Casida and Parker (2011), Hutchinson and Jackson (2012), Tinkham (2013), Ross et al. (2014), Lavoie-Tremblay et al. (2015), Weng et al. (2015), Swanwick and McKimm (2017), and Jones and Bennett (2018) also indicate that transformational leadership is a suitable leadership approach for empowering health professionals or supporting them within an organisation. In addition, Weng et al. (2015) suggest, in a substantial Taiwanese research study, that there is a significant correlation between transformational leadership and innovation within the nursing workforce. Casida and Parker (2011), in a study in the United States, likewise propose that leaders who demonstrated a transformational style were seen to be making an extra effort, achieving greater satisfaction and being more effective. Moreover, Lavoie-Tremblay et al. (2015) found that supportive leadership practices were able to have an impact on increasing retention and improving patient care.

Transformational leadership is strongly connected to the process of addressing the needs of followers, so that the process of interaction increases their motivation and energy (Bass 1990; Jones and Bennett 2018). While this is significant, transformational leadership has also gained favour because it is related to the establishment of a vision and adapting to change. Nevertheless, as Hutchinson and Jackson (2012) state, the attachment of nursing (and other healthcare disciplines) to transformational leadership theory without robust critical review or empirical exploration limits how leadership may be conceptualised in healthcare. Rafferty (1993, p. 8) warns that the 'charismatic' element of transformational leadership can be 'potentially exploitative' if the leader takes advantage of conflict in the needs or values system of followers. However, it is in this area of potential weakness that Kakabadse and Kakabadse (1999) see the power of transformational leadership, as it offers the leader the opportunity to penetrate the soul and psyche of others, increasing the level of awareness that motivates people to strive for greater ends.

Reflection Point

You may think this a little odd, but ask a child what they think leadership means. Then ask some older members of your family or society. Do they differ? If so, how do they differ? Why might these people take the perspectives they do?

Transactional Theory: Running a Tight Ship

Burns (1978) describes 'transactional leadership' as the antithesis of transformational leadership, indicating that transactional leadership exists where there is an exchange relationship between leader and followers (Jones and Bennett 2018). Here, the role of the transactional leader is to focus on the purpose of the organisation and to assist people to recognise what needs to be done in order to reach a desired outcome through a reward/punishment motivator (Jones and Bennett 2018). Kakabadse and Kakabadse (1999) describe transactional leadership as the skill and ability to deal with the mundane, operational and day-to-day transactions of organisational life. 'Keeping meetings to their time limits, ensuring the agenda is adhered to, and conducting appraisals of subordinates' (Kakabadse and Kakabadse 1999, p. 5) are but a few examples of what they call 'transactional management'. Transactional leaders, in order to lead, need to effectively manage the more routine tasks, partly in order to retain their credibility but also to keep the organisation on track (Burns 1978).

Criticism of this approach is that it relies on procedures, technicality and hard data to inform decision making, with Day et al. (2000, p. 4) describing it as a form of 'scientific managerialism' that relies on the assumption that leaders are in a position to control rewards. It is also criticised by Rafferty because it relies on the assumption that human behaviour is driven by motivation for reward and an incentive system, and because it is prone to being 'more conservative than creative' (1993, p. 8). The rationale behind transactional leadership is that in order for leaders to function effectively they should be able to control the context within which they are required to lead; in effect, managing their environment and limiting change.

Authentic/Breakthrough Leadership: True to Your Values

'Authentic leadership' (Bhindi and Duignan 1997; George 2003; Avolio and Gardner 2005; Cantwell 2015) and 'breakthrough leadership' (Sarros and Butchatsky 1996) are more recent leadership theories. Both of these perspectives on leadership point to an approach where leaders are thought to be true to their own values and beliefs, and the leader's credibility rests on their integrity and ability to be seen as a role model, because of these values and beliefs (James et al. 2021). The 'breakthrough' leader and the 'authentic' leader respect and listen to others and are guided by their passion and meaning, purpose and values (Sarros and Butchatsky 1996; Bhindi and Duignan 1997; George 2003; Avolio and Gardner 2005; Cantwell 2015).

In 2005, the American Association of Critical-Care Nurses published a statement aimed at helping establish healthy work environments. The basis for this was a list of six 'standards':

- skilled communication
- true collaboration
- effective decision making
- appropriate staffing
- meaningful recognition
- authentic leadership

In addition, Alilyyania et al. (2018, p. 35) suggest that authentic leadership has four principles at its core requiring 'balanced processing, relational transparency, internalized moral perspective, and self-awareness.' Authentic leadership is described as the 'glue' used to hold a healthy work environment together (Shirley 2006), with leaders being encouraged to engage with employees and promote positive behaviours. Wong and Cummings (2009) and Wong and Walsh (2020), writing from a nursing perspective, also suggest that authentic leadership is a suitable theory for aligning future nursing leadership practice. Writers such as Gonzalez (2012) have taken authentic leadership further and describe what they call mindful leadership, where leaders employ self-awareness and self-leadership principles while being mindful of their impact on others.

Alkharabsheh and Alias (2018) proposed that the application of authentic leadership within an organisation resulted in reduced stress in nurses and encouraged a commitment to remain in the profession. Baek et al.'s (2019) research supported these findings, identifying the positive effects of job satisfaction and commitment to the organisation when managers exhibited authentic leadership and were considered to bring greater 'citizenship' behaviours to the work environment, exhibited through politeness, dignity and respect (Qui et al. 2020).

Servant Leadership: A Follower at the Front

In keeping with some of the key elements of authentic leadership, 'servant leadership' focuses on the leader's stewardship role and encourages leaders to 'serve' others while staying in tune with the organisation's goals and values (Swanwick and McKimm 2017; Jones and Bennett 2018; James et al. 2021). The concept of servant leadership was coined and defined by Robert Greenleaf (1977), who stated that servant leaders rely less on hierarchical position and more on collaboration, trust, empathy and the use of ethical power.

A number of nursing authors have emphasised the relevance of servant leadership as a model to support the development of nursing and healthcare leadership, because its focus is both on promoting user involvement and on patients as the foundation of the health service and the most important group that leaders 'serve' (Anderson 2003; Kerfoot 2004; Swearingen and Liberman 2004; Campbell and Rudisill 2005; Peete 2005; Robinson 2006; Thorne 2006; Walker 2006; Swanwick and McKimm 2017; Jones and Bennett 2018; Ellis 2019; Lee et al. 2019; Vasudeva 2020). It is also valued as a model to support staff and influence current staff retention issues that are producing nursing workforce shortages (Swearingen and Liberman 2004). Hanse et al. (2016, p. 232), in a significant Swedish study, were able to show that nurse managers who demonstrated servant leadership had stronger 'exchange relationships' in terms of 'empowerment', 'humility' and 'stewardship' with followers. Their results reinforced the notion that servant leadership was relevant and suited to service-orientated organisations, with benefits for supporting, valuing and developing people.

Servant leadership is also valued because its key principles (Spears 1995; Box 2.3), which support caring and compassion, seem to fit appropriately within current and dominant values that are parallel with healthcare and nursing. Eicher-Catt (2005), however, believes that servant leadership is a myth that is unworkable in the real world, that it fails to live up to its promise of being gender neutral and in fact – because of the paradoxical language and apposition of 'servant' and 'leader' – that it accentuates gender bias, so that it ends up supporting androcentric patriarchal norms. There is also an argument put forward by Avolio and Gardner (2005) that servant leadership has not been developed from an empirical base and is therefore purely theoretical. Mostafa and El-Motalib (2019) and Hanse et al. (2016) found high-quality social exchanges and mutual trust were enhanced by servant leadership.

Box 2.3 Ten Key Principles of Servant Leadership	
Listening	Conceptualisation
Empathy	Foresight
Healing	Stewardship
Awareness	Commitment to the growth of people
Persuasion	Building community

Reflection Point

Reflect on the ward, unit, clinic or clinical area that you are on now. What management/ leadership style does the ward manager, clinical manager, therapy team leader (or whatever they are called) adopt? Discuss this (tactfully) with them. What style do they feel they have adopted? Are you both in agreement?

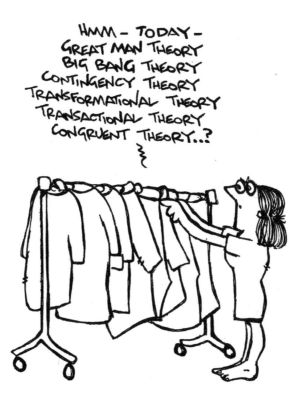

Clinical Leader Stories: 2 A Busy Shift

I was working with a Clinical Nurse Specialist (CNS) on a morning shift. Our four patients were handed over, but because a staff member had not yet arrived, we took handover for an additional four patients and initiated care for them as well. The CNS was then able to give an accurate handover when the late nurse arrived later. Our care planner looked very busy. We had one patient fasting, one going for a surgical proce- dure, one for an ECHO and another going for an X-ray. The orderly came a lot earlier for our patients than they had been booked for. The CNS directed me to fill in my planner, to start taking vital signs and fill out transfer forms for patients going for procedures. While juggling our patients the CNS assisted less-experienced nurses with other tasks,

(Continued)

Clinical Leader Stories: 2 A Busy Shift   (Continued)

for example the insertion of an IDC and administration of medications another nurse had never administered before. Under pressure, the CNS effectively delegated tasks to me (and others) that were within our scope of practice. They assisted me with tasks requiring supervision and assisted inexperienced nurses whilst staying calm and patient focused. The CNS handed over the four patients, helped care for our four patients, assisted less-experienced nurses and delegated tasks all while modelling a calm, confident demeanour. The CNS demonstrated her clinical leadership attributes through her clinical competence, her effective communication and decision-making skills, her visibility and approachability in practice, her adaptability and her calm inspiring ability. All despite the chaotic environment. They did all this while making leadership look effortless and always with a focus on quality patient care. I believe the CNS demonstrated congruent leadership – her focus was always on providing high-quality person-centred care, and despite having no official leadership role, she took charge as necessary and supported colleagues. I was sure that those around the CNS saw her clinical competence and her ability to motivate others to grow in confidence. Junior staff did not hesitate to seek her guidance and support. Senior staff frequently sought advice from her in terms of clinical decision making. The whole healthcare team around her saw her as a leader who was approachable, supportive and an excellent role model.

Elvina: Student Nurse.

Other Perspectives

Shared Leadership/Collaborative Leadership

A relatively new approach to considering leadership is the concept of shared or, more recently, collaborative leadership (Pearce and Conger 2003). Shared leadership occurs when two or more members engage in the leadership of the team in an effort to influence and direct fellow members to maximise team effectiveness (Bergman et al. 2012). Shared leadership occurs when a group of individuals lead each other to achieve successful outcomes (Carson et al. 2007). Towler (2019) suggests that it is important to distinguish shared leadership from team leadership because shared leadership describes how team members influence each other and share responsibility for tasks, rather than the concept of a team being led by a specific leader. However, shared leadership and collaborative leadership are sometimes called distributed leadership with all three having the same basic components of leadership (Northouse 2007). Carson et al. (2007), suggest that shared leadership is based on a shared purpose, social support and a voice for the team.

Compassionate Leadership

In 2017, the King's Fund proposed in a document called 'Caring to change: how compassionate leadership can stimulate innovation in healthcare' that compassionate leadership activities have many positive outcomes, at all levels of the health sector. It proposed that staff are more likely to find new and improved ways of doing things if they feel they are listened to, valued and supported as this provides a sense of psychological safety. They also suggested that giving staff autonomy in their work is important, along with developing a shared responsibility as shared leadership is more effective than a hierarchical approach. The document proposed that positive attitudes to diversity, inclusion and creativity and innovation need to be nurtured at every level of the organisation and that innovation is often spurred on by a challenge or a problem. It also proposed that a compassionate approach to leadership might be a powerful facilitator for problem solving within the health service. These views were supported by West (2021) (who contributed to the King's Fund document), who describes compassionate leadership as a strategy based on the core human value of compassion, showing that by sustaining compassion in health and social care, health professionals can cultivate wisdom, humanity, presence and high-quality care delivery in health and care services.

Compassion is the quality of having positive intentions and real concern for others. Compassion in leadership creates stronger connections between people. It improves collaboration, raises levels of trust, and enhances loyalty. In addition, studies find that compassionate leaders are perceived as stronger and more competent (Hougaard et al. 2020).

There is another leadership theory that supports a values-based healthcare leadership approach called **Congruent Leadership**. This is covered in greater detail in the next chapter.

The Right Leader at the Right Time

The essence of the great man, trait and style theories of leadership is that the individual leader is critical, but the context is not. Therefore, as long as the right leader with the appropriate leadership qualities is found or selected, the leader will be able to lead, under any circumstances. These theories imply that organisations, businesses, the military and other groups should concern themselves with the search for and development of leaders rather than be preoccupied with the context within which they have to operate. Indeed, this has been the approach taken by many organisations, and much of the literature related to leadership from a military, political, spiritual and business base revolves around describing the lives and achievements of highly regarded military generals (Fest 1974; Grabsky 1993; D'Este 1996; Hibbert 1998; Useem 1998; Grint 2000; Krause 2000; Adair 2002a); political juggernauts (Mandela 1994; Harvey 1998; Danzig 2000; Adair 2002a; Carwardine 2003; Gallagher et al. 2003); religious figureheads (Carson 1999; Grint 2000; Adair 2002a); and captains of industry (Banks 1982; Lacey 1986; Clemmer and McNeil 1989; Allan 1992; Branson 1998; Useem 1998; Danzig 2000; Grint 2000; Krause 2000; Kouzes and Posner 2003).

Situational or contingency theory and, to a small degree, the big bang theory of leadership imply that both the individual and the context are fundamental. These theories describe the leader as being aware of their own leadership skills and of the context within which they lead, so that they can plan for the degree of alignment between their leadership approach and the situation they are in. For example, where a crisis occurs and a strong leader is available, this leader can step forward to lead and only step back (if required) when the situation changes and the context is no longer conducive to their vigorous approach. Leadership is arrived at by supporting the leader in being self-aware and by situational analysis, so that, in effect, certain situations demand certain types of leader. Skilful leaders may be able to adapt their style to suit particular situations and, as such, the leader's behaviour or actions may change to suit the situation at hand. These theories of leadership found favour in, and developed from, research and literature derived from management and business perspectives (Blanchard et al. 1994; Adair 1998; Adair 2002b; Northouse 2007) and transformational and transactional theories of leadership also developed as researchers sought to explore the differences between leadership and management (Bennis and Nanus 1985; Bass 1990).

If leadership is seen to be about unifying people around values, and then constructing the social world for others around those values and helping people get through change, identifying a leadership theory that will facilitate people or practitioners to understand the application of leadership in their clinical environment or situation is important. To this end, Chapter 4 explores the elements of leadership as they relate to the practice of clinical nurse leadership and leadership for health professionals. In support of this, another theory, congruent leadership, is proposed and explored further.

It is proposed that leadership theories can also be grouped as a way of understanding their significance. For example, the great man theory, heroic leadership, the big bang theory, trait theory and the styles theories can all be understood as theories that look at the attributes of leaders and describe or outline the leadership from the perspective of the leader's personality or leadership traits. Situational or contingency theory, transformational or transactional and shared/collaborative leadership theories focus on visionary or change focused leadership with an exchange-based relationship at the heart of the theories. However, authentic, servant, congruent (see Chapter 4) (James et al. 2021) and compassionate leadership theories are all values driven– or values-focused theories. Considering leadership theories in these groups may also help gain a better insight into which theory will best support the leader's intentions or motives for leadership.

Case Study 2.1   Elizabeth I

Elizabeth I is known as a leader who survived and prospered because she was able to blend her style and approach to leadership over the course of her life. In a time when female leaders were uncommon and held in low regard, Elizabeth stood out as a resourceful and determined leader. Read about Elizabeth I and consider the challenge that follows.

Arguably England's greatest queen (notwithstanding a full assessment of the current reigning monarch, Elizabeth II), Elizabeth I (1533–1603) took her country from domestic turmoil into an age of empire that saw it rise to prominence as a world power. Elizabeth's mother, Anne Boleyn, was herself a formidable woman, but it was Elizabeth who emerged from the conflict of Henry VIII's reign, her brother Edward VI's short and turbulent stint as king and the religious fervour of her sister Mary's brief occupation of the crown, to become queen in 1558.

(Continued)

And she faced many problems. The religious differences between Protestants and Catholics domestically and across Europe, issues of succession and marriage, internal politics and division within the English court, attempts on her life by Mary Queen of Scots and sedition from foreign powers all threatened her reign.

In terms of religious tensions, Elizabeth favoured a cautious brief. To appease Catholics, she imprisoned Mary Queen of Scots but kept her alive for many years. She established the Church of England that, although principally Protestant, had the veneer of a blend of both Catholic and Protestant practices. In this way she acted with apparent tolerance towards all religious groups, minimising conflict. However, Pope Pius V was not appeased and had Elizabeth excommunicated in 1570. Mary, although in prison, was encouraged by European allies to continue to plot against Elizabeth, and in 1587 Elizabeth's patience's expired and she had Mary tried and executed for treason. Religious tensions in Europe remained high and the execution of the Scottish queen, raids by English privateers, often with royal approval, together with Elizabeth's support for Protestant rebels in the Spanish Netherlands prompted Philip II of Spain to attempt an invasion of England.

Warned of the imminent invasion, the English fleet waited in the Channel for the Spanish Armada. Elizabeth, with her army at Tilbury, addressed the men with these famous words:

> I am come amongst you . . . in the midst and heat of the battle, to live or die amongst you all; to lay down, for my God, and for my kingdom, and for my people, my honour and my blood, even the dust. I know I have but the body of a weak and feeble woman; but I have the heart of a king, and of a king of England, too.

The Spanish never landed, as history records that the valour of English sailors and the ferocity of the Channel weather scattered the Spanish fleet and cemented the glory of English seamanship.

Elizabeth faced many other enemies, but throughout her 45-year reign she demonstrated great personal courage, cunning, religious tolerance and intelligent leadership, so that she was able to retain almost absolute control of her throne, bringing England to a 'Golden Age'. She was often under pressure to marry and produce a child, but she claimed shrewdly that she was wedded to her kingdom and that she could not give her love or obedience to any one man. Known as 'Gloriana' throughout her reign, Elizabeth I smoothed England's transition to a modern seafaring nation, supported and oversaw the growth of an artistic awakening, and held the nation together in the face of a powerful and determined foreign power. As far as female leaders go, Elizabeth I proved to be a dominant force in national and domestic politics, and she can rightly be credited with setting England on a course to becoming a world power.

Challenge: Reflect on how Elizabeth was able to adapt her leadership style to hold the nation of England together through turbulent and troubling times, and how she helped establish a 'Golden Age'. How important are flexibility and adaptability to a leader? There is a saying, 'When it comes to fashion, bend like the wind, when it comes to principles, stand like a stone'. If it is important to know when to bend, it is also important to know when to stand firm. The trick might be in knowing when to do which. How do you know? Might it relate to your values, what you believe and what is important to you? Does it relate to the type of leadership theory you subscribe to?

Summary

- Leadership can be understood and defined in a number of different ways and from a number of different perspectives.
- Leadership can be defined by considering the leader's personality, by the leader's relationship to power, authority or influence over a group, as an instrument of goal achievement or viewed from the perspective of directing or setting a group's values.
- Leadership is considered to be an important instrument in effecting change.
- Leadership can also be said to involve unifying people around values and then constructing the social world for others around those values and helping people get through change.
- There are a number of leadership theories. These include the great man theory, big bang theory, trait theory, style theory, situational or contingency theory, transformational leadership, transactional leadership, authentic leadership, breakthrough leadership and servant leadership.
- There are many different styles of leadership, including autocratic, democratic, paternalistic and laissez-faire.
- Many of the theories and definitions overlap or focus on the individual leader or the context within which the leadership takes place, or both.
- In healthcare there is a growing focus on values-based leadership theories.
- There is a wide range of views, beliefs and ideas about what leadership means, what types of leadership there are and how the types of leadership might be employed to build relationships; establish and communicate a vision; and promote, challenge and bring about change to unify people around values and organisational culture.

Mind Press-Ups

Exercise 2.1

Having considered these theories of leadership, do any of them feel as if they 'fit' the clinical environment you work within, in terms of explaining what you understand leadership to be about? Why or why not?

Exercise 2.2

Using a general internet search engine, look for 'leadership styles'. See what comes up. Identify any styles that you feel will help you and note down the positive and negative aspects of each, or any characteristics that will help you use these when describing or applying leadership styles in practice.

Exercise 2.3

Look at the 10 principles of servant leadership (Box 2.3). How do these principles fit within your approach to work? Do you employ any of them in your day-to-day activities?

Exercise 2.4

Transformational leadership is associated with leaders who lead change as a definitive aspect of their role. Think about the characteristics of a transformational leader. Can you reflect on times when you could have employed a transformational leadership approach? Why would this have been appropriate?

Exercise 2.5

Authentic leadership, servant leadership, compassionate leadership and congruent leadership are all types of values-based leadership theories (James et al. 2021). Read James's article and think about how people you identify as leaders apply their values to their leadership role. Think about the characteristics of a values-based leader. Can you reflect on times when you have employed a values-based leadership approach? Why would this have been appropriate?

References

Adair, J. (1998). *Effective Leadership*. London: Pan.

Adair, J. (2002a). *Inspirational Leadership*. London: Thorogood Books.

Adair, J. (2002b). *Effective Strategic Leadership: An Essential Path to Success Guided by the World's Greatest Leaders*. London: Pan.

Alilyyania, B., Wong, C.A., and Cummings, G. (2018). Antecedents, mediators, and outcomes of authentic leadership in healthcare: a systematic review. *International Journal of Nursing Studies* 83: 34–36.

Alkharabsheh, O.H. and Alias, R.B. (2018). Authentic leadership: theory building for veritable sustained performance. *Journal of Economic & Management Perspectives* 12 (3): 19–35.

Allan, J. (1992). Fordism and modern industry. In: *Political and Economic Forms of Modernity* (ed. J. Allan, P. Abraham and P. Lewis), 229–260. Cambridge: Polity Press.

American Association of Critical-Care Nurses (2005). AACN standards for establishing and sustaining healthy work environments: a journey to excellence. *American Journal of Critical Care* 14 (3): 187–197. http://ajcc.aacnjournals.org/content/14/3/187.short (accessed 1 July 2016).

Anderson, R.J. (2003). Building hospital–physician relationships through servant leadership. *Frontiers of Health Service Management* 20 (2): 43.

Avolio, B.J. and Gardner, W.L. (2005). Authentic leadership development: getting to the root of positive forms of leadership. *Leadership Quarterly* 16 (3): 315–338.

Baek, H., Han, K., and Ryu, E. (2019). Authentic leadership, job satisfaction and organizational commitment: the moderating effect of nurse tenure. *Journal of Nursing Management* 27: 1655–1663.

Banks, H. (1982). *The Rise and Fall of Freddie Laker*. London: Faber & Faber.

Bass, B.M. (1985). *Leadership and Performance beyond Expectations*. New York: Free Press.

Bass, B.M. (1990). From transactional to transformational leadership: learning to share the vision. *Organisational Dynamics* 18: 19–31.

Bell, D. and Ritchie, R. (1999). *Towards Effective Subject Leadership in Primary School.* Buckingham: Open University Press.

Bennis, W. and Nanus, B. (1985). *Leaders: The Strategies for Taking Charge.* New York: Harper & Row.

Bennis, W., Parikh, J., and Lessem, R. (1995). *Beyond Leadership: Balancing Economics, Ethics and Ecology.* Oxford: Blackwell Business.

Bergman, J.Z., Rentsch, J.R., Small, E.E. et al. (2012). The shared leadership process in decision-making teams. *The Journal of Social Psychology* 152 (1): 17–42.

Bernhard, L.A. and Walsh, M. (1990). *Leadership: The Key to the Professionalization of Nursing.* London: Mosby.

Bhindi, N. and Duignan, P. (1997). Leadership for a new century: authenticity, intentionality, spirituality and sensibility. *Educational Management and Administration* 25 (4): 117–132.

Blake, R.R. and McCanse, A.A. (1991). *Leadership Dilemmas: Grid Solutions.* Houston, TX: Gulf.

Blake, R.R. and Mouton, J.S. (1964). *The Managerial Grid.* Houston, TX: Gulf.

Blanchard, K., Zigarmi, P., and Zigarmi, D. (1994). *Leadership and the One-Minute Manager.* London: HarperCollins Business.

Branson, R. (1998). *Losing My Virginity.* London: Virgin.

Burns, J.M. (1978). *Leadership.* New York: Harper & Row.

Campbell, P.T. and Rudisill, P.T. (2005). Servant leadership: a critical component for nurse leaders. *Nurse Leader* 3 (3): 27–29.

Cantwell, J. (2015). *Leadership in Action.* Carlton, VA: Melbourne University Press.

Carson, C. (ed.) (1999). *The Autobiography of Martin Luther King, Junior.* London: Little, Brown.

Carson, J.B., Tesluk, P.E., and Marrone, J.A. (2007). Shared leadership in teams: an investigation of antecedent conditions and performance. *Academy of Management Journal* 50 (5): 1217–1234.

Carwardine, R.J. (2003). *Lincoln: Profiles in Power.* Harlow: Pearson Longman.

Casida, J. and Parker, J. (2011). Staff nurse perceptions of nurse manager leadership styles and outcomes. *Journal of Nursing Management* 19: 478–486.

Clemmer, J. and McNeil, A. (1989). *Leadership Skills for every Manager.* London: Piatkus.

Covey, S.R. (1992). *Principle-Centred Leadership.* London: Simon & Schuster.

Danzig, R.J. (2000). *The Leader within you.* Hollywood, FL: Frederick Fell.

Day, C., Harris, A., Hadfield, M. et al. (2000). *Leading Schools in Times of Change.* Buckingham: Open University Press.

D'Este, C. (1996). *A Genius for War: A Life of General George S. Patton,* London: HarperCollins.

Downton, J.V. (1973). *Rebel Leadership: Commitment and Charisma in a Revolutionary Process.* New York: Free Press.

Dublin, R. (1968). *Human Relations in Administration,* 2e. Englewood Cliffs, NJ: Prentice-Hall.

Duke, D.L. (1986). The aesthetics of leadership. *Educational Administration Quarterly* 22 (1): 7–27.

Eicher-Catt, D. (2005). The myth of servant leadership: a feminist perspective. *Women and Language* 28 (1): 17–26.

Ellis, P. (2019). What it means to be a servant leader. *Wounds UK* 15 (5): 76–77.

Fest, J. (1974). *Hitler*. London: Weidenfeld & Nicolson.

Fiedler, F.E. (1967). *A Theory of Leadership Effectiveness*. New York: McGraw-Hill.

Freshwater, D., Graham, I., and Esterhuizen, P. (2009). Educating leaders for global health care. In: *Leadership for Nursing and Allied Health Care Professions* (ed. V. Bishop). Maidenhead: Open University Press/McGraw-Hill Education, pp. 120–41.

Fuda, P. (2014). *Leadership Transformed: How Ordinary Managers Become Extraordinary Leaders*. London: Profile.

Gallagher, G.W., Engle, S.D., Krick, R.K., and Glatthaar, J.T. (2003). *The American Civil War: This Mighty Scourge of War*. Oxford: Osprey.

Galton, F. (1869). *Hereditary Genius*. New York: Appleton.

George, B. (2003). *Authentic Leadership: Rediscovering the Secrets to Creating Lasting Value*. San Francisco, CA: Jossey-Bass.

Goertz Koerner, J. (2010). Reflections on transformational leadership. *Journal of Holistic Nursing* 28 (1): 68.

Goleman, D. (1996). *Emotional Intelligence*. New York: Bloomsbury.

Goleman, D., Boyatzis, R., and McKee, A. (2002). *The New Leaders*. London: Time Warner.

Gonzalez, M. (2012). *Mindful Leadership*. Ontario: John Wiley & Sons.

Grabsky, P. (1993). *The Great Commanders*. London: Boxtree.

Greenfield, T.B. (1986). Leaders and school: wilfulness and non-natural order in organizations. In: *Leadership and Organizational Culture: New Perspectives on Administration Theory and Practice* (ed. T.J. Sergiovanni and J.E. Corbally). Chicago, IL: University of Chicago Press, pp. 142–69.

Greenleaf, R.K. (1977). *Servant Leadership: A Journey into the Nature of Legitimate Power and Greatness*. Mahwah, NJ: Paulist Press.

Grint, K. (2000). *The Arts of Leadership*. Oxford: Oxford University Press.

Grossman, S. and Valiga, T.M. (2021). *The New Leadership Challenge: Creating the Future of Nursing*, 5e. Philadelphia, PA: FA Davis.

Handy, C. (1999). *Understanding Organisations*, 3e. London: Penguin.

Hanse, J.J., Harlin, U., Jarebrant, C. et al. (2016). The impact of servant leadership dimensions on leader–member exchange among health care professionals. *Journal of Nursing Management* 24 (2): 228–234. https://doi.org/10.1111/jonm.12304.

Harvey, A.D. (1998). Napoleon – the myth. *History Today* 48 (1): 27–32.

Hersey, P. and Blanchard, K. (1988). *Management of Organisational Behaviour*. Englewood Cliffs, NJ: Prentice-Hall.

Hibbert, C. (1998). *Nelson: A Personal History*. London: Penguin.

Hougaard, R., Carter, J. and Hobson, N. (2020). Compassionate Leadership is necessary – but not sufficient. https://hbr.org/2020/12/compassionate-leadership-is-necessary-but-not-sufficient (accessed 11 Apirl 2022).

House, R. J. (1976). 'A 1976 theory of charismatic leadership', *Working paper series 76-06*, Toronto, ON: University of Toronto. http://eric.ed.gov/?id=ED133827 (accessed 1 July 2016).

House, R.J. and Mitchell, T.R. (1974). Path–goal theory of leadership. *Journal of Contemporary Business*, Autumn 305–309.

Hutchinson, M. and Jackson, D. (2012). Transformational leadership in nursing: towards a more critical interpretation. *Nursing Inquiry* 20 (1): 11–22.

James, A.H., Bennett, C.L., Blanchard, D., and Stanley, D. (2021). Nursing and values-based leadership: a literature review. *Journal of Nursing Management* 29 (5): 916–930.

Jones, L. and Bennett, C.L. (2018). *Leadership in Health and Social Care: An Introduction for Emerging Leaders*, 2e. Banbury: Lantern.

Kakabadse, A. and Kakabadse, N. (1999). *Essence of Leadership*. London: International Thomson Business Press.

Kerfoot, K. (2004). The shelf life of leaders. *Medical Surgical Nursing* 13 (5): 348–351.

Khan, Z.A., Nawaz, A., and Khan, I. (2016). Leadership theories and styles: a literature review. *Journal of Resources Development and Management* 16: 1–7.

Kibbe, M.R. (2019). Leadership theories and styles. In: *Leadership in Surgery. Success in Academic Surgery* (ed. M. Kibbe and H. Chen). Cham: Springer https://doi.org/10.1007/978-3-030-19854-1_3.

Kirkpatrick, S.A. and Locke, E.A. (1991). Leadership: do traits really matter? *Academy of Management Executive* 5: 48–60.

Kotter, J.P. (1990). What leaders really do. In: *Harvard Business Review on Leadership*, 37–60. Boston, MA: Harvard Business School Press.

Kouzes, J.M. and Posner, B.Z. (2003). *The Leadership Challenge*, 3e. San Francisco, CA: Jossey-Bass.

Krause, D.G. (2000). *The Way of the Leader*. London: Nicholas Brealey.

Lacey, R. (1986). *Ford*. London: Heinemann.

Lavoie-Tremblay, M., Fernet, C., Lavigne, G.L., and Austin, S. (2015). Transformational and abusing leadership practices: impacts on novice nurses, quality of care and intention to leave. *Journal of Advanced Nursing* 73 (3): 582–592.

Lee, H.-F., Chiang, H.-Y., and Kuo, H.-T. (2019). Relationship between authentic leadership and nurse's intent to leave: the mediating role of work environment and burnout. *Journal of Nursing Management* 27 (1): 52–65.

Leigh, A. and Maynard, M. (1995). *Leading Your Team: How to Involve and Inspire Teams*. London: Nicholas Brealey.

Lett, M. (2002). The concept of clinical leadership. *Contemporary Nurse* 12 (1): 6–20.

Lewin, K. (1948). *Resolving Social Conflicts: Selected Papers on Group Dynamics* (ed. G.W. Lewin). New York: Harper & Row.

Lipman, J. (1964). Leadership and administration. In: *Behavioral Science and Educational Administration* (ed. D.E. Griffiths), 119–141. Chicago, IL: University of Chicago Press.

Lowney, C. (2003). *Heroic Leadership: Best Practices from a 450-Year-Old Company that Changed the World*. Chicago, IL: Loyola Press.

Man, J. (2010). *The Leadership Secrets of Genghis Khan*. London: Bantam.

Mandela, N. (1994). *Long Walk to Freedom*. London: Little, Brown.

Mann, R.D. (1959). A review of the relationship between personality and performance in small groups. *Psychological Bulletin* 56: 402–410.

Marshall, E. (2011). *Leadership in Nursing: From Expert Clinician to Influential Leader*. New York: Springer.

Maxwell, J. (2002). *The 21 Irrefutable Laws of Leadership Workbook*. Nashville, TN: Thomas Nelson.

McPherson, J. (1988). *Battle Cry of Freedom: The American Civil War*. London: Penguin.

Morgan, G. (1986). *Images of Organization*. Beverly Hills, CA: Sage.

Mostafa, A.M.S. and El-Motalib, E.A.A. (2019). Servant leadership, leader-member exchange and proactive behavior in the public health sector. *Public Personnel Management* 48 (3): 309–324.

Northouse, P.G. (2007). *Leadership: Theory and Practice*, 4e. London: Sage.

Pearce, C.L. and Conger, J.A. (2003). *Shared Leadership: Reframing the how's and why's of Leadership*. London: SAGE.

Pedler, M., Burgoyne, J., and Boydell, T. (2004). *A Manager's Guide to Leadership*. Maidenhead: McGraw-Hill Professional.

Peete, D. (2005). Needed: servant leaders. *Nursing Homes* 54 (7): 8–10.

Pondy, L.R. (1978). Leadership is a language game. In: *Leadership: Where Else Can We Go?* (ed. M.W. McCall Jr. and M.M. Lombardo). Durham, NC: Duke University Press, pp. 88–99.

Qui, S., Dooley, L.M., Deng, R., and Li, L. (2020). Does ethical leadership boost nurses' patient-orientated organisational citizenship behaviours? A cress sectional study. *Journal of Advances Nursing* 76: 1603–1613.

Rafferty, A.M. (1993). *Leading Questions: A Discussion Paper on the Issues of Nurse Leadership*. London: King's Fund.

Rigolosi, E. (2013). *Management and Leadership in Nursing and Health Care: An Experimental Approach*, 3e. Berlin: Springer.

Robinson, C.A. (2006). The leader within. *Journal of Trauma Nursing* 13 (1): 35–37.

Ross, E.J., Fitzpatrick, J.J., Click, E.R. et al. (2014). Transformational leadership practices of nurse leaders in professional nursing associations. *Journal of Nursing Administration* 44 (4): 201–206.

Sarros, J. and Butchatsky, O. (1996). *Leadership: Australia's Top CEOs Finding Out What Makes Them the Best*. Pymble, NSW: Harper Business.

Shirley, M.R. (2006). Authentic leaders creating healthy work environments for nursing practice. *American Journal of Critical Care* 15 (3): 256–268.

Smith, D. (1999). Leadership is a hard act to follow. News Review. *Sunday Times* (18 July) p. 6.

Sofarelli, D. and Brown, D. (1998). The need to leadership in uncertain times. *Journal of Nursing Management* 6: 201–207.

Spears, L.C. (ed.) (1995). *Reflections on Leadership: How Roberts Greenleaf's Theory of Servant Leadership Influenced Today's Top Management Thinkers*. New York: John Wiley & Sons.

Stanley, D. (2006). Recognising and defining clinical nurse leaders. *British Journal of Nursing* 15 (2): 108–111.

Stanley, D. (2011). *Clinical Leadership: Innovation into Action*. South Yarra, VIC: Palgrave Macmillan.

Stanton, E., Lemer, C., and Mountford, J. (2010). *Clinical Leadership: Bridging the Divide*. London: Quay Books.

Stogdill, R.M. (1948). Personal factors associated with leadership: a survey of the literature. *Journal of Psychology* 25: 35–71.

Stogdill, R.M. (1950). Leadership, membership and organisation. *Psychological Bulletin* 47 (1): 1–47.

Stogdill, R.M. (1974). *Handbook of Leadership*. New York: Free Press.

Swanwick, T. and McKimm, J. (2017). *ABC of Clinical Leadership*, 2e. Oxford: Wiley Blackwell.

Swearingen, S. and Liberman, A. (2004). Nursing leadership: serving those who serve others. *Health Care Manager* 23 (2): 100.

Tannenbaum, R. and Schmidt, W.H. (1958). How to choose a leadership pattern. *Harvard Business Review* 36: 95–101.

Tayeb, M.H. (1996). *The Management of a Multicultural Workforce.* Chichester: John Wiley & Sons.

The King's Fund (2017). Caring to change: how compassionate leadership can stimulate innovation in healthcare. www.kingsfund.org.uk/publications/caring-change?gclid=EAIaIQ obChMI1eLNj5mM8wIVVqmWCh0KRwKxEAAYASAAEgK1VPD_BwE (accessed 11 Apirl 2022).

Thorne, M. (2006). What kind of leader are you? *Topics in Emergency Medicine* 28 (2): 104–110.

Thyer, G. (2003). Dare to be different: transformational leadership may hold the key to reducing the nursing shortage. *Journal of Nursing Management* 11: 73–79.

Tinkham, M.R. (2013). The road to magnet: encouraging transformational leadership. *ACRN Journal* 98 (2): 186–188. https://doi.org/10.1016/j.aorn.2013.05.007.

Towler. A. (2019). Shared Leadership, Fundamentals benefits and implementation. https://www.ckju.net/en/dossier/shared-leadership-fundamentals-benefits-and-implementation (accessed on 10 December 2021).

Useem, M. (1998). *The Leadership Moment.* Toronto: Times Business Books/Random House.

Vasudeva, S. (2020). Influence of leaders and servant leadership. *American Medical writers Association Journal* 35 (1): 24–25.

Vroom, V.H. and Yetton, P. (1973). *Leadership and Decision Making.* Pittsburgh, PA: University of Pittsburgh Press.

Walker, T. (2006). Servant leaders. *Managed Healthcare Executive* 16 (3): 20–26.

Weberg, D. (2010). Transformational leadership and staff retention: an evidence review with implications for healthcare systems. *Nursing Administration Quarterly* 34 (3): 246.

Wedderburn-Tate, C. (1999). *Leadership in Nursing.* London: Churchill Livingstone.

Welford, C. (2002). Matching theory to practice. *Nursing Management* 9 (4): 7–11.

Weng, R.-H., Huang, C.-Y., Chen, L.-M., and Chang, L.-Y. (2015). Exploring the impact of transformational leadership on nurse innovation behaviour: a cross-sectional study. *Journal of Nursing Management* 23: 427–439.

West, M. (2021). *Compassionate Leadership: Sustaining Wisdom, Humanity and Presence in Health and Social.* London: Swirling Leaf Press.

Wong, C. and Cummings, G. (2009). Authentic leadership: a new theory for nursing or back to basics? *Journal of Health Organisations and Management* 23 (50): 522.

Wong, C.A. and Walsh, E.J. (2020). Reflections on a decade of authentic leadership research in healthcare. *Journal of Nursing Management* 28 (1): 1–3.

Yoder-Wise, P.S. (2015). *Leading and Management in Nursing,* 6e. St Louis, MO: Mosby.

Zaleznik, A. (1977). Managers and leaders: are they different? In: *Harvard Business Review on Leadership,* 61–88. Boston, MA: Harvard Business School Press.

3

Values-Based Leadership: Congruent Leadership

David Stanley

> *We are what we think,*
> *All that we are arises with our thoughts.*
> *With our thoughts we make the world.*
> *Speak or act with a pure mind*
> *and happiness will follow you as your shadow, unshakable*

The Dhammapad

Introduction: A New Theory

The previous chapter outlined a number of leadership theories and styles. This chapter goes further by focusing on theories that derive from a focus on leaders who lead by virtue of their values. The chapter will reconsider three values-based theories (Authentic Leadership/Servant Leadership and Compassionate Leadership) before outlining a new leadership theory called **congruent leadership**. This theory grew from the results of a substantial research project undertaken in the UK and has been supported in subsequent studies that were developed specifically explore the concept of clinical leadership in the health service (Stanley 2006a, b, 2008, 2010, 2011, 2012; Stanley and Sherratt 2010; Stanley et al. 2012, 2014b, 2015; Stanley et al. 2017; Stanley and Stanley 2018; Stanley and Stanley 2019). Congruent leadership is proposed as a framework to support an understanding of clinical leadership and offers the new hypothesis that clinical leaders are more appropriately seen and recognised because of a match between their values and beliefs, and their actions (Stanley 2008, 2011, 2012, 2019, 2020).

The first part of the chapter outlines the main theories that relate to a values-based leadership approach before focusing on how the theory of congruent leadership was developed (or discovered). Then the chapter will elaborate on the theory, what it means, how it is defined and what constitutes congruent leadership. The chapter suggests that clinically focused leaders who display their values and beliefs may be able to effectively foster support, lead clinically and drive change, even if they are not initially aware that this is

Clinical Leadership in Nursing and Healthcare, Third Edition.
Edited by David Stanley, Clare L. Bennett and Alison H. James.
© 2023 John Wiley & Sons Ltd. Published 2023 by John Wiley & Sons Ltd.

possible or that they are even being followed. The chapter also highlights how congruent leadership is related to power, quality processes, innovation and change and why it offers a solid foundation for clinical professionals to develop and gain leadership potential. The strengths and limitations of congruent leadership are also explored.

Values-Based Leadership

Values-based leadership approaches offer a relatively new way of considering leaders and leadership. Copeland (2014, p. 105) suggests that these theories have emerged in response to 'excessive evasive and disheartening ethical leadership failures' and that they have grown from a lack of ethical leadership, other authors concur (Viinamaki 2009; Ahn et al. 2011; Baloglu 2012; Peregrym and Wolf 2013; Stanley 2019). Values are recognised as the 'key components of effective leadership and an essential trait for leaders to possess' (Graber and Kilpatrick 2008, p. 180).

It is proposed that in order to restore hope and redirect an organisation's moral compass, values should be placed at the core of the leader's approach to leading. Wynia and Bedzow (2019) support this and claim that a new focus on values-based leadership is mirrored in nursing and healthcare. Values such as care, compassion, courage and commitment, supported by effective communication and clinical competence, are needed if a 'culture of care is to survive' (Faith 2013 p. 6). As such, values-based leadership can be described as providing a strong underlying moral and ethical foundation with values-based leadership anchoring the leader's behaviour in positive ethical and moral practice (Bass and Avolio 1993; Bass and Steidlmeier 1999; Brown and Treviño 2006).

Values-Based Leadership Theories Applied in Healthcare

1. Authentic Leadership
The concept of authentic leadership developed within scholarship from the increasing focus on ethics and organisational behaviours and the move towards transformational models of leadership (Avolio et al. 2004). Considered as a core paradigm for progressive forms of leadership, focusing on self-awareness and moral perspectives, authentic leadership refers to a process aligned from positivity of psychological aptitudes and organisational contexts, leading to self-awareness and self-regulated positive behaviours among leaders (Avolio and Gardner 2005) taking three perceptions into consideration: the intrapersonal, developmental and interpersonal. Authentic leadership accepts that self-knowledge and personal concepts drive individual leadership, that leadership may be developed, that relationships are important, and that leaders may both influence and be influenced by their values (Cairns-Lee 2015). With four principles at its core, authentic leadership requires 'balanced processing, relational transparency, internalized moral perspective, and self-awareness' (Alilyyani et al. 2018 p. 35). While it is a relatively new theoretical concept and critical views of this include a lack of empirical data of its effectiveness, it has an alliance with the professional values of leading within healthcare. Transparency, moral perspective, balance and self-awareness are key to this approach; however, further critique

proposes the authentic leader could function without moral maturity and align to corrupt values (Avolio and Gardner 2005).

Authentic Leadership grew from the immoral business practices seen in the ENRON collapse and the corrupt and profit-driven behaviours of the ENRON company in the United States (George 2003). Authentic leadership was seen as a leadership approach that called on company executives and business leaders to behave in ways that promoted moral and ethically sound practices focused on clients and consumers, rather than just profits. From a nursing perspective the application of an authentic leadership approach is described as the 'glue' to hold a healthy work environment together (Shirley 2006, 2009), with leaders being encouraged to engage with employees and promote positive behaviours. Wong and Cummings (2009) and Wong and Walsh (2020), also writing from a nursing perspective, suggest that authentic leadership is a suitable theory for aligning future nursing leadership practice.

Bhindi and Duignan (1997), George (2003) and Cantwell (2015) suggest that Authentic Leadership points to an approach where leaders are thought to be true to their own values and beliefs, and the leader's credibility rests on their integrity and ability to be seen as a role model, because of these values and beliefs (James et al. 2021).

Authentic leadership theory has become popular in healthcare literature in Canada, with authors such as Laschinger and Wong applying authentic leadership when addressing issues of workplace empowerment, work-life balance and self-efficacy, the new graduate experience, burnout and mental health. James et al. (2021) were able to show that authentic leadership is seen as a valuable leadership theory for considering how ethically sound and morally appropriate leadership can be applied in healthcare.

2. Servant Leadership

In Chapter 2 it was suggested that servant leadership focuses on the leader's stewardship role and encourages leaders to 'serve' others while staying in tune with the organisation's goals and values (Swanwick and McKimm 2017; Jones and Bennett 2018; James et al. 2021). The concept of servant leadership grew from the American 'Bible Belt' and the writing of Robert Greenleaf (1977), who stated that servant leaders rely less on hierarchical position and more on collaboration, trust, empathy and the use of ethical power.

Servant leadership is also valued because its key principles, which support caring and compassion, seem to fit appropriately within current and dominant values that are parallel with healthcare and nursing (Spears 2004). Mostafa and El-Motalib (2019) and Hanse et al. (2016) found high-quality social exchanges and mutual trust were enhanced by servant leadership while Savel and Munro (2017) assert that premodern concepts of servant leadership are rooted in Christianity and ancient Chinese writings with beliefs about leadership centering on the need for leaders to place prominence on serving others. In the modern context, Greenleaf (1970, 1998) developed the concept of servant leadership, arguing that the servant-leader has an innate desire to serve first and at some later point decides to lead, contrasting this with the individual who is a leader first. The servant leader prioritises others' needs and nurtures others in their professional development. An emphasis is placed on listening to colleagues and shared decision making.

A number of nursing authors have emphasised the relevance of servant leadership as a model to support the development of nursing and healthcare leadership, because its focus is both on promoting user involvement and on patients as the foundation of the health service and the most important group that leaders 'serve' (Anderson 2003; Kerfoot 2004; Swearingen and Liberman 2004; Campbell and Rudisill 2005; Peete 2005; Robinson 2006; Thorne 2006; Walker 2006; Swanwick and McKimm 2017; Jones and Bennett 2018; Ellis 2019; Lee et al. 2019; Vasudeva 2020). Others are explored here in more detail. Mahon (2011) and Neill and Saunders (2008) argue that a servant leadership approach to nurse leadership can lead to greater job satisfaction and morale, stronger collegial relationships and professional growth. Jackson (2008) asserts that servant leadership can create greater research capacity and Ellis (2019) and Neill and Saunders (2008) claim servant leadership can enhance the quality of patient care. Savel and Munro (2017) also argue that servant leadership offers the potential for non-stereotypical 'quiet' leaders to lead.

Mostafa and El-Motalib's (2019) research investigated the relationship between servant leadership and proactive behaviours in the context of leader–member exchange (LMX) among nurses (with the LMX referring to the quality of the dyadic relationship between leaders and their followers and the level of reciprocal social exchange and mutual trust). The study proposed three hypotheses: (i) that servant leadership will be positively related to LMX; (ii) that LMX will be positively related to employee proactive behaviours; and (iii) that LMX will mediate the relationship between servant leadership and employee proactive behaviours. The authors assert that the study findings provide evidence of the importance of servant leadership in the public sector. They also argue that the study provides an insight into why servant leadership could lead public sector employees to engage in behaviours that contribute to long-term organisational effectiveness.

Hanse et al. (2016) also undertook a cross-sectional study in Sweden. Their study also aimed to investigate the impact of servant leadership on LMX among 240 health-care professionals. The authors assert that the findings of this study indicate that a servant leadership style positively influences high-quality LMX among healthcare professionals, the majority of whom were nurses. Another Nordic study, situated in four regional hospitals in Iceland, is reported by Gunnarsdóttir (2014). The aim was to explore the attitudes of Nordic health-care staff towards servant leadership and to investigate whether there was a link between elements of servant leadership and enhanced staff outcomes. The authors argue that since patient safety and staff dissatisfaction persist as risks to the sustainability of healthcare, the findings of this research support the importance of servant leadership for sustainable healthcare services with its potential to reinforce trust, social cohesion, shared goals and social capital. Jooste and Jordaan (2012) conducted a survey which addressed the impact of servant leadership on empowerment, compassion, trust and role modelling. The findings of their study suggest that the student nurses perceived that the nurse manager 'never' or only 'sometimes' acted as a servant leader to students in primary healthcare clinics.

Another study by Garber et al. (2009) explored servant leadership and collaboration and suggested that nurses' attitudes towards collaboration were generally more positive than physicians' and that nurses had a more positive perception of themselves as servant leaders than physicians. The nurses, physicians and residents perceived themselves as role models for collaboration but, when asked if nurses and physicians in the organisation were role models for collaboration, their perceptions were less positive. Likewise, physicians' and nurses' self-perceptions regarding servant leadership were more positive than their perceptions of organisational leadership practices with regards to servant leadership.

However, there is a significant paucity of empirical literature which examines the benefits and limitations of servant leadership in the context of nursing or healthcare. Eicher-Catt (2005) believes that servant leadership is a myth that is unworkable in the real world, that it fails to live up to its promise of being gender neutral and in fact – because of the paradoxical language and apposition of 'servant' and 'leader' – that it accentuates gender bias, so that it ends up supporting androcentric patriarchal norms. There is also an argument put forward by Avolio and Gardner (2005) that servant leadership has not been developed from an empirical base and is therefore purely theoretical

In summary, the current body of empirical research into servant leadership, particularly qualitative research, is limited in scope, quality and quantity. However, the limited research that is available suggests that the application of servant leadership principles can enhance job satisfaction, professional practice and organisational effectiveness by building and strengthening relationships among staff. Interestingly though, individuals' perceptions of themselves as servant leaders can be incongruent with their perceptions of leadership styles at the organisational level.

3. Compassionate Leadership

Compassionate leadership was first proposed by the King's Fund in 2017 as a way for National Health Service (NHS) staff to feel a sense of psychological safety and find new and improved ways of doing things by feeling they are listened to, valued and supported. The Kings Fund (2017) also suggested that developing a shared sense of responsibility, shared leadership and giving staff autonomy in their work was more important than a traditional hierarchical leadership approach. The document proposed that positive attitudes to diversity, inclusion, creativity and innovation needed to be nurtured at every level of the organisation and that innovation is often spurred on by a challenge or a problem. It also proposed that a compassionate approach to leadership might be a powerful facilitator for problem solving within the health service. West (2021) supported these views and went on to describe compassionate leadership as a strategy based on the core human value of compassion, showing that by sustaining compassion in health and social care, health professionals can cultivate wisdom, humanity, presence and high-quality care delivery in health and care services.

Compassion is the quality of having positive intentions and real concern for others. Compassion in leadership creates stronger connections between people. It is thought to improve collaboration, raise levels of trust and enhance loyalty. In addition, Hougaard et al. (2020) found that compassionate leaders are perceived as stronger and more competent, but they add that a sole focus on compassionate in leadership is not enough, and that for leadership to be effective, compassion must be combined with wisdom. They go on to add that by 'wisdom' they mean leadership competence, or a deep understanding of what it is that motivates people and how to manage them to deliver on agreed priorities. Therefore for compassionate leadership to be effective, it requires 'pushing agendas, giving tough feedback, making hard decisions that disappoint people, and, in some cases, laying people off' (Hougaard et al. 2020, https://hbr.org/2020/12/compassionate-leadership-is-necessary-but-not-sufficient) Showing compassion in leadership can't come at the expense of wisdom and effectiveness. You need both. Wise compassionate leadership means doing hard things in a human way.

West and Chowla (2017) suggest that collective leadership is required to create the right culture for healthcare organisations to be effective and that caring in the healthcare field requires compassion for others and acts of attending, understanding, empathising and helping.

Compassion is a human value and as such compassionate leadership sits within the frame of a values-based approach to leadership. But it is proposed here in keeping with Hougaard et al. (2020) view, that its singularity means that a focus on compassion alone neglects other vital values followers seek when searching for leaders to lead effectively and responsibly.

Congruent Leadership: Another View

The theory of congruent leadership developed from the results of my doctoral research and a series of subsequent studies that explored clinical leadership from the perspective of a number of health professional disciplines. The initial research was undertaken with nurses at a large acute hospital in the UK between 2001 and 2004. This was followed up with five further research projects that explored the phenomenon of clinical leadership from the perspective of paramedics (in 2008); senior registered nurses and managers in the aged care arena (in 2012); ambulance volunteers (in 2013); allied health professionals, mainly dietetists, occupational therapists, physiotherapists, social workers, podiatrists and speech therapists (between 2014 and 2015); and remote and rural area nurses (in 2017). All the studies since the doctorate took place in Australia. It was soon clear that none of the previously established leadership theories described or supported the results that began to emerge from the research. As such, a new leadership theory was needed.

Congruent leadership is proposed as a new theory to frame and understand leadership in the health service (although it is highly likely that the theory can be extrapolated to other domains). As it has emerged from studies with input from health professionals, it is proposed that congruent leadership better explains and understands leadership predominantly located in the clinical area, at the bedside, in the clinic, for the paramedic at the roadside and across all healthcare-related disciplines. Beyond this, congruent leadership can be used to explain leadership in education, at the chalkboard or whiteboard; in industry and business, at the coalface or in the office; and in the military, on the battlefield. This introduction sets out to explain what congruent leadership is and how it came into being.

It All Started with Clinical Leadership

At the time that I started to explore clinical leadership (about 1999 when I was a nurse practitioner), the dominant theory supporting clinical and healthcare leadership was transformational leadership (Freshwater et al. 2009; Marriner-Tomey 2009; Weberg 2010; Marshall 2011; Tinkham 2013; Ross et al. 2014; Jones and Bennett 2018). The theory became more prominent with Kotter's (1990, p. 40) publications that proposed and supported the idea that 'leadership is all about coping with change'. This theory had been established for some time but came to prominence in the NHS after the electoral victory of the Blair, Labour Government in 1997. The Labour victory initiated a raft of changes across the UK, and specifically in the NHS. Change was the watch word, and as everything was being reconceptualized, what the government wanted were leaders who could champion change and generate innovations; hence, a leadership theory that supported change was pushed and everyone started applying 'transformational' leadership theory as change swept the NHS. The plans for leadership development were set out in the 'Making a Difference' document (DOH 1999), and the clinical leaders were described as being nurse managers and nurse consultants. However, transformational leadership theory is based on the leader's vision and how their vision is communicated to those who see them as leaders (or are told they are their leaders, e.g. managers). In the course of the clinical leadership research I have undertaken, having a vision or being visionary was seldom identified by respondents as being relevant or significant. Instead, clinically focused leaders were rarely described as having or requiring the attribute of being visionary. This led to a conclusion that established leadership theories, which rested on 'vision' as their basis, were unable to describe the type of leadership displayed by clinically focused leaders. It also led me to wonder if the NHS's ideas of who the clinical leaders were was correct.

There were other theories to consider too. Australian authors Bhindi and Duignan (1997) described what they called 'authentic leadership', where in order to lead, leaders were required to be true to themselves, with this approach to leadership based on the leader's personal credibility and integrity. This was followed by George (2003), who also described 'authentic leadership' in which leaders served others through their leadership and by focusing on their values. These views run parallel to Pondy's (1978) description of leadership where leaders were encouraged to explore their values and lead from recognition of what was identified as important, a view further supported by Scully (2015), who asserted the importance of positive values in leadership.

In the research studies described shortly, time and time again, what stood out as important were values in action, and respondents made comments that supported or pointed to the idea that clinically focused leaders or those who were described as clinical leaders were rarely seen to be driven by or heard to be articulating a vision. Respondents commonly said something like 'That one' (as they pointed from the interview room when a particular health professional passed the door), 'that one, she/he is a clinical leader . . . if my mother becomes sick, she's the one I'd want to look after her'. Or as one allied health professional said, 'a clinical leader is an expert in their field . . . approachable, effective communicators and empowered, are able to act as a role model, motivating others by matching their values and beliefs about care to their practice'.

It was evident that it was the leaders' actions that drew people to identify them as clinical leaders, and it was the synergy of values between the person identifying the leader and the leaders' actions that prompted these leaders to be seen as such. Considering these things, I set out to ask these questions: Who are the clinical leaders? And how do we recognise them?

Over the following 20 years I have undertaken six research studies (often with collaborators) that have led to and support the development of congruent leadership theory. They are offered in outline in Boxes 3.1–3.6.

Box 3.1	Clinical Leadership Study 1

Study title
  In Command of Care: Clinical Nurse Leadership (Doctoral thesis)

Aim
To identify who the clinical leaders are in a large NHS Trust in the English Midlands and to explore and critically analyse the experience of being a clinical nurse leader.

Location	Dates
Worcestershire in the English Midlands	Feb 2001–Dec 2004
Methodology	**Methods**
Qualitative – grounded theory (Interviews and Questionnaires)	Questionnaire and interviews
Target group	**Analysis**
Registered/qualified Nurses (D–H Grade) on 36 clinical areas (in three hospitals) across one NHS Acute Trust	Interviews = NVivo 0.6 and manual
	data configuration
	Questionnaire = SPSS

Sample	Gender mix	Ethics
Interviews n = 50 (42 RNs/8 clinical leaders)	Questionnaire	West Midlands South Strategic Health Authority: Hereford and Worcester Local Research Ethics Committee; LREC 02/43 and permission from Worcester Royal Hospital DON
Questionnaires 850 sent out, 188 returned [22.6%]	Female = 95%	
	Male = 5%	
	Interviews	
	Female = 100%	

Results
Clinical leaders were recognised because they were approachable, clinically competent, visible in practice, made effective decisions and communicated well. They were seen to be empowered and positive clinical role models who, most importantly, displayed their values and beliefs and held fast to their guiding principles about care and nursing. The results indicated that the attribute least likely to be associated with clinical leadership was 'controlling' (78%). The data pointed to another leadership theory that supported clinically focused leadership. This was called congruent leadership. This grew from both the questionnaire and interview results, which suggested that clinical leaders were followed because their colleagues and peers saw the leader's actions as a translation of their values and beliefs into practice.

Clinical leaders were evident in large numbers and represented a wide range of levels of staff, but most commonly it was the most senior clinically focused nurses and rarely the ward managers who were selected or identified as clinical leaders. In

(Continued)

addition, the clinical leaders seemed to be more commonly identified in specialist areas of practice, such as accident and emergency and intensive care areas.

Clinical leaders were often unaware that they had followers, and commonly clinical leaders were not 'tagged' to a titled or senior position. The common theme was that clinical leaders had their values on show, and these were based on a foundation of care. Moreover, many of the clinical leaders identified suggested that they faced issues of role conflict and struggled to maintain their 'clinical focus' in the face of 'management demands'.

Related Publications

Bishop, V. (ed.) (2009). *Leadership in Nursing and Allied Health Care Professions*, Buckingham: Open University Press.

Chapter 2: Leadership and management: A new mutiny?

Chapter 7: Clinical leadership and the theory of congruent leadership

Lawrence, J., Perrin, C. & Kierman, E. (2015). *Building Professional Nursing Communication*, Cambridge: Cambridge University Press.

Part of Chapter 8: Professional skills for nurses and other health professionals: Context and capability of practice.

Stanley, D. (2004). 'Clinical leadership: A pilot study explored', *Paediatric Nursing*, vol. 16, no. 3, pp. 39–42.

Stanley, D. (2006a). 'Part 1: In command of care: Clinical nurse leadership explored', *Journal of Research in Nursing*, vol. 2, no. 1, pp. 20–39.

Stanley, D. (2006b). 'Part 2: In command of care: Towards the theory of congruent leadership', *Journal of Research in Nursing*, vol. 2, no. 2, pp. 132–44.

Stanley, D. (2006c). 'Role conflict: Leaders and managers', *Nursing Management*, vol. 13, no. 5, pp. 31–7.

Stanley, D. (2006d). 'Recognising and defining clinical nurse leaders', *British Journal of Nursing*, vol. 15, no. 2, pp. 108–11.

Stanley, D. (2007). 'Lights in the shadows', *Contemporary Nurse*, vol. 24, no. 1, pp. 45–51.

Stanley, D. (2008). 'Congruent leadership: Values in action', *Journal of Nursing Management*, vol. 64, pp. 84–95.

Stanley, D. (2009). 'Leadership: Behind the mask', *ACORN*, vol. 22, no. 1, pp. 14–20.

Stanley, D. (2010). 'Clinical leadership and innovation', *Connections*, vol. 13, no. 4, pp. 27–8.

Stanley, D. (2011). *Clinical Leadership: Innovation into Action*, Melbourne: Palgrave Macmillan.

Stanley, D. (2012). 'Clinical leadership and innovation', *Journal of Nursing Education and Practice*, May, pp. 119–26.

Stanley, D. (2014). 'Clinical leadership characteristics confirmed', *Journal of Research in Nursing*, vol. 19, no. 2, pp. 118–28.

Stanley, D. & Sherratt, A. (2010). 'Lamp light on leadership: Clinical leadership and Florence Nightingale', *Journal of Nursing Management*, vol. 18, pp. 115–21.

Box 3.2   Clinical Leadership Study 2

Study title
  Perceptions of Clinical Leadership in the St John Ambulance Service in Western Australia

Aim
To identify how clinical leadership is perceived by paramedics and ambulance person-nel in the course of their everyday work and the effectiveness and consequences of the application of clinical leadership in pre-hospital care delivery.

Location	Dates
Western Australia (metropolitan, rural and remote areas of practice)	Feb–Nov 2010

Methodology	Methods
Qualitative – phenomenology	Questionnaire

Target group	**Analysis**
250 paramedic (non-volunteer) and ambulance officers who attended in-service education between February and November 2010 in Perth, Western Australia	Questionnaire = SPSS and spreadsheet

Sample	**Gender mix**	
250 questionnaires distributed, 104 returned = 41.6% return rate	Questionnaires Female = 36% Male = 64%	**Ethics** Ethical approval was sought and secured through the Curtin University Human Research Ethics Committee (Nu: SON&M 1–2010)

Results
In relation to the characteristics of a clinical leader, most respondents suggested that clinical leaders needed to be clinically competent (96%), a role model for others (93%), an effective communicator (89%), inspire confidence (85%), be approachable (96%) have integrity (93%), be supportive (91%), be a decision maker (87%), be visible in prac-tice (86%) and set direction (87%). Just over 84% indicated (in keeping with Study 1) that 'controlling' was the attribute least associated with clinical leadership. Under half (42%) saw themselves as clinical leaders, although over one-third (35%) felt that they could not engage in leadership activities for a range of reasons, including a lack of encouragement, lack of training opportunities, work pressures and a lack of opportunity to be leaders. Almost 60% indicated that they faced barriers to becoming or deploying clinical leadership, with many indicating that they faced resistance from colleagues, no opportunities, the current management culture and a lack of experience.
  Of the 104 respondents, their average length of service with the St John Ambulance Service was just under 7 years (6.9 years), with the longest service of any respondent

(Continued)

being 30 years. In terms of formal leadership training, only 40.6% indicated that they had some sort of formal leadership training (although it was not clear what constituted this). In terms of formal management training, 26% indicated that they had some sort of management training. The gender make-up of the respondents was in keeping with the wider ambulance service, with 64% male. The age distribution showed that the majority (68%) were under the age of 41.

A large number of respondents were from metropolitan centres, with only 7.4% of respondents indicating that they were based in rural or regional areas. Most respondents did not care where their experience was from or what sort of experience it was as long as they had valid roadside experience. Most did not value research insights or qualifications. What mattered was that the values of the clinical leaders were matched by their actions and abilities. Many did not see themselves as clinical leaders and few thought that they could influence organisational issues. Most respondents thought that they should have an influence on clinical care and valued team working. Clinical leaders (in keeping with Study 1) were seen to be visible role models, leaders in clinical practice, skilled, experienced, clinically focused, approachable, knowledgeable, driven by their desire to provide high-quality care, of high moral character and practised in change. They were seen to be team members who made decisions, often under pressure.

Related Publications

Stanley, D. (2011) *Cliniial Leadership: Innovation into Action*, Melbourne: Palgrave Macmillan.

Stanley, D., Cuthbertson, J. & Latimer, K. (2012) 'Perceptions of clinical leadership in the St. John Ambulance Service in WA. Paramedics Australasia', *Response*, vol. 39, no. 1, pp. 31–7.

Stanley, D. (2013). Perceptions of clinical leadership in the St John Ambulance Service in WA: A research Report. http://www.sph.uwa.edu.au/__data/assets/pdf_file/0003/2272647/Report-Perceptions-of-clinical-leadership-in-the-St.pdf

The results from the six studies outlined have led to and supported the development of a new leadership theory: **congruent leadership**. This theory suggests that leaders demonstrate a match (congruence) between the leader's values and beliefs, and their actions.

The research results indicated that clinically focused nurses and a range of health professionals who have moved decisively and clearly in the direction of their values and beliefs can be seen expressing congruent leadership. They may have simply stood by their values, working not because they wanted to change the world but because they knew that what they were doing was the right thing and that their actions were making a difference.

When acting out or role modelling their values and beliefs (even subconsciously), something was happening in their relationships with their clients, patients or colleagues that gave a clear signal about what they believed or what their values were. This linked congruent leadership with the expression of emotional intelligence and values-based relationship building and caring/compassionate engagement.

The research studies indicated that others responding to the expression of the leaders' values and beliefs in action saw these leaders as such because they were approachable,

Box 3.3   Clinical Leadership Study 3

Study title
  Leadership at Home: Perceptions of Clinical Leadership at Swan Care Group Bentley Park

Aim
To investigate perceptions of leadership and approaches to leadership development of senior nurses and care home managers in an aged care residential facility in Western Australia.

Location	Dates
Swan Care residential facility in Bentley	Mar–Sept 2012
Park, Perth, Western Australia	

Methodology	Methods
Qualitative – phenomenology	Questionnaire and interviews

Target group	Analysis
Senior clinical nurses and residential	Interviews = NVivo 0.6 and manual data
care home managers in a residential	configuration
care home in Western Australia	Questionnaire = SPSS

Sample	Gender mix	Ethics
20 staff were sent questionnaires: 10 with a return rate of 50%	Questionnaires Female = 100% Male = 0%	Ethical approval was sought and secured with the University of Western Australia Human Research Ethics Office (RA/4/1/5084) and the study had the consent of the management of Swan Care Bentley Park
Eight senior nurses or care home staff were interviewed (some had also completed the questionnaire)	Interviews Female = 100% Male = 0%	

Results
Results of the study indicated that the attributes and characteristics of clinical leaders identified by the senior nurses and care home managers who participated in the study were consistent with the results of the two previous studies. The vast majority of respondents suggested that clinical leaders were identified because they were approachable (100%), had sound clinical skills and knowledge (100%), were honest, had integrity (100%), supported others (100%) and were visible in the clinical area (100%).

It was also noted that participants saw a distinction between leadership and management and that their more clinically focused roles led them towards a

(Continued)

leadership-centred approach. However, few had any leadership instruction beyond clinical 'experience' and almost all saw barriers that hindered their development or application of leadership in the care home environment. In order to play a more effective part in service improvement and care provision and have a positive impact on resident care and staff support, it was considered essential that senior nursing and care home managers be better supported to recognise the significance of developing clinical leadership attributes and applying them in the care home environment.

As with the two previous studies, few participants saw themselves as clinical leaders, although they recognised that clinical leaders were evident at all levels in the care home, and again, the 'manager' was less likely to be seen as a clinical leader than the more senior clinically focused nursing staff. As with the previous studies, the attribute least likely to be associated with clinical leadership was 'controlling' (80%). Again, leaders seemed to be recognised because they had their values on show, rather than because of any affinity with their vision.

Related Publications

Stanley, D. (2013) 'Leadership at home: Perceptions of clinical leadership at Swan Care Group, Bentley Park: A pilot study report', http://www.sph.uwa.edu.au/__data/assets/pdf_file/0004/2272639/Leadership-At-Home-Swan-Care-Group-report.pdf (accessed 1 July 2016).

Stanley, D., Latimer, K. & Atkinson, J. (2014b) 'Perceptions of clinical leadership in an aged care residential facility in Perth, *Western Australia', Health Care Current Reviews*, vol. 2, pp. 122. doi:10.4172/hccr.1000122

Box 3.4   Clinical Leadership Study 4

Study title
Volunteer Ambulance Officers' Perceptions of Clinical Leadership in St John Ambulance Services Western Australia Incorporated

Aim
To identify how clinical leadership skills were perceived by volunteer ambulance officers in the course of their everyday work and the effectiveness and consequences of such skills in pre-hospital care delivery.

Location	Dates
Western Australia (metropolitan, rural and remote areas of practice)	Sept 2012–Apr 2013
Methodology	**Methods**
Qualitative – phenomenology	Online and paper-based questionnaires
Target group	**Analysis**
Volunteer ambulance officers (VAO) in Western Australia	Questionnaire (paper-based and online) with SPSS

(Continued)

Box 3.4   (Continued)

Location		Dates

Sample	Gender mix	Ethics
Approximately 500 VAO were sent questionnaires (although there were estimated to be 2787 VAO in the service in WA at the time of the study) and 61 were returned, a return rate of only 12.2%	Questionnaire Female = 49% Male = 51%	Ethical approval was sought and secured with the University of Western Australia Human Research Ethics Office (RA/4/1/5451) and had the consent of the management of the St John Ambulance Service WA Inc.

Results

Respondents' average length of service with the St John Ambulance Service was just under 10 years (9.9 years), with the longest service of any respondent being over 40 years. In terms of formal leadership training, only 32.7% indicated that they had some sort of formal leadership training (although it was not clear what constituted this). A further 60.7% indicated that they had not had any formal leadership training and 6.6% were not sure. In terms of formal management training, a similar 31.2% indicated that they had had some sort of management training, while 65.5% indicated that they had not, and 3.3% were unsure.

The gender make-up of the respondents was interesting, in that there was almost a 50:50 split, men making up 50.8% of the sample. The age distribution showed that the majority (73.1%) were over the age of 41. A large number of respondents were from regional centres, with only 8.2% of respondents indicating that they were based in metropolitan areas. In relation to the characteristics of a clinical leader, most suggested that clinical leaders needed to be clinically competent (90%), a role model for others (89%), an effective communicator (87%), to inspire confidence (85%), be approachable (84%), have integrity (79%), be flexible (77%) and set direction (75%). Almost 84% indicated (in keeping with all the studies) that 'controlling' was the attribute least associated with clinical leadership. Most did not care where their experience was from or what sort of experience it was as long as they had valid roadside experience. Most did not value research insights or qualifications. What mattered was that the values of the clinical leaders were matched by their actions and abilities.

Many respondents did not see themselves as clinical leaders and few thought that they could influence organisational issues. Most thought that they should have an influence on clinical care and valued team working. Clinical leaders were seen to be visible role models, leaders in clinical practice, skilled, experienced, clinically focused, approachable, knowledgeable, driven by their desire to provide high-quality care, have high moral character and practised in change. They were seen to be team members who made decisions, often under pressure.

Related publications

Stanley, D., Metcalfe, H., Gallagher, O. & Cuthbertson, J. (2013) 'Volunteer ambulance officers' perceptions of clinical leadership in the St. John Ambulance Service in WA: A research report', http://www.sph.uwa.edu.au/__data/assets/pdf_file/0003/2272647/Report-Perceptions-of-clinical-leadership-in-the-St.pdf (accessed 1 July 2016).

Box 3.5   Clinical Leadership Study 5

Study title
  Western Australian Allied Health Professionals' Perceptions of Clinical Leadership

Aim
To identify how the concept and application of clinical leadership are perceived by allied health professionals (AHPs) and the implications for service improvement, the adoption of quality initiatives and innovations for change.

Location	Dates
Western Australia (metropolitan, rural and remote areas of practice)	Nov-Dec 2014

Methodology	Methods
Mixed methods with quantitative data dominating the mix	Online SurveyMonkey questionnaire

Target group	Analysis
AHPs employed within the Western Australian Department of Health Main professional disciplines included dietetics, occupational therapy, physiotherapy, podiatry, social work and speech pathology	Questionnaire = SPSS (version 21) with qualitative data analysed by spreadsheet and Word documents

Sample size	Gender mix	Ethics
311 online questionnaires were returned, with 307 offering relevant data	Female = 86.5% Male = 13.5%	Ethical approval was sought and secured through the Government of Western Australian Department of Health South Metropolitan Health Service Human Research Ethics Committee (No: HREC 14/45 Code: EC00265)

Results
Participants in this study represented only 6.1% of the total AHP workforce of the WA Department of Health. The data indicated that the respondents had been AHPs for an average of 14.6 years. The vast majority of respondents came from the six targeted allied health professions groups of dietetics (11.2%), occupational therapy (17.8%), physiotherapy (19.7%), podiatry (3.0%), social work (18.4%) and speech pathology (15.5%). The majority of respondents were at Health Service Union Award (HSU) Level P1 (base-grade clinician) or P2 (senior clinician) (68.1%), with only about 15% of respondents at Level P4 or beyond. The majority of respondents (86.5%) were female and the median respondent age was 38.9 years, with the majority of AHP respondents being between 21 and 40 years (54.3%). Moreover, the majority of respondents worked in acute hospital environments (59.9%) and in a metropolitan location (73.7%).

(Continued)

Box 3.5 (Continued)

In terms of the respondents' perceptions of clinical leadership, the majority of respondents (79.2%) saw themselves, and thought they were seen by others (76.2%), as clinical leaders. The main attributes identified as being attributed to clinical leaders were effective communicator, sets direction, is clinically competent, has integrity and is honest, is approachable, acts as a role model for others, copes well with change, is supportive, is a mentor and is a motivator. The main attribute identified as being least associated with a clinical leader was 'is controlling' (83.7%). In support of this, when asked if a clinical leader needed to be in a management position to be effective, only 22.2% agreed that they did. However, when asked if having a clinical focus was important for an effective clinical leader, 85.3% suggested that it was. Other attributes seen as central to effective clinical leadership were to have the skills and resources to perform tasks effectively, possess team working skills, be visible in the clinical environment, express appreciation to colleagues, be an initiator, have a high moral character, communicate well or be an 'excellent communicator' and be flexible.

Clinical leaders were also perceived as having an impact on how clinical care is delivered, supporting staff, being innovative, leading change and service improvement, participating in professional development and (although to a lesser extent) influencing organisational policy.

A large number of respondents (81.4%) indicated that there were barriers hindering their effectiveness as a clinical leader. The barriers included a lack of time and a high clinical demand on their time, having to deal with bureaucracy, a lack of opportunities to be a clinical leader, limited funding and resources, a lack of mentorship, working part time and problems with the whole health system.

Related publications

Stanley, D., Hutton, M. & McDonald, A. (2015) *Western Australian Allied Health Professionals'*

Perceptions of Clinical Leadership: A Research Report, http://www.ochpo.health.wa.gov. au/docs/WA_Allied_Health_Prof_Perceptions_of_Clinical_Leadership_Research_ Report.pdf (accessed 1 July 2016).

Stanley, D., Blanchard, D., Hohol, A., Hutton, M. & McDonald. (2017). Health professionals' perceptions of clinical leadership. A pilot study. Cogent Medicine. vol. 4, No. 1 https://doi.org/10.1080/2331205X.2017.1321193

Box 3.6   Clinical Leadership Study 6

Study title

There where the 'bullets can fly': Clinical Leadership in Rural and Remote North-Western New South Wales.

Aim

To explore how clinical leadership is perceived by nurses in rural and remote areas of New South Wales, Australia.

(Continued)

Location		Dates
New South Wales Australia (Rural and remote areas of practice)		April - Nov 2017

Methodology		**Methods**
Qualitative		Interviews
Target group		**Analysis**
Nurses working in rural and remote areas of the north-western parts of New South Wales, Australia.		Questionnaire = recorded and transcribed interviews then with spreadsheet and word documents
Sample size	**Gender mix**	**Ethics**
56 nurses interviewed across 14 different health facilities (rural hospitals, multipurpose service centres community health services).	Female = 94.6% Male = 5.5%	Ethical approval was sought and secured through the Hunter New England Health Service Human Research Ethics Committee on the 28th of June 2017 code: (No: HREC 17/06/21/5.02)

Results

A thematic analysis resulted in the development of five themes and findings that supported an understanding of clinical leadership in a rural and remote practice context. The themes were leadership in rural and remote areas; the impact of clinical leadership in rural and remote areas; barriers in rural and remote practice; training and development needs; and rural and remote practice challenges. Clinical leader characteristics were compatible and consistent with the previous studies. They were valued if they had good clinical skills, were approachable, could communicate effectively, and if their values aligned with those expected by their colleagues. Values seen as desirable were being trustworthy, honest, caring, compassionate and having respect for others. Clinical leaders were evident in significant numbers and seen to be have a considerable impact on the quality of care and the initiation of change in practice or the delivery of quality care. They also faced barriers, if the health facility was poorly staffed, if they felt bullied, or lacked support and if the community was strongly co-dependent.

Related publications

Stanley, D. & Stanley K. (2018). Report: There where the "bullets can fly": Clinical Leadership in rural and remote north-western New South Wales. Research Report UNE Print ISBN: 978-64467-203-7

Stanley, D. & Stanley, K. (2019). Clinical leadership and rural and remote practice: A qualitative study. *Journal of Nursing Management*. vol. 27, no. 6. pp. 1314-24.

Stanley, D. (2020). Bullying and threats to belonging in rural and remote practice. *Australian Nursing and Midwifery Journal*. vol. 26, No.11, p. 26.

clinically knowledgeable and competent. They were visible in practice, were role models for the behaviour they espoused and communicated well. They were able to make effective decisions, were empowered, were compassionate and caring and could motivate others, and, because their actions were evident or matched their values and beliefs, they were seen as passionate and committed leaders. This was rarely because they were visionaries, were in powerful positions or wielded great authority.

The studies were undertaken with a range of different health professionals, used a range of methodologies and were conducted in different countries, with different genders and over a wide span of years, although all three of the studies with nurses as subjects employed interviews while the remaining studies used only questionnaires. The study results have been presented in a number of countries (Thailand, Singapore, Tanzania, Canada, the UK, Australia and Ireland), all with resounding endorsements of the principles of congruent leadership theory. In addition, three replica studies have been undertaken in the UK, Australia, and South Africa. The results from the study in Australia were published in 2021 by Coventry and Russell (2021). While exploring the attributes of clinical nurse educators, Coventry and Russell (2021) suggested that their findings support the findings evident in the original studies with clinical nurse educators seen as visible, approachable, and related to colleagues with clearly identified values and passionate patient-centred principles – pointing to their application of a congruent leadership approach.

Each of the six studies and Coventry and Russell's (2021) study focused on capturing data about clinically focused leaders. The results point to a new way of understanding leadership that suggests that leaders are followed not for their vision, for being visionary, for being creative or for being transformational, but because there is a match between their values and beliefs, and their actions.

The various research studies indicated that followers were attracted to or followed congruent leaders because of the principles they stood by. The leaders carried these like a standard or banner that they may not intentionally show or be conscious that others saw. However, it was their values and their application through their actions that followers recognised and rallied to. The congruent leader's metaphorical banner or standard was usually a statement of what they believed was important to them. It might say 'I care for patients like they were my family', 'I teach these children as if they were my own', 'I'll be here at the bedside with you', 'I know what it's like, I'm on your side' or 'Together we can do it'. Whatever it was, it was the demonstration of the leaders' values and beliefs that prompted others to see them as leaders and follow them, even if the leader was not aware of this.

These clinically focused leaders capture what it means to be a congruent leader: standing by their values in the execution and drive of their actions, putting their hands where their heart is, walking their talk and acting out and following through with what they believe to be right.

Reflection Point

Look around your organisation, ward or healthcare team. Think about the results from the studies outlined in Boxes 3.1–3.6. Who are the clinical leaders where you work, and do they fit the results from the studies?

Should the results of these studies matter? Why might they be relevant or not?

These leaders are not selling a vision or communicating a path for others to follow; they are living their vision and walking the path themselves, role modelling with commitment, conviction and determination what they believe is the right thing to do. They are congruent leaders.

Congruent Leadership Theory Explored

Congruent leaders are skilled and experienced nurses and other health professionals. Congruent leaders may have a vision and idea about where they want to go, but this is not why they are followed – it is because they are driven by their values and beliefs about care and high-quality nursing or health practice. Congruent leadership is based on the leader's values, beliefs and principles and is about where the leader stands, not where they are going (Stanley 2019). This approach to leadership is paralleled by Kouzes and Posner's description of leadership, which suggests that 'values drive commitment' and that 'people want to know what you stand for and believe in' (2010, p. xxii). Congruent leaders are motivational, inspirational, organised, effective communicators and they build relationships. They commonly have no formal, structured or hierarchical position in an organisation, and even if they do, it is not their position that motivates the follower, but their values and beliefs as evidenced by their actions.

Congruent leaders appear to be guided by passion, compassion, commitment, courage and respect for others. They build enduring relationships, stand the test of their principles and they are more concerned with supporting the empowerment of others than with power or their own prestige. Kouzes and Posner support this view, suggesting that 'if you are ever to become a leader whom others willingly follow, you must be known as someone who stands by his or her principles' (2010, p. 34).

In contrast to congruent leaders, transformational leaders are commonly found in positions called leadership or management, have hierarchical or titled positions or fulfil a leadership role as an expectation of their job description (see Table 3.1).

Not all leadership is about changing or challenging people's vision of the future. Some leaders in the research interviews were seen as leaders because they demonstrated where their values lay and were followed because others identified with these values and stood with them. One research participant said:

> I think you've got to have respect for that person because of the way they nurse, you identify with them, identify with the way they nurse and agree with that.

Another commented:

> I am not only able to empathise with patients and their relatives, but with staff as well . . . trying to think 'what would they be going through?' . . . it makes my ability to communicate with them much better.

Another added:

> I think people know that I am quite passionate about what I do and I also like to support others . . . to achieve the best they can achieve and very strongly centred on patient care and good standards of care.

Table 3.1 Comparison of the features of transformational and congruent leadership.

Transformational leadership features	Congruent leadership features
Driven by establishing direction and aligning people	Driven by acting on values and beliefs
Motivating and inspiring	Motivating and inspiring
Produces change, often dramatic	Approachable/open
About where you are going (vision)	Actions based on values and beliefs
Effective communicators	About where you stand (principles)
Creative/initiative	Effective communicators
Recognised leadership/management, hierarchical or titled positions	Visible
	Empowered
	Any level, not necessary to have a title or hierarchical position
	Guided by passion, compassion
	Build enduring relationships

Note: Although there are some similarities, the key differences relate to what motivates or drives the leaders: vision or values and principles.

Congruent leadership explains why and how nurses and other health professionals and non-titled leaders at all levels can function and be effective without formal influence in the clinical area and without formal deference to the organisation's vision. As such, the qualities of a congruent leader include honesty, loyalty and integrity.

Leadership comes from having respect for another person's 'way they nurse', 'approach to care', 'therapeutic skills' or 'clinical knowledge'. Other health professionals identify with these values and beliefs and with the clinician's capacity to empathise with colleagues and clients.

A Solid Foundation

If nursing and other clinically focused health disciplines are to develop effective leaders, they need to do so without losing the core values and principles that guide their professional, client-focused core (Scully 2015; Stanley 2019). Congruent leadership establishes a foundation from which all good or effective clinically focused leaders can start, because it grounds the leader's principles within the core values of their profession's principles and values. This will ensure that the dominant cultural narrative of these professional disciplines is one of patient-centred or person-centred care, therapy or treatment. In this way, the profession's core values and care-centred attributes are placed ahead of those associated with previously dominant values, which commonly stem from groups that may sometimes be in conflict with professional values (e.g. financial or economic or even managerial goals and directives). In an effort to achieve their vision, transformational leaders may at times move from positions of influence and power to positions of control. As such, they run the risk of potential exploitation (Rafferty 1993) and may seek to secure more control in an effort to achieve their goals. Unwittingly, in doing so, they run the risk of losing their connection to the professional discipline's core values and guiding principles, or at best they become embroiled in a state of conflict as their managerial (controlling) demands conflict with their professional and often personal desire to remain focused on patient care, therapy and treatment (Gentile 2010).

In the UK, the whole National Health Service (NHS) has embraced the 6Cs established by the UK Chief Nurse in 2013. These are care, compassion, communication, courage, commitment and competence (Stephenson 2014; Taylor and Bradbury-Jones 2014) and represent the collective understanding (values) of what the NHS sees as central to the ethos and culture that is being developed. However, words and slogans are not enough. In April 2014, a blog on nursingtimes.net, which followed an article announcing the roll-out of the 6Cs, prompted an online discussion on the *Nursing Times* website. The article suggested that porters, caterers, doctors and Trust chief executives were to be asked to embrace the 6Cs in an effort to extend the core values to all staff working in the NHS. One anonymous blogger noted:

> I am involved in a complaint we have made to a Mental Health Trust. Our family has been treated appallingly by the Chief Executive during the process of the complaint, causing immense upset and stress. That same Chief Executive, a nurse, blogs and twitters about compassion and being open and honest. Words and silly slogans mean nothing unless they practice what they preach.

Clearly, this chief executive was not regarded as a congruent leader by the anonymous blogger who made the complaint. This or issues like it sit behind the call for senior NHS managers to embrace compassionate leadership. It also reminds us that talking about our values and putting them into action are two very different things. Have nurses and the NHS lost sight of the values that matter? Had these remained in clear focus, might the issues discussed in the Francis Report (Francis 2013) have occurred?

The recognition and application of congruent leadership may offer clinically focused health professionals an opportunity to develop greater influence in the leadership stakes. However, until nurses, physiotherapists, ambulance officers and other clinically focused health professionals can themselves influence and initiate this and, importantly, recognise themselves as congruent leaders, others may continue to see clinical nursing and other clinically focused health professionals as secondary, subsidiary or of low status (Antrobus and Kitson 1999).

This said, a healthy 80% of allied health professionals in our studies did indicate that they saw their potential to be clinical leaders. This was less well demonstrated by the other health professionals, with only 40% of ambulance officers, 47.5% of volunteer ambulance officers and 30% of senior nursing home staff able to recognise themselves as clinical leaders.

In the nursing literature, nurses have in the past been described as 'invisible' and 'dirty' (Roberts 1983; Robinson 1991; Davies 1995; Wilkinson and Miers 1999) and, while the references are somewhat dated, it is possible that the remnants of these views persist. In *From Silence to Voice*, Buresh and Gordon (2013) indicate that nurses remain at risk if they are not able to find their voice and offer clear communication about their profession. Views are supported in the Paradoxes in Nurses' Identity, Culture and Image by McAllister and Brien (2020). These views further support the notion that some clinically focused health professionals continue to hold the view that they have only a limited stake in leadership or being seen as leaders.

Also associated with the recognition of congruent leadership is the realisation that values, as well as standards, need to become the focus of development in the health service in general (Scully 2015). Government documents and other literature released over recent years (Curtis et al. 2011; NHS Leadership Academy 2013; DoH UK 2015a,b; DoH WA 2015; Rafferty et al. 2015; The King's Fund 2017) may have focused more on what is important (values) than in the past. While considerable consultation has taken place, directives and directions are not always in keeping with the values and guiding principles of the nursing profession, ideal nursing practice or the professional practices of other health disciplines. Indeed, consultation with nursing groups is not always clearly demonstrated.

This has led to the clash of values that O'Reilly and Pfeffer (2000) found likely to disrupt the development, success and performance of companies in the business world. Clinically focused health professionals, it should be remembered, make up a huge percentage of the body of any health service. Nurses constitute the largest single group in the health services of America, Australia and the UK (Grosios et al. 2010; Australian Institute of Health and Welfare 2014; American Association of Colleges of Nursing 2016), and allied health professionals are a significant proportion of other health professions, with 6% in the UK (Oliver 2015) and approximately 17% in Australia (Australian Institute of Health and Welfare 2014). If clinically focused health professionals are unable to express their core values and beliefs, or are inhibited from doing so, the negative impact on leadership for the health service is likely to be considerable. West (2021) makes this point in calling for compassionate leadership. Nurses and other health professionals contribute too much to patient care and the health service to remain unrecognised (and unheard), because their contribution, values and leadership are sorely needed.

Reflection Point

Consider the clinical leaders stories throughout the book. There is one in most chapters. Do they demonstrate the attributes of clinical leaders or actions that display congruent leadership? If not, why not? If so, then why? Relate one of the stories to a clinical colleague and ask them if they feel that the actions discussed refer to a congruent leader. Does this even matter?

Why might these stories be relevant, or if not, why not, when considering the theory of congruent leadership?

The Strengths of Congruent Leadership

There are a number of strengths afforded by an understanding and application of congruent leadership, outlined in what follows.

Grassroots Leaders

One of the main strengths of congruent leadership is that it supports the promotion of 'grassroots' (Roberts 1983, p. 29) leaders. If, as Roberts and others have suggested, nurses (and possibly other health professionals) are an oppressed group, then finding ways to liberate leaders within the core group of health professionals without plucking them out or removing them from the rank and file will ensure that leaders can develop who remain focused on the core issues, values and beliefs that are relevant in a patient-focused environment. The congruent leader's credibility is recognised and established when their actions match their values and beliefs. It is their ability to demonstrate or display their actions and not their position, title or role that facilitates their ability to lead.

Historically, Mary Seacole (see Case Study 3.1) offers an example of a congruent leader. Mary felt so strongly about nursing and her need to help others that she travelled independently, as an 'unofficial nurse' (Bostridge 2004, p. 19) to the Crimean War to provide care and treatment to British soldiers, where at great personal and financial risk she stood by her principles with definitive action (Bostridge 2008).

Another example in support of congruent leadership is offered in the research studies, where an identified clinical leader, when discussing a change in the type of clients for whom her ward would cater, indicated:

> I had to take a long hard look at my values and beliefs and look at the values and beliefs of the team and . . . I decided that although I wanted to champion the cause of older people I didn't necessarily think that putting them all together in one place did that and I think it didn't put over the picture of what normal society is about and we realised that we could still fight things like ageism or whatever in . . . a general ward.

Congruent leadership helps grassroots leaders, clinical leaders and clinical staff who lead on an everyday basis. Giving clinical leaders a name for their leadership approach with which they can identify can only lead to an increase in grassroots leaders or clinical leaders *actually* seeing themselves as leaders. Many of the research interviewees described what they saw as the qualities and characteristics of clinical leaders but failed to recognise these qualities or attributes in themselves, even when others could. Current leadership theories that emphasise 'vision' as the key attribute of leadership or that link leadership and management responsibilities close down avenues of expression or understanding for leaders who lead without formal authority, recognised power or titles that encompass leadership (Welford 2002; Thyer 2003; Goertz Koerner 2010; Man 2010; Weberg 2010; Casida and Parker 2011; Marshall 2011; Hutchinson and Jackson 2012; Tinkham 2013; Ross et al. 2014; Weng et al. 2015; Swanwick and McKimm 2017; Jones and Bennett 2018; Stanley 2019).

Foundation for Other Theories

Another strength of congruent leadership is that it offers a foundation on which other theories can be constructed (Figure 3.1). From this foundation, clinical leaders, nurses and grassroots leaders can build an understanding of and connection with the core values and beliefs about healthcare. From a foundation that recognises and values the contribution that clinically focused health professionals make, clinical work is identifiable and named.

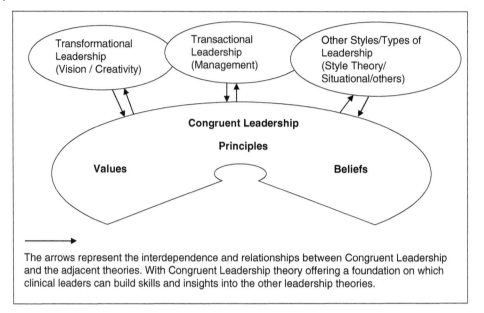

The arrows represent the interdependence and relationships between Congruent Leadership and the adjacent theories. With Congruent Leadership theory offering a foundation on which clinical leaders can build skills and insights into the other leadership theories.

Figure 3.1 The relationship of congruent leadership to other leadership theories/models.

No longer invisible, clinical work is recognised and clinical leaders who are approachable, knowledgeable, clinically competent, effective communicators, visible, positive role models, empowered, decision makers and who stand and hold fast to their guiding principles can have a positive impact on healthcare and lead clinical care forward by holding to the principles central to each profession.

Strong Link between Values and Actions

A significant strength of congruent leadership is that it builds a strong link between values and beliefs and actions. In this regard it is not static, but dynamic with congruent leadership making explicit the link between purpose, meaning and values and the leader's commitment to acting on them and in accordance with them. Congruence is a statement of agreement, of consistency, and using this word to describe this type of leadership helps promote the link among values, beliefs, meaning and action. In effect, having beliefs and recognising your own values and knowing where you stand are of little merit if they are not employed when you are faced with challenges, or if they are not displayed and congruent with your actions. Authors in support of authentic leadership (Bhindi and Duignan 1997; George 2003; Wong and Cummings 2009) recognise this to some extent, with George indicating that authentic leadership is about 'being yourself; being the person you were created to be' (George 2003, p. 11).

Nevertheless, congruent leadership is more than just being. It is about acting, displaying, demonstrating and living the leader's values and beliefs. Although similar to authentic leadership, congruent leadership emphasises the translation of values and beliefs into action, for it is in the action that leadership is evident and effective. Clinical leaders employing a congruent leadership approach are recognised and feel valued for the contribution they make to care and for the value they add to nursing's therapeutic benefit for patients (Freshwater 2002). Clinical leaders are also recognised because the actions and activities they employ are based on and guided by the values and beliefs they hold passionately, not only for the vision, creativity and clinical expertise they may bring to clinical practice.

Supports Further Understanding of Clinical Leadership

One of the main benefits of congruent leadership is in advancing an understanding of clinical leadership. Indeed, in any environment where leaders are not invested with authority or a title to lead; where leaders function in the trenches, at the front line, at the coalface or in direct proximity to the patient, client, child or service user; understanding, promoting and developing congruent leadership may be of benefit.

One of the common themes from the research that supports this book was the conflict that clinically focused health professionals felt when trying to reconcile leadership and management tensions (Stanley 2006d). When health professionals gave voice to their values (Gentile 2010) or lived them in their actions (Stanley 2006a, b, 2008, 2011, 2019), they commonly ran the risk of coming into conflict with organisational or management goals or objectives. Therefore, congruent leadership facilitates and supports an approach to leadership focused on clinically based values.

Anyone Can Be a Congruent Leader

Congruent leaders are found in a range of positions and across the spectrum of an organisation (Stanley 2019). The application of congruent leadership is not limited to people in leadership, titled or senior positions. Anyone can apply or demonstrate congruent leadership, if they are encouraged and supported to see the significance of their values and beliefs.

Reflection Point

Can anyone be a congruent leader? The study results indicate that clinical leaders who display congruent leadership attributes can be found in large numbers right across the health service. What do you think? Are you a clinical leader? And if so, does the theory of congruent leadership resonate with you?

The Limitations of Congruent Leadership

There are limitations to congruent leadership theory, to which the discussion now turns.

New Theory

Congruent leadership is a new theory that was confirmed as a valid theory to support clinical leadership (Stanley 2019). The research undertaken to support the concept is valid and now extensive and made explicit in this chapter. I have exposed the theory to a large number of qualified health professionals at conferences and in leadership courses, in different countries and contexts. The resounding conclusion is that it resonates with their experience of leading in practice and fits with and supports their understanding of clinical leadership.

Similar to Other Values-Based Leadership Theories

Authentic leadership, breakthrough leadership, servant, compassionate leadership and congruent leadership all focus on values as the driving force for which the leader is recognised. Nevertheless, similar is not the same, and it may be because congruent leadership has grown from a health professional focus that it rests on a firmer base to help support an understanding of clinical leadership.

Not Driven by a Focus on Change

Significantly from a health service perspective, congruent leadership is not obvious in its focus on the promotion of leaders who are directed to change practice and lead change (Stanley 2019). This does not mean that congruent leaders do not engage in innovation and change, just that they are not driven by this focus. It is noted that health reform across the globe is focused on better leadership for the improvement of patient care and leadership that can support and help promote change and stimulate innovation. The NHS Leadership Centre was specifically directed at promoting leadership that focused very firmly on 'change' rather than values-based leadership (NHS Leadership Centre 2002), and the development of clinical leaders who can influence people and lead change is a significant focus of much of nurse education and health service training.

However, as congruent leadership is focused on translating values and meaning into action, it can be assumed with confidence that many of the leaders' actions will result in change and innovation, as clinical leaders seek to influence and improve the quality of care provision. I acknowledge that organisations specifically seeking to promote leaders who drive and foster change may find congruent leadership too obscure for their purposes. I would assert, though, that focusing on people's values and beliefs and clarifying these remains a crucial first step in any change process.

Not Suitable for Leaders with 'Control' as an Objective

Leaders who are required to exercise control over others (managers), or who are not visible or engaged in the process of doing the 'work' of the people or groups they lead, will struggle to employ a congruent leadership approach. Congruent leaders do not talk through their values or beliefs or order others to adopt them, they display them. They stand by them and make them evident to others, sometimes unconsciously. If clinical leaders are in a position where they are unable to engage in the 'work' of their colleagues, or if they are required to exercise control over (manage) their colleagues – or those they lead – congruent leadership may not be evident and will be of limited value. I would argue these same challenges are faced by those trying to institute compassionate leadership. In the research results, 'controlling' was specifically seen as a characteristic not associated with clinical leadership and, as such, a leader functioning in a position of control, if it results in a clash of values, will find the application of congruent leadership difficult or inappropriate (Stanley 2019).

Congruent Leadership, Change and Innovation

Mahatma Gandhi, the Hindu religious and political leader and social reformer, once said, 'We must be the change we wish to see in the world'. In many ways this sits at the core of what congruent leadership means. In the study used to expose congruent leadership, no assumptions were made about who the clinical leaders were or what their characteristics might be. Instead, these matters were rigorously explored.

As indicated in the Gallup Report (2010) on nursing leadership, clinical leaders make a significant contribution to the quality of patient care. This is confirmed by Stanton et al. (2010), who add that the clinical leader's time has come (although they imagined the clinical leader was a doctor). This is driven by a need to engage clinicians in policy developments, as the emphasis on quality increases, as the need for front-line clinical staff to engage in change and innovation grows and, finally, as clinicians are recognising themselves as stakeholders in the health industry. However, clinical leaders can do so much more if they are recognised (by themselves and others) as leaders and encouraged to see that leadership does indeed exist at many levels. If clinical leaders are shown to display congruent leadership, their passion is for participation in hands-on patient care and they are driven to improve and deliver a high-quality service, then the pool from which nursing and the health service can draw future leaders is greatly enhanced.

As well as allowing others to see these aspects, they need to recognise them themselves. If change and innovation are to be supported and promoted from the clinical environment, it will be the nurse or health professional who intervenes, who takes action, or who responds to challenges because they stand by what they believe, who will make a significant contribution. Indeed, they are as valuable, as important and as effective as the leader with a grand plan.

Recognising the significance of values and beliefs and their impact on actions is vital, but in terms of influencing innovation and change it is also essential that clinically focused health professional leaders understand the tools that can be used to facilitate change. Nurses and other health professionals in countries all over the world can be heard sitting in tearooms or at the lunch table discussing what is wrong with the health service, or how 'the recent changes in care delivery will have this or that impact' and 'if only they could do this or the other' or 'if only someone would listen to my view'. Complaining, suggesting, theorising and proposing – these ideas and opinions often go no further than the tearoom or lunch table.

It could be that whining is the natural state of the hard-pressed health professional, but I don't believe it. Sometimes change or innovation is slow or resisted because health professionals have not learnt to listen to their 'true' or inner voice (Buresh and Gordon 2013) or simply because they have not learnt the skills associated with effectively managing or driving change and innovation or the liberation of empowerment. The ideas and suggestions are there – just listen in to any tearoom or lunch table conversation. It may also be that health professionals are not clear about what leadership means, who leaders can be, or who are recognised as leaders in clinical practice.

While managers might have the authority to support change, they may not have the practice focus or clinical insights to see what change is needed in practice (Stanley 2006d). Thus, it is clinically focused health professional leaders who are in an ideal position to see the change that is needed, and the value and impact that change and innovation can have for patient or client care. However, they may feel that they lack the authority to take their ideas and suggestions further.

Change and innovation can be affected by the congruent leader, but first the clinically focused health professional leader needs to understand the significance of their own values and beliefs. Second, they need to recognise that they have followers, because these followers have realised the match between the clinically focused leader's values and beliefs and their actions. People look to clinically focused health professional leaders for leadership even if the leader is not aware of it. The third point is that change can occur even without power or formal authority. Therefore, clinically focused health professional leaders need to understand that, used effectively, reflection and change management techniques, creativity, evidence-based approaches, networks and delegation can be powerful tools to support, motivate and inspire others and to minimise conflict.

Congruent leaders in clinically focused positions can exercise considerable influence over clinical change and support substantial innovation, if they only recognise that leadership is not tied to positions of power, titles, badges, big offices and authority. Leaders in clinically focused practice-related positions do not need to have the 'big picture' or exercise 'vision', or be in powerful and authoritarian positions, or hold budgetary control. Clinically focused leaders are the front-line, coalface, roadside, bedside decision-makers (Stanton et al. 2010; Stanley 2019) and when they employ (or can learn to employ) collaborative strategies to limit conflict, develop the motivation and influence of others and implement change management techniques, they can be the force that will help deliver high-quality, more effective care and shape a better tomorrow for the health service.

Congruent Leadership and Power

Congruent leadership is not power neutral. The power of congruent leadership comes from unifying groups and individuals around common values and beliefs. This is not a strategy as such, but the results from my research demonstrate that nurses and other health professionals seek out or follow leaders who are more inclined to display or hold values and beliefs that they themselves hold. Manley found that when she displayed her values and beliefs, others began to share them and the clinical area united as colleagues began to identify with the common purpose of 'providing patient-centred care' (Manley 2000b, p. 38). One of the statements made by a participant in Manley's research supports this by saying, 'sometimes I feel like an evangelist trying to spread [the] word to other people in other areas' (2000b, p. 37). A clinically focused leader, operating within the core professional principles, or by a set of standards or guiding principles of a professional body or registration authority – for instance, the Australian Nursing and Midwifery Council's (2016a) Code of Professional Conduct or (2016b) Registered Nurse Standards of Practice – is more likely to be recognised for their consideration of patients' rights and needs and their caring attitude than a nurse or health professional who functions outside of these guiding principles or who is not engaged in direct patient care. Therefore, a nurse or health professional seeking to lead in the clinical environment will find greater success if their values and beliefs are consistent with the dominant values and beliefs of their colleagues, or if they are able to bring their colleagues to a point where their values and beliefs about care, therapy and professional behaviour coincide. Conflict (Stanley 2006c; Gentile 2010) can result if the principles and values of one group or individual are at odds with others, and power and influence in terms of leading often fall to the dominant group or leader.

A congruent leader's power and influence derive from being able to articulate and display their values, beliefs and principles, as the examples in Box 3.6 and Manley's (2000a, b) research was able to illustrate. Followers recognised or aligned themselves with these same values or beliefs and, by supporting and promoting them, increased the leader's credibility and worth. By promoting the significance of this leader's values and beliefs over any others, the leader would be able to influence or change practice or generate innovation. Change, while often not the intention (although it was for Manley), results when values and beliefs are displayed, promoted and then adopted by followers.

Berwick (1994), a US medical practitioner, and Schneider (1999), writing from a pharmacological viewpoint, indicate that clinical expertise sits at the core of clinical leadership potential. Although being clinically competent and knowledgeable are included in the characteristics identified in my studies, being a 'clinical expert' was not a central characteristic of clinical leadership (Stanley 2019). This may add support to the argument that clinically focused leaders employ congruent leadership that is based on their values and beliefs rather than on their clinical skills, clinical knowledge and technical abilities. Pendleton and King feel that medical practice and healthcare are suffused with values, although they tend to be expressed as standards. Both are similar, they say, and both act as guiding principles, although 'values state what is important . . . and tend not to vary', while 'standards state what is good or acceptable . . . and may well vary' (2002, p. 1353).

In the business world too, O'Reilly and Pfeffer (2000) and Gentile (2010) see values as crucial. In comparing the performance of a number of companies with superior results in their area of specialism, the more successful companies had an approach to leadership that was based on values. Values came first and acted as guiding principles that helped these companies to make crucial and difficult decisions. O'Reilly and Pfeffer (2000) also noted that the values these successful companies held were not prioritised as such, but that the companies operated in such a way as to aim to function so that their values were shown, and they worked hard to resolve clashes of values. Focusing on values meant that the businesses were able to build trust, motivation and commitment (O'Reilly and Pfeffer 2000). Hall (2005) supports this view, suggesting that companies who addressed and followed sound ethical practices were much more likely to be profitable and successful, by a considerable margin. Kouzes and Posner (2010) offered similar research where they demonstrated that employees who were clear about the organisation's values and also had a high degree of clarity about their own personal values had a greater commitment to the organisation. Significantly, it was a correlation between a person's personal values and their match to the organisation's values that drew the strongest commitment. Their conclusion was that people cannot commit fully to anything unless it fits with their own beliefs or values (Kouzes and Posner 2010). This is a powerful concept for the health service to grasp, as many health professionals enter their profession because they value 'making a difference' (Stanley et al. 2014a) or want to work with people and help make a difference for people.

Successful clinically focused leadership is therefore proposed to rest on a model of congruent leadership that, as with the business view of O'Reilly and Pfeffer (2000), Kouzes and Posner (2010), Gentile (2010) and Hall (2005) and the healthcare view of Pendleton and King (2002), is based on leaders who respond to challenges and critical problems with actions and activities in accordance with (congruent with) their values and beliefs.

Clinical Leader Stories 3:   A Ward Leader

Leadership is required to give direction and align interprofessional teams within primary healthcare areas to deliver effective healthcare. Congruent leadership is a leadership theory directly linked to the clinical domain. In a recent placement experience, I was buddied with a nurse who showed excellent leadership skills and attributes which helped to deliver effective care to all patients as well as making the working environment inviting and positive. Her leadership aligned with congruent leadership theory, where her passion for patient care drove her leadership. Anyone can become a leader, and I feel leadership involves taking responsibility for management activities, being a role model to more inexperienced healthcare professionals and ensuring best practice is implemented. The role also involves working in collaboration with and on behalf of other clinicians to improve the healthcare system.

Clinical leadership is a very important aspect in healthcare. Along with ensuring that the workplace runs smoothly, clinical leadership is essential in implementing best practice for the care of patients, leading to improved patient outcomes. With regards to this, safety and quality of healthcare are also increased due to the tasks and procedures involved in clinical leadership. This is because leadership ensures all patients are adequately cared for by ensuring that the qualification or skill set of nursing staff match the requirements of the shift.

Along with this, clinical leadership leads to an increase in patient satisfaction, decrease in patient mortality, fewer medication errors and fewer hospital-acquired infections. During a recent placement, I was fortunate enough to be buddied with a senior RN who demonstrated excellent clinical leadership on the ward. Each day, this nurse would spend time to create a shift planner for the shift, with all the tasks that needed to be completed. Once completed, she would talk to myself and others and delegate tasks that were to be completed. She also took time out of her busy schedule to walk through clinical procedures that I was not confident in; she explained the theory behind the procedures and allowed me to be part of the practical component. Her perseverance allowed me to gain confidence in completing the skills. This was very beneficial in my nursing practice as theoretical knowledge is best learnt through practice rather than observing the skill. This RN also became the voice for all the nurses during the handover safety talk regarding an issue that a variety of nurses had identified and were seeking to change. The outcome was positive.

(Continued)

During this placement, I learned the importance of leadership and how to become an effective leader. The passion, support and care my buddy nurse demonstrated through-out her leadership role on placement allowed me to understand these concepts which I will endeavour to achieve throughout my career as a nurse. I have also learnt how to become an effective leader for future students that I may be placed with, including allowing them to get as many hands-on experiences as possible, rather than just observing to further develop their understanding and confidence. Continuing to develop positive leadership attributes will allow me to be involved in improving the quality and sustainability of healthcare systems for the future and encourage further leadership opportunities for new nurses. Clinical leadership is an important aspect for the operation of every ward. During placement, I was fortunate enough to be buddied with a nurse who showed excellent clinical leadership.

Annalise: Student Nurse.

Congruent Leadership and Quality

Clinical leaders are able to make a significant contribution to the quality of patient care and initiate innovation and quality in front-line clinical services (see Chapter 16). This can be enhanced if clinical leaders are encouraged to recognise that leadership occurs and needs to be evident at many levels in an organisation (Stanley 2019).

If health professionals focus on the values that are central to their professions' core and on patient-centred care, they will also be drawn towards focusing on improving patient outcomes, client care, therapeutic improvements and quality processes. It is clear that safety and quality issues are paramount to governments, public policy and decision makers at health department and senior health organisation levels, to the media and, most impor-tantly, to consumers of healthcare (Francis 2013). It is proposed here that the key to having the most effective impact on safety and quality processes is to focus on the development of leadership skills at all levels, but specifically on clinically focused leaders who function at the 'coalface' in the clinical area and in close proximity to clients and patients (Mahoney 2001; Rich 2008; Murphy et al. 2009).

It is clinically focused leaders who operate in daily contact with clients and patients, and who are more likely to recognise and be able to respond to deficits in patient care or lapses in quality. If healthcare organisations and institutions are to deliver safe, high-quality healthcare to patients, clients or consumers, then governance systems and processes need to be robust and operate throughout the organisation. For this to be the case, communica-tion systems and leadership systems need to be likewise robust and acknowledge the criti-cal place that clinically focused health professionals play in implementing quality processes or reporting faults in those processes.

The Australian Victorian Quality Council (2005) has also suggested that clinically focused leaders play a significant role in quality processes by participating in establishing strategic safety objectives and in setting, and taking responsibility for implementing, the safety agenda. They also suggest that clinical leaders should foster the allocation of resources to support best practice; that they should act as 'champions' for service improve-ment; and that they should raise the status of safety and quality activities, contribute to clinical practice improvement initiatives and educate their fellow clinicians. Mahoney (2001) and Rich (2008) support these suggestions and add that clinically focused health professional leaders should act as role models for quality, provide expert evidence-based care, collaborate with others to facilitate best practice, take responsibility for quality initiatives and advocate for changes that will benefit clients and patients. If these aspirations are central to how clinical leaders practise, then congruent leadership will be evident.

Cook (2001), Baker et al. (2004), Sirola-Karvinen and Hyrkas (2006), Alleyne and Jumaa (2007), Wong and Cummings (2007) and Murphy et al. (2009) all agree with the proposition that clinically focused leaders are recognised as vital for the provision of good patient care, the promotion of creative and productive work environments and the development of excellent nursing practice. Murphy et al. (2009) also suggest that clinical leadership offers a cost-effective way of improving patient care outcomes in times of financial contraction.

The characteristics identified as being consistent with congruent health professional leaders (clinically competent, clinically knowledgeable, effective communicators, decision makers, empowered motivators, open and approachable, role models and visible in practice) underpin the role that clinically focused leaders can play in promoting quality improvement initiatives and the implementation of evidence-based practice. Indeed, it is arguable that it is because clinically focused leaders are driven by their values and beliefs that these leaders, displaying congruent leadership, are ideally placed to have positive impacts on safety and quality processes.

Debate and further research may be needed to establish or even rediscover what the core values of the nursing profession or other health professions may be (examples are given in Box 3.7). However, the Gallup Report (2010) on nursing leadership suggests that the US public rated nurses as having the highest standards of honesty and ethical practice (at 83%) of any professional group.

Understanding professional values may not be as simple as proposing a list of characteristics or attributes. The Australian Nursing and Midwifery Council's (2018) Code of Professional Conduct and National Competency Standards (2016) offer further insights into what are thought to be minimum standards (a type of expression of professional values) for nursing professionals. These offer significantly more detail about the issues of both values and ethically based professional practice and behaviour.

Box 3.7   Top 10 Health Professional Values

Honesty/truthfulness/fairness	Clear interpersonal skills/listening skills
Integrity	Organised
Trustworthiness	Professionalism
Compassion/care	Clinical knowledge
Respect	*Others mentioned, but not as constantly cited, are*
Reliability	*Creativity, Self-Control and Humility*

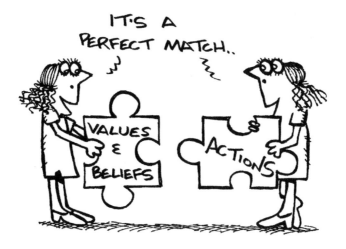

To conclude, clinical nurse leadership is commonly demonstrated in the ward or unit by a clinical leader who is directly involved in providing healthcare. Clinical leaders are visible to their colleagues and considered to be knowledgeable, competent clinicians (although not necessarily experts), who motivate and inspire others because their values, beliefs and guiding principles are on show and are recognised as such. These principles and values motivate and guide the clinical leader to act in ways that support patients' rights and address issues of confidentiality, dignity, privacy and advocacy. When they deal with critical problems, face challenges and direct or provide care, it is the clinical leader's employment of a congruent leadership approach, based on values, beliefs and principles, that is evident. Leaders who 'control' and manage from within offices, or who fail to display values and beliefs in congruence with their actions, are rarely seen as clinical leaders.

Case Study 3.1   Mary Seacole's: 'Mother Seacole'

Mary Seacole's story is offered as an example of how a clinically focused health professional was able to exercise power, bring about change and innovation and have an impact on quality healthcare in the nineteenth century. If Mary could do it, then how much more likely are congruent leaders now to be able to support health professional innovation and change? Read the outline of Mary's achievements and consider the challenge that follows.

Mary Seacole was born Mary Jane Grant in Kingston, Jamaica in 1805. She had a mixed-race (free Creole) mother and a Scottish-born officer for a father. Her mother ran a boarding house for sick and injured soldiers and sailors and it was here that Mary began to learn her nursing skills. Mary's mother was a noted 'doctress' who used traditional Caribbean and African herbal remedies to heal and tend the sick in her care. As a Creole, Mary saw herself as lucky, almost privileged, compared to the fortunes of the slave community that dominated the island.

Mary was educated and supported by an elderly woman whom she referred to as 'her kind patroness'. In 1821 she travelled to London for the first time. In this era about a

---

(Continued)

Case Study 3.1 (Continued)

third of all Britain's trade was with Caribbean islands and travel across the Atlantic was relatively common. When Mary returned to Jamaica she nursed her 'old indulgent patroness' before returning to their family home. Mary continued to learn much from her mother and also travelled about the Caribbean and parts of Central America, where she ran a series of taverns and boarding houses, all the while learning more about medicine and caring for ill people.

In 1836 she married Edwin Horatio Hamilton Seacole (rumoured to be an illegitimate son of Horatio Nelson and Emma, Lady Hamilton), but he died in 1844 after a series of financial and domestic disasters overcame them. Following a time of deep grief, Mary turned a 'bold front to fortune' and assumed the management of her mother's hotel. She threw herself into her work, declining many offers of marriage. In 1850 she treated patients suffering from a cholera epidemic that killed an estimated 32 000 Jamaicans. With great insight into the transmission of disease, she recognised that the outbreak of the epidemic was likely to be attributed to a steamship that had arrived from New Orleans, Louisiana. Her experience in dealing with cholera was to prove vital later in her life.

In 1851 she travelled to visit her half-brother in Panama, Central America and arrived in time to treat the first victim of a cholera outbreak there. The patient survived and Mary's reputation as a healer was cemented. Other patients came to her for care and while the rich paid, she treated the poor for free. Mary remained in Panama for a time, becoming ill herself, but she made a speedy recovery and went on to open a hotel and tavern and continued to care for the ill and injured. In 1853 she returned to Jamaica and was immediately recruited by medical authorities to help deal with an outbreak of yellow fever. Mary's response was to recruit a number of other Afro-Caribbean woman and to set up a hospital outside Kingston where they cared for victims of the disease. After the outbreak subsided, Mary travelled back to Panama to finalise her business dealings and it was here that she learnt about the escalating conflict in the Crimea. She decided to volunteer and set off to enlist as a nurse in London.

Mary travelled with letters of recommendation from various doctors in Jamaica and Panama, but she was unable to convince the British medical or military authorities to use her. Even though the Nightingale nurses who travelled to the Crimean were understaffed, due to her skin colour Mary was refused an interview and the opportunity to go with the Nightingale nurses. Not put off, Mary applied to the publicly subscribed Crimean Fund to travel independently but was again refused. Once more undaunted, she raised her own funds with the help of a doctor from Panama and set off for the Crimea on a Dutch ship, the SS *Hollander*.

On the way she stopped at Malta, and a doctor returning from the Crimea wrote a letter of recommendation and introduction to Florence Nightingale for Mary to use on her arrival. In Constantinople, Mary arranged to travel to Scutari and meet with Florence, but she was again rejected.

Having come this far, Mary transferred her supplies to another ship and set off for the seat of the fighting on the Crimean Peninsula, arriving at Balaclava early in 1855. Here

(Continued)

she built a 'hotel' at a place she called Spring Hill. The 'hotel' was built from driftwood, packing cases, iron sheets and house parts scavenged from the nearby town of Kamara. She used local labour and opened the newly christened 'British Hotel' in March 1855. The 'hospital' provided provisions and food for French and British soldiers. It was little more than a collection of huts, one of which served as a small hospital ward. Mary provided tea and coffee and dealt with common medical complaints in the mornings and then set off to visit casualties around the battle area in the afternoons.

Florence Nightingale made a number of references to Mary Seacole in various correspondence, referring to her as 'a woman of bad character' whom she accused of running a 'bad house' or brothel. Yet there is no evidence to support this and Nightingale is also recorded as saying that Mary Seacole 'had done a great deal of good for the poor soldiers'. Mary made a point of visiting the battlefields and treating wounded and ill men, often under fire. A *Times* newspaper special correspondent said of Mary that she was a 'warm and successful physician, who doctors and cures all manner of men with extraordinary success. She is always in attendance near the battlefield to aid the wounded and has earned many a poor fellow's blessing'. A soldier said of her, 'she had the secret of a recipe for cholera and dysentery, and liberally dispensed the specific, alike to those who could pay and those who could not. It was bestowed with an amount of personal kindness which, though not an item of the original prescription, she deemed essential to the cure'.

So closely involved in the front-line care of soldiers was Seacole that she was the first woman into Sevastopol after the siege was lifted. The war's conclusion brought ruin, though, as the trade at the British Hotel diminished and she returned to England poorer than she had left. Soon she was declared bankrupt and a fund was set up (the Seacole Testimonial Fund) to offer support. In July 1857 the Seacole Fund Grand Military Festival was held to contribute to her Testimonial Fund. The event was supported by many military men and over 1000 artists performed, including 11 military bands, and the attendance was over 40 000. Mary also produced an autobiography, *The Wonderful Adventures of Mrs. Seacole in Many Lands*, the first book written by a black woman in Britain. Gradually she regained her financial footing and when she died in 1881, in London, she was financially independent again.

Her many achievements in the Crimean War were somewhat overshadowed by Florence Nightingale's fame and while well known in her lifetime, Mary has since faded from the pages of history. She remains well known in the Caribbean and there has been a resurgence of interest in her contribution to nursing in recent years. In 2004, Mary Seacole was voted into first place in an online poll of 100 Great Black Britons, and her contribution to nursing and medical care in Central America, the Caribbean and the Crimea solidifies her place as a supreme clinically focused and congruent leader. In 2016 a statue of Mary was unveiled opposite St Thomas's Hospital in London.

Challenge: Mary lived an extraordinary life, yet it was based on simple principles. Like any other congruent leader, when she was needed she stood tall. Her contribution to the health and welfare of the French and British fighting men in the Crimea was no less personal, and often more so, than the care offered by Florence Nightingale, yet like

(Continued)

Case Study 3.1   (Continued)

so many people in the health service it has gone unnoticed and unrecognised in the shadow of other forces and issues. Think about what you have achieved in the past week or month. How many lives have you touched in the course of your work? These achievements may not have got into the papers or been seen on the evening news, but they matter very much to the people whose lives you have touched. Reflect on when you have stood tall, stood out or advocated for the people in your care. How have your actions affected the personal life or influenced the history of a patient, client or their family? What might have occurred if you had not spoken up or acted on their behalf? When were you last a congruent leader?

Summary

- Congruent Leadership developed from the results of research specifically exploring healthcare-related clinical leadership.
- Congruent Leadership is based on a number of research studies undertaken within a range of different health professional disciplines, using a range of methodologies, in different countries, with different genders and over a wide span of years.
- Congruent leaders match their values and beliefs to their actions.
- Congruent leaders are not consciously selling a vision or communicating a path for others to follow. Instead, they are recognised because they are living their values and walking their path with conviction, commitment and determination.
- Congruent leadership is proposed as a framework to support an understanding of clinically focused leadership.
- A new hypothesis is offered that suggests that clinical leaders may be more appropriately seen and recognised by the match between their values and beliefs and their actions.
- Congruent leadership offers a solid foundation on which clinical professionals can develop and gain leadership potential.
- Congruent leadership is not power neutral. The power of congruent leadership comes from unifying groups and individuals around common values and beliefs.
- If health professionals focus on the values that are central to their professions' core, they will also be drawn towards focusing on improving patient outcomes, client care and quality processes.
- The strengths of congruent leadership are that it supports a focus on grassroots leadership, it offers a foundation on which other theories can be built, it builds a strong link between values and beliefs and it supports the advancement of the clinical leader's place in health service development.
- The limitations of congruent leadership are that it is a new theory, that it is similar to other value-based leadership theories, that it is not suitable for leaders where 'controlling' is a key function of their role and that it does not have 'change' as its primary focus.
- Congruent leaders are focused on quality, innovation and change by acting out their values and beliefs.

- Clinical leaders are found in great numbers and across the spectrum of the health service.
- Clinical leaders are practitioners who have gone to the edge and flown, stepped boldly in the direction of their values and beliefs or confidently stood by them and demonstrate congruent leadership.

Mind Press-Ups

Exercise 3.1

Think about your personal values and take some time to make a list them. Are the things you listed similar to the values offered in Box 3.7?

Exercise 3.2

Discuss your values list with a professional colleague. Find out if they have similar values, what their values are or how they might express them.

Exercise 3.3

Congruent leadership describes a leader who is recognised because their actions match their values and beliefs. Can you think of healthcare practitioners whom you would identify as congruent leaders?

References

Ahn, M.J., Ettner, L.W., and Loupin, A. (2011). From classical to contemporary leadership chalelenges: a values-based leadership view. *Journal of Leadership Studies* 5 (1): 6–22.

Alilyyani, B., Wong, C.A., and Cummings, G. (2018). Antecedents, mediators, and outcomes of authentic leadership in healthcare: a systematic review. *International Journal of Nursing Studies* 83: 34–64.

Alleyne, J. and Jumaa, M.O. (2007). Building the capacity for evidence based clinical nursing leadership: the role of executive co-coaching and group clinical supervision for quality patient services. *Journal of Nursing Management* 15 (2): 230–243.

American Association of Colleges of Nursing (2016) *Media Relations, Nursing Fact Sheet*, http://www.aacn.nche.edu/media-relations/fact-sheets/nursing-fact-sheet (accessed 11 January 2016).

Anderson, R.J. (2003). Building hospital–physician relationships through servant leadership. *Frontiers of Health Services Management* 20 (2): 43.

Antrobus, S. and Kitson, A. (1999). Nursing leadership: influencing and shaping health policy and nursing practice. *Journal of Advanced Nursing* 29 (3): 746–753.

Australian Institute of Health and Welfare (2014) *Australia's Health 2014, Australia's Health System*, http://www.aihw.gov.au/australias-health/2014/health-system (accessed 11 January 2016).

Australian Nursing and Midwifery Council (2016a). *National Competency Standards for Nurse Practitioners*. Canberra: Australian Nursing and Midwifery Council.

Australian Nursing and Midwifery Council (2016b). *Code of Professional Conduct*. Canberra: Australian Nursing and Midwifery Council.

Avolio, B.J. and Gardner, W.L. (2005). Authentic leadership development: getting to the root of positive forms of leadership. *The Leadership Quarterly* 16: 315–338.

Avolio, B.J., Gardner, W.L., Walumbwa, F.O. et al. (2004). Unlocking the mask: a look at the process by which authentic leaders impact follower attitudes and behaviors. *The Leadership Quarterly* 15 (6): 801–823.

Baker, G.R., Norton, P.G., and Flintoff, V. (2004). The Canadian adverse events study: the incidence of adverse events among hospital patients in Canada. *Canadian Medical Association* 17 (10): 1678–1686.

Baloglu, N. (2012). Relations between value-based leadership and distributed leadership: a casual research on school principle behaviours. *Educational Sciences Theory & Practice* 12 (2): 1375–1378.

Bass, B. and Avolio, B. (1993). *Multifactor Leadership Questionnaire*. Palo Alto, CA: Consulting Psychologists Press.

Bass, B. and Steidlmeier, P. (1999). Ethics, character, and transformational leadership behavior. *The Leadership Quarterly* 10 (2): 81–217.

Berwick, D. (1994). Eleven worthy aims for clinical leadership of health care reform. *JAMA* 272 (10): 797.

Bhindi, N. and Duignan, P. (1997). Leadership for a new century: authenticity, intentionality, spirituality and sensibility. *Educational Management and Administration* 25 (4): 117–132.

Bostridge, M. (2004) 'The ladies with the lamps', *BBC History*, Oct., pp. 18–19.

Bostridge, M. (2008). *Florence Nightingale: The Woman and Her Legend*. London: Penguin/Viking.

Brown, M. and Treviño, L. (2006). Ethical leadership: a review and future directions. *The Leadership Quarterly* 17 (3): 595–616.

Buresh, B. and Gordon, S. (2013). *From Silence to Voice: What Nurses Know and Must Communicate to the Public*, 3e. Ithaca, NY: IRL Press.

Cairns-Lee, H. (2015). Images of leadership development from the inside out. *Advances in Developing Human Resources* 17 (3): 1–16.

Campbell, P.T. and Rudisill, P.T. (2005). Servant leadership: a critical component for nurse leaders. *Nurse Leader* 3 (3): 27–29.

Cantwell, J. (2015). *Leadership in Action*. Carlton, VA: Melbourne University Press.

Casida, J. and Parker, J. (2011). Staff nurse perceptions of nurse manager leadership styles and outcomes. *Journal of Nursing Management* 19: 478–486.

Cook, M.J. (2001). The renaissance of clinical leadership. *International Nursing Review* 48 (1): 38–46.

Copeland, M.K. (2014). The emerging significance of values-based leadership: a literature review. Business faculty publications, St. John Fisher College. Fisher Digital Publications. *International Journal of Leadership Studies* 8 (2): 105–135.

Coventry, T.H. and Russell, K.P. (2021). The clinical nurse educator as a congruent leader: a mixed method study. *Journal of Nursing Education and Practice* 11 (1): 8–18.

Curtis, E.A., de Vries, J., and Sheerin, F.K. (2011). Developing leadership in nursing: exploring core factors. *British Journal of Nursing* 20 (5): 306–309.

Davies, C. (1995). *Gender and the Professional Predicament in Nursing*. Buckingham: Open University Press.

Department of Health (1999). *Making a Difference*. London: HM Stationery Office.

Department of Health (2015a). *Changing the NHS for the Better*. London: HM Stationery Office.

Department of Health (2015b). *Culture Change in the NHS: Applying the Lessons of the Francis Inquiries*. London: HM Stationery Office.

Department of Health Western Australia (2015) *Strategic Intent 2015–2020*, Perth: Department of Health, http://www.health.wa.gov.au/HRIT/docs/publications/WA_Health_Strategic_Intent_2015-2020.pdf (accessed 1 May 2016).

Eicher-Catt, D. (2005). The myth of servant leadership: a feminist perspective. *Women and Language* 28 (1): 17–26.

Ellis, P. (2019). What it means to be a servant leader. *Wounds UK* 15 (5): 76–77.

Faith, K.E. (2013). The role of values-based leadership in sustaining a culture of caring. *Healthcare Management Forum* 26: 6–10.

Francis, R. (2013). *Report of the Mid Staffordshire NHS Foundation Trust Public Inquiry*. London HM: Stationery Office.

Freshwater, D. (ed.) (2002). *Therapeutic Nursing*, 120–141. London: Sage.

Freshwater, D., Graham, I., and Esterhuizen, P. (2009). Educating leaders for global health care. In: *Leadership for Nursing and Allied Health Care Professions* (ed. V. Bishop). Maidenhead: Open University Press/McGraw-Hill Education.

Gallup Report (2010). *Nursing Leadership from Bedside to Boardroom: Opinion Leaders' Perceptions*. Princeton, NJ: Robert Wood Johnson Foundation.

Garber, J.S., Madigan, E.A., and Fitzpatrick, J.J. (2009). Attitudes towards collaboration and servant leadership among nurses, physicians and residents. *Journal of Interprofessional Care* 23 (4): 331–340.

Gardner, W. and Avolio, B. (ed.) (2005). Authentic leadership theory and practice: origins, effects and development: vol. 3. In: *Monographs in Leadership and Management*. New York: Elsevier Science.

Gentile, M.C. (2010). *Giving Voice to Values: How to Speak Your Mind When You Know What's Right*. New Haven, CT: Yale University Press.

George, B. (2003). *Authentic Leadership: Rediscovering the Secrets to Creating Lasting Value*. San Francisco, CA: Jossey-Bass.

Goertz Koerner, J. (2010). Reflections on transformational leadership. *Journal of Holistic Nursing* 28 (1): 68.

Graber, D.R. and Kilpatrick, A.O. (2008). Establishing values-based leadership and values systems in healthcare organizations. *Journal of Health & Human Services Administration* 31 (2): 179–197.

Greenleaf, R.K. (1970). *The Servant as Leader*. South Orange, NJ: Greenleaf Publishing Center.

Greenleaf, R.K. (1977). *Servant Leadership: A Journey into the Nature of Legitimate Power and Greatness*. Mahwah, NJ: Paulist Press.

Greenleaf, R.K. (1998). *The Power of Servant Leadership*. San Francisco, CA: Berrett-Koehler Publishers.

Grosios, K., Gahan, P.B., and Burbridge, J. (2010). Overview of healthcare in the UK. *EPMA Journal* 1 (4): 529–534.

Gunnarsdóttir, S. (2014). Is servant leadership useful for sustainable Nordic health care? *Nordic Journal of Nursing Research and Clinical Studies* 34 (2): 53–55.

Hall, M.L. (2005). Shaping organisational culture: a practitioner's perspective. *Peak Development Consulting* 11 (1): 1–16.

Hanse, J.J., Harlin, U., Jarebrant, C. et al. (2016). The impact of servant leadership dimensions on leader-member exchange among health care professionals. *Journal of Nursing Management* 24 (2): 228–234.

Hougaard, R., Carter, J. & Hobson, N. (2020) Compassionate Leadership is necessary – but not sufficient. https://hbr.org/2020/12/compassionate-leadership-is-necessary-but-not-sufficient

Hutchinson, M. and Jackson, D. (2012). Transformational leadership in nursing: towards a more critical interpretation. *Nursing Inquiry* 20 (1): 11–22.

Jackson, D. (2008). Servant leadership in nursing: a framework for developing sustainable research capacity. *Collegian* 15: 27–33.

James, A.H., Bennett, C.L., Blanchard, D., and Stanley, D. (2021). Nursing and values-based leadership: a literature review. *Journal of Nurse Management* 29 (5): 916–930.

Jones, L. and Bennett, C.L. (2018). *Leadership in Health and Social Care: An Introduction for Emerging Leaders*, 2e. Banbury: Lantern.

Jooste, K. and Jordaan, E. (2012). Student nurse's perceptions of the nurse manager as a servant leader. *Africa Journal of Nursing and Midwifery* 14 (1): 76–88.

Kerfoot, K. (2004). The shelf life of leaders. *Medical Surgical Nursing* 13 (5): 348–351.

Kotter, J.P. (1990). What leaders really do. In: *Harvard Business Review on Leadership*, 37–60. Boston, MA: Harvard Business School Press.

Kouzes, J.M. and Posner, B.Z. (2010). *The Truth about Leadership: The No-Fads, Heart of the Matter Facts You Need to Know*. San Francisco, CA: Jossey-Bass.

Lee, H.-F., Chiang, H.-Y., and Kuo, H.-T. (2019). Relationship between authentic leadership and nurse's intent to leave: the mediating role of work environment and burnout. *Journal of Nursing Management* 27 (1): 52–65.

Mahon, K. (2011). In praise of servant leadership – horizontal service to others. *Dynamics (Pembroke, Ont.)* 22 (4): 5–6.

Mahoney, J. (2001). Leadership skills for the 21st century. *Journal of Nursing Management* 9: 269–271.

Man, J. (2010). *The Leadership Secrets of Genghis Khan*. London: Bantam Books.

Manley, K. (2000a). Organisational culture and consultant nurse outcomes. Part 1: Organisational culture. *Nursing Standard* 14 (36): 34–38.

Manley, K. (2000b). Organisational culture and consultant nurse outcomes. Part 2: Nurse outcomes. *Nursing Standard* 14 (37): 34–39.

Marriner-Tomey, A. (2009). *Guide to Nursing Management and Leadership*, 8e. St Louis, MO: Mosby Elsevier.

Marshall, E. (2011). *Leadership in Nursing: From Expert Clinician to Influential Leader*. New York: Springer.

McAllister, M. and Brien, D.L. (2020). *Paradoxes in Nurses' Identity, Culture, and Image.* in The Shadow Side of Nursing, New York: Routledge.

Mostafa, A.M.S. and El-Motalib, E.A.A. (2019). Servant leadership, leader–member exchange and proactive behavior in the public health sector. *Public Personnel Management* 48 (3): 309–324.

Murphy, J., Quillinan, B., and Carolan, M. (2009). Role of clinical leadership in improving patient care. *Nursing Management* 16 (8): 26–29.

National Health Service Leadership Academy (2013). *Healthcare Leadership Model: The Nine Dimensions of Leadership Behaviour.* Leeds: NHS Leadership Academy.

National Health Service Leadership Centre (2002). *NHS Leadership Qualities Framework.* London: NHS Leadership Centre.

Neill, M.W. and Saunders, N.S. (2008). Servant leadership. Enhancing quality of care and staff satisfaction. *Journal of Nursing Administration* 38 (9): 395–400.

Oliver, D. (2015) 'Allied health professionals are critical to new models', King's Fund blog, http://www.kingsfund.org.uk/blog/2015/11/allied-health-professionals-new-models-care (accessed 1 May 2016).

O'Reilly, C. and Pfeffer, J. (2000). *Hidden Power.* Cambridge, MA: Harvard Business School Press.

Peete, D. (2005). Needed: servant leaders. *Nursing Homes* 54 (7): 8–10.

Pendleton, D. and King, J. (2002). Values and leadership: education and debate. *BMJ* 325: 1352–1355.

Peregrym, D. and Wolf, R. (2013). 'Values-based leadership: the foundation of transformational servant leadership. *The Journal of Values-Based Leadership* 6 (2): 1–13.

Pondy, L.R. (1978). Leadership is a language game. In: *Leadership: Where Else Can we Go?* (ed. M.W. McCall Jr. and M.M. Lombardo), 87–99. Durham, NC: Duke University Press.

Rafferty, A.-M. (1993). *Leading Questions: A Discussion Paper on the Issues of Nurse Leadership.* London: King's Fund.

Rafferty, A.-M., Philippou, J., Fitzpatrick, J. M. & Ball, J. (2015) Culture of Care Barometer: Report to NHS England on the Development and Validation of an Instrument to Measure Culture of Care in NHS Trusts, London: National Nursing Research Unit, King's College London, http://www.england.nhs.uk/wp-content/uploads/2015/03/culture-care-barometer. pdf (accessed 1 July 2016).

Rich, V.L. (2008). Creation of a patient safety culture: a nurse executive leadership imperative. In: *Patient Safety and Quality: An Evidence-Based Handbook for Nurses* (ed. R.G. Hughes). Rockville, MD: Agency for Healthcare Research and Quality, Chapter 20c, http://www.ncbi. nlm.nih.gov/books/NBK2642 (accessed 1 July 2016).

Roberts, S.J. (1983). Oppressed group behaviour: implications for nursing. *Advances in Nursing Science* 5: 21–30.

Robinson, J. (1991). Introduction: beginning the study of nursing policy. In: *Policy Issues in Nursing* (ed. J. Robinson, A. Gray and R. Elkan), 1–8. Milton Keynes: Open University Press.

Robinson, C.A. (2006). The leader within. *Journal of Trauma Nursing* 13 (1): 35–37.

Ross, E.J., Fitzpatrick, J.J., Click, E.R. et al. (2014). Transformational leadership practices of nurse leaders in professional nursing associations. *Journal of Nursing Administration* 44 (4): 201–206.

Savel, R.H. and Munro, C.L. (2017). 'Servant leadership: the primacy of service. *American Journal of Critical Care* 26 (2): 97–99.

Schneider, P. (1999). Five worthy aims for pharmacy's clinical leadership to pursue in improving medication use. *American Journal of Health System Pharmacy* 56 (24): 2549–2552.

Scully, N.J. (2015). Leadership in nursing: the importance of recognising inherent values and attributes to secure a positive future for the profession. *Collegian* 22 (4): 439–444.

Shirey, M.R. (2009). Authentic leadership, organizational culture, and healthy work environments. *Critical Care Nurse Quarterly* 32 (3): 189–198.

Shirley, M.R. (2006). Authentic leaders creating healthy work environments for nursing practice. *American Journal of Critical Care* 15 (3): 256–268.

Sirola-Karvinen, P. and Hyrkas, K. (2006). Clinical supervision for nurses in administrative and leadership positions: a systematic literature review of the studies focusing on administrative clinical supervision. *Journal of Nursing Management* 14 (8): 601–609.

Spears, L.C. (2004). 'Practicing servant-leadership. *Leader to Leader* no. 34: 7–11.

Stanley, D. (2006a). Part 1: in command of care: clinical nurse leadership explored. *Journal of Research in Nursing* 2 (1): 20–39.

Stanley, D. (2006b). Part 2: in command of care: towards the theory of congruent leadership. *Journal of Research in Nursing* 2 (2): 132–144.

Stanley, D. (2006c). Recognising and defining clinical nurse leaders. *British Journal of Nursing* 15 (2): 108–111.

Stanley, D. (2006d). Role conflict: leaders and managers. *Nursing Management* 13 (5): 31–37.

Stanley, D. (2008). Congruent leadership: values in action. *Journal of Nursing Management* 64: 84–95.

Stanley, D. (2010). Clinical leadership and innovation. *Connections* 13 (4): 27–28.

Stanley, D. (2011). *Clinical Leadership: Innovation into Action*. Melbourne: Palgrave Macmillan.

Stanley, D. (2012). Clinical leadership and innovation. *Journal of Nursing Education and Practice* 2 (2): 119–126.

Stanley, D. (2019). *Values-Based Leadership in Healthcare: Congruent Leadership Explored*. London: Sage.

Stanley, D. (2020). 'Bullying and threats to belonging in rural and remote practice. *Australian Nursing and Midwifery Journal* 26 (11): 26.

Stanley, D. and Sherratt, A. (2010). Lamp light on leadership: clinical leadership and Florence nightingale. *Journal of Nursing Management* 18: 115–121.

Stanley, D. & Stanley K. (2018). Report: There where the "bullets can fly": Clinical Leadership in rural and remote north-western New South Wales, Research Report UNE Print ISBN: 978-64467-203-7.

Stanley, D. and Stanley, K. (2019). 'Clinical leadership and rural and remote practice: a qualitative study. *Journal of Nursing Management* 27 (6): 1314–1324.

Stanley, D., Cuthbertson, J., and Latimer, K. (2012). Perceptions of clinical leadership in the St. John ambulance service in WA. Paramedics Australasia. *Response* 39 (1): 31–37.

Stanley, D., Beament, T., Falconer, D. et al. (2014a). *Profile and Perceptions of Men in Nursing in Western Australia: Research Report*. Perth: UWA Print.

Stanley, D., Latimer, K., and Atkinson, J. (2014b). Perceptions of clinical leadership in an aged care residential facility in Perth, Western Australia. *Health Care Current Reviews* 2: 122. https://doi.org/10.4172/hccr.1000122.

Stanley, D., Hutton, M. and McDonald, A. (2015) Western Australian Allied Health Professionals' Perceptions of Clinical Leadership: A Research Report, http://www.ochpo. health.wa.gov.au/docs/WA_Allied_Health_Prof_Perceptions_of_Clinical_Leadership_ Research_Report.pdf (accessed 1 July 2016).

Stanley, D., Blanchard, D., Hohol, A. et al. (2017). Health professionals' perceptions of clinical leadership: a pilot study. *Cogent Medicine* 4 (1): https://doi.org/10.108 0/2331205X.2017.1321193.

Stanton, E., Lemer, C., and Mountford, J. (2010). *Clinical Leadership: Bridging the Divide.* London: Quay Books.

Stephenson, J. (2014) 'NHS England to rollout '6Cs' nursing values to all health service staff', Nursing Times, 23 April, http://www.nursingtimes.net/roles/nurse-managers/ exclusive-6cs-nursing-values-to-be-rolled-out-to-all-nhs-staff/5070102.fullarticle (accessed 1 May 2015).

Swanwick, T. and McKimm, J. (2017). *ABC of Clinical Leadership*, 2e. Oxford: Wiley Blackwell.

Swearingen, S. and Liberman, A. (2004). Nursing leadership: serving those who serve others. *Health Care Manager* 23 (2): 100.

Taylor, J. and Bradbury-Jones, C. (2014). Editorial: writing a helpful journal review: application of the 6 Cs. *Journal of Clinical Nursing* 23: 2695–2697. https://doi.org/10.1111/jocn.12643.

The King's Fund. (2017) Caring to change: how compassionate leadership can stimulate innovation in healthcare. https://www.kingsfund.org.uk/publications/caring-change?gclid= EAIaIQobChMI1eLNj5mM8wIVVqmWCh0KRwKxEAAYASAAEgK1VPD_BwE.

Thorne, M. (2006). What kind of leader are you? *Topics in Emergency Medicine* 28 (2): 104–110.

Thyer, G. (2003). Dare to be different: transformational leadership may hold the key to reducing the nursing shortage. *Journal of Nursing Management* 11: 73–79.

Tinkham, M.R. (2013). The road to magnet: encouraging transformational leadership. *ACRN Journal* 98 (2): 186–188. https://doi.org/10.1016/j.aorn.2013.05.007.

Vasudeva, S. (2020). 'Influence of leaders and servant leadership. *American Medical writers Association Journal* 35 (1): 24–25.

Victorian Quality Council (2005). *Developing the Clinical Leader's Role in Clinical Governance: A Guide for Clinicians and Health Services.* Melbourne: Victorian Department of Health.

Viinamaki, O.-P. (2009). 'Intra-organizational challenges of values-based leadership. *Electronic Journal of Business Ethics and Organisational Studies* 14 (2): 6–13.

Walker, T. (2006). Servant leaders. *Managed Healthcare Executive* 16 (3): 20–26.

Weberg, D. (2010). Transformational leadership and staff retention: an evidence review with implications for healthcare systems. *Nursing Administration Quarterly* 34 (3): 246.

Welford, C. (2002). Matching theory to practice. *Nursing Management* 9 (4): 7–11.

Weng, R.-H., Huang, C.-Y., Chen, L.-M., and Chang, L.-Y. (2015). Exploring the impact of transformational leadership on nurse innovation behaviour: a cross-sectional study. *Journal of Nursing Management* 23: 427–439.

West, M. (2021). *Compassionate Leadership: Sustaining Wisdom, Humanity and Presence in Health and Social.* London: Swirling Leaf Press.

West, M. & Chowla, R. (2017) 'Compassionate Leadership for Compassionate Health Care' (Chapter 14), in P. Gilbert (ed), Compassion, New York: Rutledge.

Wilkinson, G. and Miers, M. (ed.) (1999). *Power and Nursing Practice*. London: Macmillan.

Wong, C. and Cummings, G. (2007). The relationship between nursing leadership and patient outcomes: a systematic review. *Journal of Nursing Management* 15 (5): 508–521.

Wong, C. and Cummings, G. (2009). Authentic leadership: a new theory for nursing or back to basics? *Journal of Health Organisations and Management* 23 (50): 522.

Wong, C.A. and Walsh, E.J. (2020). 'Reflections on a decade of authentic leadership research in healthcare. *Journal of Nursing Management* 28 (1): 1–3.

Wynia, M. and Bedzow, I. (2019). Values based leadership during the transformation of health care. *People and Strategy* 42 (3): 28–33.

4

Followership

David Stanley

We don't need any more leadership training; we need some followership training.
Maureen Carroll, in Lewis 2001, p. 358

Introduction: From behind They Lead

According to Hersey et al. (1996), 'followership' is the flip side of leadership. Followers, they feel, are vital because they accept or reject the leader and determine the leader's personal power. Kellerman (2012), Raffo (2013), Malakyan (2014), Uhl-Bien et al. (2014), Smith-Trudeau (2017), Hanks (2020) and Varpio and Teunissen (2021) agree, adding that the interaction between followers and leaders occurs on a multitude of levels, and that followers should be considered when trying to define or understand leadership (Peters and Haslam 2018). Uhl-Bien et al. (2014) and Smith-Trudeau (2017) suggest that the outcomes that leaders achieve are very much dependent on the attributes of their followers, with Grint commenting that followers make the leader and that 'it only requires the good follower to do nothing for leadership to fail' (2000, p. 133). As such, understanding followership is vital if leaders are to understand the perspectives of followers and lead successfully.

Leaders cannot function without followers, who often act as their eyes and ears and moral compass (in the business world this may even involve customers, and in the health arena it must include clients and patients), a view supported by Hanks (2020). Leaders cannot achieve much without the 'permission' of followers. Indeed, as any culture is based on the people within it, it is often because of their followers that leaders achieve their goals (Malakyan 2014; Varpio and Teunissen 2021). Leaders frequently get the praise for the work that followers do, and leaders should be aware that much of the credit that rests on their shoulders was first carried on those of their followers. This chapter considers what it means to be a follower and addresses the responsibilities and characteristics of followers.

Clinical Leadership in Nursing and Healthcare, Third Edition.
Edited by David Stanley, Clare L. Bennett and Alison H. James.
© 2023 John Wiley & Sons Ltd. Published 2023 by John Wiley & Sons Ltd.

Defining Followership

As Crossman and Crossman (2011) point out, definitions of followership have been intrinsically linked to definitions of leadership, particularly in terms of links to words such as 'subordinate'. More recently, authors have used terms such as collaborators, partners, participants and even constituents to describe the changing relationship of followers to leaders (Uhl-Bien 2006; Varpio and Teunissen 2021). Writing from a radiology perspective, Penny (2017, p. 607) suggests that, 'in the clinical setting, followership relates to how the follower supports the leader while simultaneously meeting the mission of the organization and the professional directives or standards of ethics placed upon the individual by the profession'. Definitions commonly focus on a dependent follower–leader relationship, a leader-member exchange (Xu et al. 2019) or a process in which 'subordinates' recognise their responsibilities to those who are in authority or have recognised leadership roles. Most definitions focus on a hierarchical relationship, although some focus on the interactive nature of the follower–leader relationship (Smith-Trudeau 2017), with followers seen as enthusiastic, cooperative, active and engaged, as partners in the relationship rather than passive 'subordinates' waiting to be told what to do. Carsten et al. (2010) in support of these later views define followership this way:

> Followership is a relational role in which followers have the ability to influence leaders and contribute to the improvement and attainment of group and organisational objectives. It is primarily a hierarchically upward influence. (p. 559)

Followers' Responsibilities

It will be instructive to begin by considering followers' responsibilities, as, like leaders, they have many. Followers' responsibilities are no less important than those of leaders, as it is followers who enable good leadership to flourish. To be effective, followers need to recognise that they have responsibilities. These include but may not be limited to:

- developing a high degree of literacy about the institution/organisation (Penny 2017)
- taking responsibility for achieving their personal and organisational goals
- taking ownership of their work
- being active rather than passive (Raffo 2013)
- connecting themselves to the organisation in meaningful ways (Penny 2017)
- becoming loyal to the organisation's values (Penny 2017)
- recognising and being aware of their own personal and professional values
- making a personal commitment and being open to change
- asking a great deal of the leader
- demonstrating respect
- not blaming a manager or employer for unpopular decisions or policies
- if they have an opportunity to express an opinion or view, doing so honestly; 'yes men' are poor followers (Wedderburn-Tate 1999)

Offermann (2005) and Penny (2017) suggests that leaders are vulnerable to the actions of followers; Kellerman (2012) and Malakyan (2014) go further, proposing that in recent years the balance of power has shifted in favour of followers. Leadership studies and leadership training have commonly neglected the role and place of followers in supporting leadership (Kellerman 2012; Raffo 2013; Malakyan 2014; Smith-Trudeau 2017; Peters and Haslam 2018). Even good leaders can be led into making poor decisions and into ineffective leadership patterns by the actions of empowered and strong followers. Potentially worse, and more often, leaders may be hoodwinked by followers who fool them with flattery or hinder them with false realities. The case of General Sir Ian Hamilton is offered as an example of the impact of poor followership (Box 4.1).

Box 4.1   A Historical Example of a Good Leader with Poor Followers: General Sir Ian Hamilton

General Sir Ian Hamilton was appointed commander of the Allied forces responsible for the assault on the Gallipoli peninsula in 1915. According to Rhodes-James (1965), Hamilton possessed almost every conceivable qualification for a great culmination of an exceptional career. He was an elderly professional soldier with vast experience of combat, leadership and warfare (Carlyon 2010). He also had immense physical and mental courage and resilience and showed imagination and daring. Yet for all this, his leadership of the Gallipoli landings and subsequent assault on the peninsula failed utterly.

There were many contributing factors to the failure. Hamilton became ill with dysentery for some months, which left him incapacitated for years after the landings. He had difficult and independent-minded subordinate commanders. The effort of launching an assault more than a thousand miles from home and with a large percentage of untried and semi-trained soldiers against well-prepared and well-defended positions compounded his difficulties. Moreover, he was initially stationed offshore on the ship HMS *Queen Elizabeth* while many of his staff were on other transports. This led to significant communication problems.

As the campaign continued, Hamilton moved his headquarters to the island of Imbros and became increasingly removed from the commanders operating across the Aegean on the Gallipoli peninsula. Here he was further isolated by the actions of his administrative staff, in particular an officer called Braithwaite, who tended to protect Hamilton too enthusiastically from what he regarded as unimportant or inappropriate juniors; thus the general was kept in the dark about the reality of the situation on the peninsula (Rhodes-James 1965; Carlyon 2010).

Hamilton made considerable mistakes in his leadership of the Gallipoli campaign. He was out of touch with his front-line commanders for far too long, and he failed to intervene personally in the conduct of the battles or to respond speedily to requests for support or direction. However, he was also poorly served by his administrative staff, in particular Braithwaite, who painted an overly optimistic view of the developing battles and who went as far as keeping vital information from Hamilton at crucial times.

In many respects, Hamilton's failure was the result of his isolation and shelter from the realities of the campaign by his distance from the front line and by interfering administrative staff. Sir Ian Hamilton was an elderly veteran of the British Army, and his staff's respect and care actually failed to serve him with accurate and realistic information on which he could base his decisions. In this example, Hamilton's followers had a negative impact on his capacity to flourish as a leader.

To guard against the influence of ineffective or disruptive followers, leaders need support people who can relay bad news and who can communicate and act on a solid set of values. Leaders also need to encourage open debate and discourse so that they are not protected or insulated from those they lead (Offermann 2005; Smith-Trudeau 2017).

To be effective, followers must have the confidence and courage to offer unwelcome advice or information, if necessary, because leaders require the best and most relevant information if they are to make clear and accurate decisions. Penny (2017) supports this by suggesting the development of the Courageous Follower Model. This proposes that followers need to support the leader and contribute to the leader's success, assume responsibility for a common purpose and act independently, challenge constructively if the common purpose is being threatened, support change willingly and take a moral stand to prevent ethical abuses.

Being a follower is not about trailing, sheep-like, in the wake of a leader because they have authority or because they have been appointed to lead, nor is it about abdicating responsibility and waiting passively for the problems around you to be solved. Followers should be deeply involved in the fabric of an organisation/ward or team and participate by actively engaging with the tasks and duties, decisions and direction under consideration. Effective follower-ship prepares people to be effective leaders (Malakyan 2014; Penny 2017; Peters and Haslam 2018; Xu et al. 2019). Followers should seriously consider questions about their responsibilities to the organisation and the leader and be willing to honestly question their capacity to follow effectively before undertaking a followership role. Followers should think about these issues:

- How good are their followership skills?
- Are they ready to be engaged as followers?
- Are they courageous enough to offer honest and potentially unwelcome information?
- Are they ready to change or adapt along the lines the leader is heading?
- Are they perceived by their leader as a good follower?
- What style of follower do they represent?

In an article about followership in 2002, Paul Di Carlo suggests that there are five types of follower. He describes them in what he calls the 5-P follower model:

- **Participant**: followers who are actively involved and contribute to moving forward
- **Pessimist**: followers who think that change means 'we're doomed' and need to share this with everyone
- **Passenger**: followers who are only here in body, the mind is elsewhere
- **Pig**: followers who are only here for the food
- **Prisoner**: followers who are here, but not by choice

Reflection Point

Look around your organisation, ward or healthcare team. What type of follower are you? What about your fellow followers, what sort of followers are they? Where might they fit on Di Carlo's 5-P follower model?

Di Carlo's 5-P follower model is not the only way to consider the type of follower you might be. Kelley (1988) suggests that followers can be identified by five levels of activity and critical thinking: sheep; yes people; alienated followers; survivors; and effective followers. Douglas (1992) proposes that followers display a range of followership styles from 'very democratic' to 'very autocratic', and he developed a short questionnaire to explore the preferred style. The intention is that followers read a range of 16 statements about the type of employer they would prefer to be in a followership role to. Five options from 'strongly agree' to 'strongly disagree' are offered for each statement, and the score total gives an insight into the follower's preferred style. Box 4.2 is an adaptation of Douglas's Followership Style Questionnaire.

Box 4.2   Followership Style Questionnaire.

	Statements	SA	A	MF	D	SD
1	I expect my job to be very explicitly outlined for me.	1	2	3	4	5
2	When the boss says to do something, I do it. After all, he/she is the boss.	1	2	3	4	5
3	Rigid rules and regulations usually cause me to become frustrated and inefficient.	5	4	3	2	1
4	I am utterly responsible for and capable of self-discipline based on my contacts with the people around me.	5	4	3	2	1
5	My job should be made as short in duration as possible so that I can achieve efficiency through repetition.	1	2	3	4	5
6	Within reasonable limits I will try to accommodate requests from persons who are not my boss because these requests are typically in the best interests of the company anyway.	5	4	3	2	1
7	When the boss tells me to do something that is the wrong thing to do, it is their fault, not mine, when I do it.	1	2	3	4	5
8	It is up to my leader to provide a set of rules by which I can measure my performance.	1	2	3	4	5
9	The boss is the boss. And the fact of the promotion suggests that they are on the ball.	1	2	3	4	5
10	I accept orders only from my boss.	1	2	3	4	5
11	I would prefer my boss to give me general objectives and guidelines and then allow me to do the job my way.	5	4	3	2	1
12	If I do something that is not right, it is my own fault, even if my supervisor told me to do it.	5	4	3	2	1
13	I prefer jobs that are not repetitious, the kind of task that is new and different each time.	5	4	3	2	1
14	My supervisor is in no way superior to me by virtue of position. They do a different kind of job, one that includes a lot of managing and coordinating.	5	4	3	2	1
15	I expect my leader to give me disciplinary guidelines.	1	2	3	4	5
16	I prefer to tell my supervisor what I will or at least should be doing. I am ultimately responsible for my own work.	5	4	3	2	1
	Total =					

(Continued)

Box 4.2   (Continued)

Scoring: Add all the numerical values together (e.g. the total might be 70). Now divide this by 16 (the total number of questions, e.g. 70 divided by 16 = 4.37, a score in the 'very democratic' range). See the ranges below to determine your followership style.

Score	Description	Followership style
Less than 1.9	Very autocratic	Cannot function well without programmes and procedures, needs feedback
2.0–2.4	Moderately autocratic	Needs solid structures and feedback, but can also carry on independently
2.5–3.4	Mixed	Mixture of above and below
3.5–4.0	Moderately participative	Independent worker, does not need close supervision, just a bit of feedback
Greater than 4.1	Very democratic	Self-starter, likes to challenge new things by themselves

Source: Douglas (1992).

The questionnaire contains 16 statements about the type of employer/leader you prefer. Imagine yourself in a subordinate (follower) position of some kind and use your responses to indicate the preferred way in which your employer/leader might interact with or relate to you. The responses are marked on a five-point scale with ratings SA = strongly agree, A = agree, MF = mixed feelings, D = disagree and SD = strongly disagree.

Followership is not easy and can often be inhibited by a number of factors. These include:

- Leaders who are not trustworthy
- Leaders who are poor communicators
- Leaders whom the followers find they cannot respect
- Leaders who think followers should read minds (poor communication again)
- Followers who feel as if they are not 'needed' in an organisation or who are undervalued
- Poor change processes that exclude followers or neglect their needs or concerns (Xu et al. 2019)
- Leaders who make poor attempts at getting followers to participate
- Poor attention to rewards (which go far beyond monetary issues)
- Leaders who employ inequality, bias, nepotism and unfairness
- Leaders who are cynical, destructive or hard to approach

The Good Follower

Good followers do not withhold or avoid difficult options or decisions. Good followers need to be courageous (Penny 2017). They search for other points of view. They seek out the 'why' in each situation. They keep the leader honest, give opinions and offer the organisation a chance at greatness. Good followers increase both the leader's chance of getting the job done and enhancing the collaborative relationship. Good followers are the keys to leadership success and change. Understanding the needs and concerns of followers is vital for leaders if they are to engage them in supporting and working effectively together (Alwazzan 2017; Peters and Haslam 2018).

Reflection Point

When you picked up this book, I am sure you considered your role as a leader, but have you ever thought about your role as a follower? Malakyan (2014) is clear that leaders and followers are almost symbiotic in their relationship, each being dependent on the other. Peters and Haslam (2018), when studying the Royal marines, found that marines identified as leaders by the officers often did not recognise followers as leaders, but other followers saw their follower peers as emerging leaders. So that the different perspective of the assessor meant that followership and leadership were sometimes revered. What impact might the position of the follower have on the leader's capacity to lead or follow through with their change agenda and innovations? What if the characteristics of the followers determined the type of leader that emerged? Kelley (1992), for example, suggests that without his armies (followers), Napoleon was just a man with grandiose ambitions. What impact do your followers' behaviours have on your success or ability to be a leader?

Looking at the leadership–follower dyad (a group of two) from a postmodern perspective, it might be suggested that it is situational, context driven or jointly constructed. To provide some structure at this point, here are three ways in which the leadership–follower dyad has been construed:

- Leadership can be explained in terms of a leader–member exchange relationship, where leaders provide direction and support, and followers achieve agreed outcomes (Avolio and Bass 1988). Such approaches define follower characteristics as **dependent variables**, influenced by a leader (Dvir and Shamir 2003; Xu et al. 2019).
- Situational leadership theories describe follower characteristics as **moderator variables** (Vroom and Yetton 1973); that is, the characteristics of *followers* act to influence the relationship between the leader and the follower, and/or the leader and their actions.
- In general, very little effort has been expended in examining follower characteristics (as opposed to behaviours) that act as **independent variables**; that is, follower characteristics that have a direct effect on leader behaviours.

Five examples of studies that have explored follower characteristics as independent variables are those by Bass (1990), Ehrhart and Klein (2001), Dvir and Shamir (2003), Gordon et al. (2015) and Xu et al. (2019). Bass (1990) focused more on a review of follower behaviour in relation to the success of the transformational leader. Ehrhart and Klein (2001), Dvir and Shamir (2003) and Xu et al. (2019) studied follower characteristics and noted that successful transformational leadership and the leader-member exchange is not just inherent within the leader's role but is significantly influenced by the leader–follower relationship. Raffo (2013) identified the characteristics of post-industrial followers and suggested that these included self-management (Chapter 10), team spirit, a positive attitude, being a contributor, competence and being ethical. Gordon et al. (2015) explored medical trainees' conceptualisation of both followership and leadership, demonstrating a lack of clarity and indeed negativity existed around the concept of followership.

Malakyan (2014) is of the view that leaders and followers can even trade places and that this forms the basis of their co-dependence. Leadership traits are not superior to followership traits and therefore leadership and followership need to be seen as non-static and dynamic, and leaders and followers need to approach their co-dependence willingly.

In relation to congruent leadership, followers have much of the power, because if they do not align themselves with the values and beliefs of the leader, they will not follow that leader. And as with Peters and Haslam's (2018) research with marines, leaders are identified by the followers and are more likely to be seen within the follower ranks. The leader will be isolated and even if they are not aware of their lack of followers, the leader's actions will not generate motivation among followers or identification with the leader's values and beliefs. The important message to take away from these suggestions is that you do not have to assume that following a leader renders the follower powerless and passive.

Effective leadership is an active process that is affected by the characteristics of, and interaction among, the leader, the follower and the context. As such, these variables can be used both to understand these relationships and to engage more effectively as a leader and as a follower. Regardless of the theoretical model involved, this is a discussion about a relationship; that is, it would be reasonable to surmise that a leader-follower dyad works, or does not work, depending on the quality or type of relationship bonds (and values-based links) developed between a follower and a leader.

Clinical Leader Stories: 4 Learning about the ECG

When I was a third-year nursing student I was placed on a Cardiac Unit. During the pm shift, a registered nurse approached me and two other students during some down time and asked if we wanted to learn more about electrocardiograms (ECGs). Being students, we jumped at the opportunity, particularly because I was only familiar with the basics. The nurse explained a lot and shared her knowledge surrounding the ECG and particular rates, rhythms and signs to look out for. This nurse went into great detail and always asked if we needed more explanation and utilised terms that we could understand and remember She even drew diagrams on the white board whilst explaining concepts, and they were very supportive and reassuring the entire time. This was a very positive experience for me and the others as the cardiac unit can be very stressful and overwhelming at times. The registered nurse wasn't in a leadership role; however, she demonstrated many of the attributes I expected to see in a clinical leader. The registered nurse was clearly clinically knowledgeable and competent, supportive, values and beliefs focused, motivational, an effective communicator, a mentor and very

(Continued)

approachable. The registered nurse displayed all these attributes while helping us understand the ECG; therefore, I believe she was a clinical leader. She has had a strong influence on my personal professional practice, and I feel she created a safer work environment and motivated me to apply this knowledge in my future practice.

Nicholas: Student Nurse

The Not-So-Good Follower

Not all seemingly compliant followers are 'good' or useful. There has been scant research in this area of late, however, Wedderburn-Tate (1999, p. 130) suggests that 'just say yes' followers support the concept of wanting to please the leader by doing or saying what the leader wants. However, she claims that this can lead to the creation of an unhealthy relationship where the yes-sayer and the leader 'mis-serve' each other. The leader is given positive responses by the follower, who may misrepresent reality for fear of offending or appearing disloyal; while the leader – seeking more relevant information or new yes-sayers – sees the follower as superfluous. Yes-sayers are almost sycophantic in their approach to loyalty and rarely offer genuine service to the leader or the organisation.

Wedderburn-Tate (1999) proposes a list of symptoms of leaders with a tendency to prefer yes-sayers:

- They perceived followers who were not yes-sayers as troublemakers
- They perceived followers who were not yes-sayers as not team players
- They did not like people who disagreed with them
- They saw disagreement as a sign of disloyalty

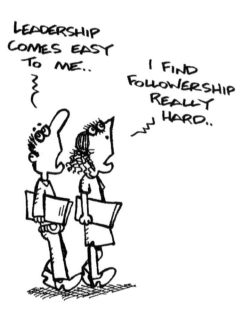

- They believed that disagreement always causes conflict
- They may tell lies to protect followers from harm (real or perceived)
- They are keen to please those in positions of power

The story of General Hamilton is an example of the negative impact on a leader of being served by followers who tried to please and protect him from reality. I believe General Hamilton wanted to be a great leader and in the end felt disserved by those few followers who professed to have his interests are heart. Leaders that promote and encourage the 'yes-sayer' follower are far more dangerous and far less likely to apply a morally sound or ethically appropriate approach in their leadership or dealings with followers (e.g. Hitler, Stalin, Trump). A leader can recognise this and should be on guard against it, though some will see it as another tool for power. Yes-saying followers tend to be:

- dismissive of comments or feedback by other followers who want to offer realistic information to the leader
- dissenting or even bullying of other followers who want to offer realistic feedback to the leader
- keen to monopolise the leader's time
- keen to offer their views and opinions without being sought
- overprotective of the leader, their vision or values, and staunchly active (almost fanatical) in defence of the leader if criticised
- 'close' to the leader, in personal terms or in proximity, standing by them or usually sitting by them in meetings or at social gatherings

---

Reflection Point

General William T. Sherman (famous during the American Civil War) said, 'We have good corporals and good sergeants and some good lieutenants and captains, and those are far more important than good generals'. If this is the case, does it apply to healthcare organisations? If so, how? Are middle- and lower- level leaders more significant in determining the success and progress of an organisation? Does Sherman's statement apply in your ward, clinical area or clinical domain? If so, what does that mean for issues like leadership/followership training or career progression?

Followership and leadership are uniquely and inextricably linked in a symbiotic relationship (Wedderburn-Tate 1999; Penny 2017; Varpio and Teunissen 2021). Dynamic leadership is dependent on and influenced by the style that followers employ and by their capacity to take followership responsibilities seriously. In the same way that effective leaders need to understand and foster their understanding of followership, followers need to recognise that they have a responsibility to the leader to be 'good' followers. Good followers increase the leader's chance of getting the task or job done, as well as offering the organisation a chance at greatness. Teams are made up of leaders and followers and ultimately, the success of the team is dependent on the collaboration and efforts of all its members. In many ways, followers are the key to an organisation's and a leader's success (Penny 2017; Varpio and Teunissen 2021).

Case Study 4.1   Dorothea Dix

Dorothea Dix was a leader who lost her followers and was soon lost to history (for a while). Read about Dorothea and consider the challenge that follows.

Known as the American Florence Nightingale, Dorothea Dix did much as a social activist and health reformer before and after the American Civil War. She was born in 1802 in Maine, grew up in Worcester, Massachusetts, and then lived with her wealthy grandmother in Boston. Her father was an alcoholic, and Dorothea, though supported by her grandmother, struggled initially in traditional female occupations: governess, teacher and writer. She refused a proposal of marriage, choosing instead to focus on her teaching career; however, unhappy with her life, in her mid-30s she suffered a debilitating breakdown. Hoping for a cure, she travelled to England. There she was fortunate to meet with a family of Quakers and notable social reformers, who suggested that the government should better support an active role in social welfare. She was exposed to the British lunacy reform movement and on finding a more useful purpose for herself, returned to America in 1840 or 1841.

Following on from what she had observed in England, Dorothea undertook an investigation into how the insane poor were cared for in Massachusetts. Her report painted a bleak picture. She described people caged, kept in stalls and pens, in chains, sometimes naked and even beaten. The outcome was a government Bill to expand the state's mental health hospitals and provide better care for the insane.

She travelled with great energy to a number of other states across the north of America, producing similar evaluations and engaging with legislators to draft reform Bills in other states. In 1854 she initiated a Bill in Congress, whereby federal land would be sold to support further facilities for the insane, but President Franklin Pierce vetoed this, arguing that the federal government should not be involved in state-related medical responsibilities. Disappointed by this setback, Dorothea left again for Europe. She took part in an evaluation of Scottish insane asylums and participated in the development of the Scottish Lunacy Commission.

On her return to America, she once more turned to social reform activities, but these were interrupted by the outbreak of the Civil War in 1861. Dorothea was soon appointed Superintendent of (Female) Union Army Nurses, and she set about recruiting nurses for the cause. She drew up a list of requirements for applicants that included (Ward et al. 1992, p. 149):

- a certificate from two physicians
- a certificate from two clergymen
- being at least 30 years old
- being of good health
- being of good moral character
- being unattractive and modest of dress

More than 3,000 women volunteers applied (many were nuns) and they served with the Union (Northern) army throughout the war. Dorothea and her nurses provided what comfort and care they could, often faced with staggering numbers of wounded from

---

(Continued)

Case Study 4.1 (Continued)

---

both armies. They did not differentiate between them; as one of the Dix nurses stated, 'though enemies, they were nevertheless helpless, suffering human beings'. The Southern army had minimal medical services, and Dorothea is fondly remembered in the Southern states for her bipartisan care of their troops during the war. Sadly, the skills she employed as a social crusader (independence, single-mindedness, passion, energy) were less useful when managing large numbers of female nurses. Although a superb organiser, she often clashed with Army doctors (who referred to her as 'Dragon Dix'), to the point where she felt she had no real authority. Dorothea's duties involved organising training facilities for nurses, purchasing supplies, recruiting nurses and setting up field hospitals. She was ill prepared for dealing with the military establishment and was often in conflict with doctors over their drinking habits and neglect of sanitation. Her nurses too commonly found her aloof and although soldiers saw her as an 'angel of mercy', she often felt alone in her efforts to deal with the female nursing service. She recalled her contribution during the Civil War years as the greatest failure of her life.

After the war Dorothea worked to help trace missing soldiers and to assist soldiers in securing their pensions, before returning to social reform activities. In 1881 she moved to New Jersey and lived at the state hospital, where she was awarded a private suite for her use, for 'as long as she lived'. Increasingly an invalid, she maintained a vital correspondence with nurses around the world until her death in 1887.

As a social reformer (she was never trained as a nurse), Dorothea Dix made significant personal contributions to the welfare of mentally ill people in both Europe and America. Her views on the treatment of the mentally ill were radical for the time and very humane, influenced by her unhappy upbringing, social advantages, education and personal passion to make legislative and social improvements for their welfare.

Challenge: Dorothea remembered her greatest contribution as her greatest failure. What might you say to someone you know who has lost sight of the great work and contribution they make in healthcare? Dorothea was unsupported by the medical men and to some extent by the Northern Army in general. What role do followers have in supporting the work of the leader? Would Dorothea's assessment of her efforts have been more sympathetic if she had been given more relevant feedback by those she led in the nursing service and in the Northern Army administration?

Summary

- Followership is the flip side of leadership.
- Understanding followership is vital for leaders to understand the perspectives of followers.
- Followers have responsibilities that are at least as important as the leader's responsibilities.
- Followers often display a preferred style. This can be determined to assess their capacity to follow or hinder a leader's course.
- Good followership can be inhibited by poor leadership.

- Followers are not powerless and good followers have the power to make good leaders great.
- Team success is dependent on leaders and followers working towards the same goals.

Mind Press-Ups

Exercise 4.1

Reflect on the relationships you have had with a past or present 'leader'. Think about the kind of working relationship you have had with them and what thought (if any) you have put into your responsibilities as a follower.

Exercise 4.2

Undertake the Followership Style Questionnaire in this chapter. What are your thoughts about the result? Have you ever been taught about followership? Yes or No. Why do you think this is?

Exercise 4.3

Does your organisation encourage the participation of followers? Do you feel that you have 'power' as a follower? If not, how could you use some of the change models offered in Chapter 7 to increase your influence as a follower?

Exercise 4.4

Who would you identify as the most effective followers in your ward/clinic/team or clinical area? Are these the same people you might identify as leaders or potential leaders?

References

Alwazzan, L. (2017). When we say. . . leadership, we must also say. . . followership. *Medical Education* 51: 560.

Avolio, B.J. and Bass, B.M. (1988). Transformational leadership, charisma and beyond. In: *Emerging Leadership Vistas* (ed. J.G. Hunt, H.R. Balgia, H.P. Dachler and C.A. Sachiesheim). Lexington, MA: Heath.

Bass, B.M. (1990). *Bass and Stogdill's Handbook of Leadership: Theory, Research and Management Applications*. New York: Free Press.

Carlyon, L. (2010). *Gallipoli*. Sydney: Picador/Pan Macmillan.

Carsten, M., Uhl-Bien, M., West, B. et al. (2010). Exploring social constructions of followership: a qualitative study. *The Leadership Quarterly* 21: 543–562.

Crossman, B. and Crossman, J. (2011). Conceptualising followership – a review of the literature. *Leadership* 7 (4): 481–497.

Di Carlo, P. (2002). *Followership, Followers and Following*, http://Bloorresearch.com, http://www.bloorresearch.com/analysis/followership-followers-and-following (accessed 1 July 2016).

Douglas, L.M. (1992). *The Effective Nurse Leader and Manager*, 4e, 25–28. St Louis, MO: Mosby.

Dvir, T. and Shamir, B. (2003). Follower developmental characteristics as predicting transformational leadership: a longitudinal field study. *The Leadership Quarterly* 14 (3): 327–344.

Ehrhart, M.G. and Klein, K.J. (2001). Predicting followers' preferences for charismatic leadership: the influence of follower values and personality. *The Leadership Quarterly* 12 (2): 153–179.

Gordon, L.J., Rees C.E., Ker, J.S. Cleland ,J. (2015). Dimensions, discourses and differences: trainees conceptualising health care leadership and followership . *Medical Education* 49 no. 12. pp.1248-62.

Grint, K. (2000). *The Arts of Leadership*. Oxford: Oxford University Press.

Hanks, S. (2020). Leadership and followership in a pandemic - where do you stand? *Journal of the Irish Dental Association* 66 (3): 111.

Hersey, P., Blanchard, K., and Johnson, D.E. (1996). *Management of Organizational Behaviour: Utilizing Human Resources*, 7e. Englewood Cliffs, NJ: Prentice-Hall.

Kellerman, B. (2012). *The End of Leadership*. London: HarperCollins.

Kelley, R.E. (1988). In praise of followers. *Harvard Business Review* 66 (6): 142–148.

Kelley, R.E. (1992). *The Power of Followership*. New York: Currency Doubleday.

Lewis, J.P. (2001). *Project Planning, Scheduling and Control: A Hands-on Guide to Bringing Projects in on Time and on Budget*. New York: McGraw-Hill.

Malakyan, P.G. (2014). Followership in leadership studies: a case of leader-follower trade approach. *Journal of Leadership Studies* 7 (4): 6–22.

Offermann, L.R. (2005). When followers become toxic. In: *Harvard Business Review on the Mind of the Leader*. Boston, MA: Harvard Business School Publishing.

Penny, S.M. (2017). Serving, following and leading in health care. *Radiologic Technology* 88 (6): 603–617.

Peters, K. and Haslam, S.A. (2018). I follow, therefore I lead: a longitudinal study of the leader and follower identity and leadership in the marines. *British Journal of Psychology* 109: 708–723.

Raffo, D.M. (2013). Teaching followership in leadership education. *Journal of Leadership Education* 12 (1): 262–273.

Rhodes-James, R. (1965). *Gallipoli*. London: Pan.

Smith-Trudeau, P. (2017). Nursing leadership and followership: reflections on the importance of followers. Vermont Nurse Connection, January, February, March. pp. 2–3.

Uhl-Bien, M. (2006). Relational leadership theory: exploring the social processes of leadership and organising. *The Leadership Quarterly* 17 (6): 654–676.

Uhl-Bien, M., Riggio, R.E., Lowe, K.B., and Carson, M.K. (2014). Followership theory: a review and research agenda. *The Leadership Quarterly* 25 (1): 83–104.

Varpio, L. and Teunissen, P. (2021). Leadership in interprofessional healthcare teams: empowering knotworking with followership. *Medical Teacher* 43 (1): 32–37.

Vroom, V.H. and Yetton, P.W. (1973). *Leadership and Decision Making*. Pittsburgh, PA: University of Pittsburgh Press.

Ward, G.C., Burns, R., and Burns, K. (1992). *The Civil War: an Illustrated History*. London: Pimlico Edition.

Wedderburn-Tate, C. (1999). *Leadership in Nursing*. London: Churchill Livingstone.

Xu, A.J., Loi, R., Cai, Z., and Linden, R.C. (2019). Reversing the lens: how followers influence leader-member exchange quality. *Journal of Occupational and Organizational Psychology* 92: 475–497.

5

Leadership and Management
Clare L. Bennett and Alison H. James

'*A man dies when he refuses to stand up for that which is right...*'

Rev. Martin Luther King (1965)

Introduction: Why Delineate?

Much ink has been spent outlining the differences between leadership and management, with arguments extending to the relative merits of each. In this chapter we argue that leadership and management are equally important, interdependent and inter-related. Yet we will also argue that leadership and management are distinct, serving different purposes and requiring different skills (St George 2012; Gumbo 2017; Nene et al. 2020).

In healthcare, at the clinical level, leadership and management roles frequently blur, with ward managers often having leadership roles and clinical leaders also holding management responsibilities (Stanley 2017). As Wood (2021 p. 284) outlines: 'Working out who leads and who manages is difficult, with the added anomaly that not all managers are leaders, and some people who lead work in management positions'. There is, therefore, a very real potential for role ambiguity (Stanley 2006; Cutcliffe and Cleary 2015; Nene et al. 2020) and conflict can occur when clinicians take on management roles without appropriate training, support or instruction (Stanley 2017; Nene et al. 2020). Likewise, tensions can occur between clinical leaders and managers, when leaders feel that their efforts are stymied by management or organisational aspirations or targets (Stanley 2006; Kerridge 2013; Orvik et al. 2015; Scully 2015; Stanley 2017; Nene et al. 2020).

This chapter, therefore, begins by delineating between management and leadership, because an awareness among clinicians as to when they are operating in leadership or management roles can help in ensuring that the most appropriate skill set is utilised, to achieve the best outcomes (Jones and Bennett 2018). It also explores the skills required for each role and the need for education. We then move on to addressing some of the controversies regarding healthcare leadership and management, and we finish by discussing the future for both roles.

Clinical Leadership in Nursing and Healthcare, Third Edition.
Edited by David Stanley, Clare L. Bennett and Alison H. James.
© 2023 John Wiley & Sons Ltd. Published 2023 by John Wiley & Sons Ltd.

Who Should Take Centre Stage?

Reflection Point

Take a moment to consider whether leadership and management are equally important in achieving safe, compassionate clinical care, or whether one is more important than the other. Make some notes to justify your response. Next, consider the following well-known account of leadership and management and evaluate whether it influences your initial response:

> The manager administers;
> the leader innovates.
> The manager maintains;
> the leader develops.
> The manager focuses on systems and structure;
> the leader focuses on people.
> The manager relies on control;
> the leader inspires trust.
> The manager has a short-range view;
> the leader has a long-range perspective.
> The manager asks how and when;
> the leader asks what and why.
> Managers have their eyes on the bottom line;
> leaders have their eyes on the horizon.
> The manager imitates;
> the leader originates.
> The manager accepts the status quo;
> the leader challenges it.
> The manager is the classic good soldier;
> the leader is his own person.
> The manager does things right;
> the leader does the right thing.

Adapted from Warren G Bennis 1989

For some time, the terms management and leadership have been used interchangeably. However, this is misleading, and although management and leadership overlap, they are not synonymous (Kotter 1990a, b; Bass 2010). Therefore, Bennis's (1989) differentiation, whilst crude, is helpful in demonstrating the different and, sometimes, competing perspectives between what leaders and managers do and their differing ways of viewing the world. However, where we disagree with Bennis is in relation to the positioning of leaders over managers, because without effective management in healthcare, service provision becomes impossible (Stanley 2017). Playing down the importance of managers in supporting staff and keeping healthcare organisations running is not our intention. Indeed, as we saw throughout the COVID-19 pandemic, the upscaling and remodelling of services to provide additional care facilities internationally and the roll out of vaccination programmes was attributable to effective management. Managers are not, therefore, secondary in importance to leadership roles, as is sometimes perceived (Stanley 2017).

However, an understanding of the difference between management and leadership can be helpful because each demands different skills in order to achieve their objectives. Managerial activities are essential to the smooth running of an organisation and the attainment of care standards and targets. An example of a fundamental management role is staff rostering. Whilst widely held as one of the more mundane aspects of clinical management, the skill involved in providing around-the-clock cover, that takes into account patient acuity, variability in admission patterns, regulations regarding staff breaks between and during shifts and staff availability, should not be underestimated (Wynendaele et al. 2021). Indeed, the challenges that this aspect of management presents are yet to be resolved through software packages underpinned by mathematical models (Wynendaele et al. 2021), but without the fulfilment of this key management role, the attainment of care standards would become impossible. Likewise, procurement is an essential management function. If there is a shortage of equipment, clinical care cannot be provided to optimal standards, as observed in the disruption to supplies of blood test tubes in England in 2021, which led to a temporary reduction in non-clinically urgent blood testing (GPOnline 2021).

Although a great deal has been written about leadership and management, much of the literature which delineates between them is underpinned by a weak evidence base (West et al. 2015), with some of the older literature not reflecting the complex systems that characterise healthcare today. Increasing complexity has shaped the development of healthcare leadership and management, with the exponential growth of health services, a blend of public and private providers, a surge in regulators, internal and external markets, technological developments and greater patient acuity making the role of the manager and leader increasingly complicated and vital (The King's Fund 2021).

Good managers bring order and consistency, which can ensure that key dimensions such as quality are maintained, whereas leadership is about coping with change and/or creating disruption (Stanley 2017). Katz's (1955) seminal work describes management as being concerned with directing a group or organisation with a focus on task-orientation, staff development, conflict resolution and the maintenance of ethics and discipline. Kotter (2001) expands this definition, claiming that management is concerned with planning, organising, budgeting, coordinating and monitoring. Likewise, Kotterman (2006) describes managers as focusing on the attainment of short-term goals, risk avoidance and standardisation to enhance efficiency.

Zaleznik's (1977) seminal paper argues that organisations require both effective managers and effective leaders to reach their goals. However, he highlights the different contributions that managers and leaders make, arguing that leaders promote change and are people-orientated, whereas managers promote stability, exercise authority and are task-orientated. He, therefore, makes the point that management and leadership positions require different types of people (Zaleznik 1977), which may be problematic in healthcare with the tendency for role overlap (Stanley 2006; Cutcliffe and Cleary 2015; Nene et al. 2020).

Watson (1983) uses the 'seven Ss' model to differentiate between managerial and leadership roles. The model proposes that managers rely on strategy, structure and systems, in other words, the operational element of organisations, requiring planning, budgeting, organising, staffing, problem solving and controlling. In contrast, Watson (1983) asserts that leaders use the 'softer' Ss – staff, style, shared goals and skills. Later, Bryman (1986) added that leadership is also concerned with strategic motivation.

The Healthcare Leadership Model (NHS Leadership Academy 2021) emphasises that leadership is not necessarily related to seniority within an organisation. In contrast, management roles tend to be dependent upon formal positions and attained through specific training schemes, such as the NHS Graduate Management Training Scheme (NHS Graduate Management Training Scheme 2021). Clinical leaders focus on motivating and inspiring others towards a common goal (Kotter 1990a). They create a passion among others to share their vision, they focus on the attainment of long-term goals, take risks, challenge the status quo and work towards adapting to change (Nene et al. 2020).

In healthcare environments, overlaps between the roles often exist, with managers leading and leaders managing. Kotterman (2006) argues that a well-balanced organisation requires a blend of leaders and managers to succeed. Bennis and Nanus (2005) asserts that 'vision' is the main difference between leadership and management. Management, he states, consists primarily of three things:

- analysis
- problem solving
- planning

whereas leadership consists of:

- vision
- values
- communication of vision and values

With change and innovation characterising modern healthcare, the role of clinical leadership has strengthened over recent years, because it is integral to initiating innovation (Stanley 2017). Innovation and change always demand more leadership (Kotter 1990b) because of its concern with aligning people, setting direction, motivating, inspiring, employing credibility, adopting a visionary position, anticipating change and coping with change (Jones and Bennett 2018).

Management and leadership are, therefore, two different, yet complementary activities (Kotter 1990b). As outlined in Table 5.1, management is a function that must be exercised in any organisation; leadership is a relationship between the leader and the led that can energise an organisation (Stanley 2017).

Reflection Point

In Table 5.1 the emphasis for each factor is presented as extremes on a continuum. For each factor, draw a line that represents each continuum and mark the point that reflects the relative emphasis that you place on leadership or management when working in your clinical area on a day-to-day basis. Repeat the exercise with a change in context, for example, imagine that you are implementing an innovation, that you are dealing with a member of staff's continued lateness, researching an alternative approach to an aspect of patient care or implementation of a maternity leave policy.

Table 5.1 Summary of the difference between factors attributable to leadership and management.

Factors	Leadership	Management
Aims	Change/innovation	Stability/status quo
Objectives	Communication of vision Expression of values	Achievement of organisational aims or objectives
Theoretical approach	Transformational or congruent	Transactional
Relationship with conflict	Uses conflict constructively	Avoids or manages conflict
Relationship to power	Personal charisma/ personality/ values	Formal authority/hierarchical position
Blame/responsibility	Takes the blame	Tends to blame others/processes
Core energy	Passion	Control
Relationship to the led/ managed	Followers	Subordinates
Creativity	Explores new roads/innovation	Travels on existing paths
Main focus	Leading people/establishing new ways	Managing work/tasks/people
Planning	Sets direction	Plans detail
Motivation from	Heart/spirit	Head/mind
Response pattern	Proactive	Reactive
Persuasion style	Sell	Tell
Personal motivation	Excitement for work/ unification of values	Money or other tangible reward/ getting job done
Relationship to rules	Breaks or explores the boundary of rules	Makes or keeps rules
Approach to risk	Takes risks	Minimises risk
Approach to the future	Creates new opportunities/ innovation	Establish systems/processes
Who within an organisation	Anyone/everyone	Those with specific senior hierarchical positions
Relationship to the organisation	Essential	Necessary

Source: Stanley (2011). Reproduced with permission of Springer Nature.

Skills

For centuries, people have debated whether leaders are born or made. Trait theories (see Chapter 2), such as the 'great man' theory, assert that certain people are born to lead and others are born to be led (cited in Morrison 1993). However, more recent research has questioned this belief, and we now know that many leadership qualities and skills can be developed over time (Mumford et al. 2000). The same is true in relation to management qualities.

Reflection Point

Consider whether effective leaders and managers are born or made.

Katz's work in the 1950s is seminal to the skills approach to leadership and management (Katz 1955). His work aimed to address leadership and management in terms of three sets of skills that he argued can be developed: technical, human and conceptual; he asserting that although the significance of each skill may vary depending on the leader's or manager's position within the organisation, each skill is important for success. Technical skills are concerned with knowledge, proficiency and competence in a specific field of work or activity. They also refer to analytical capabilities and the ability to use specialist tools and techniques (Katz 1955). Technical skills are considered more important at the lower levels of the organisational hierarchy (Katz 1955; Goleman 1998). Katz (1955) defined human skills as 'the ability to work effectively as a group member and to build cooperative effort within the team …' (Katz 1955, p. 34). Human skills are characterised by how a leader consistently perceives and behaves towards superiors, peers and followers. Leaders engage in human skills when they motivate individuals and groups, demonstrate empathy and understanding and involve others in decision-making. Human skills are essential throughout all levels of leadership (Katz 1955; Hicks and Gullett 1975). Conceptual skills encompass the 'thinking skills' needed by leaders. This set of skills involves being able to see both the bigger picture in terms of what is going on within the entire organisation, as well as the organisation in terms of its component parts and how they interact and depend on one another (Katz 1955). Conceptual skills are likely to be of most value at the higher levels of the organisational hierarchy where policy decisions and long-term actions are required (Katz 1955; Hicks and Gullett 1975). Whilst dated, this literature is still of relevance today (Jones and Bennett 2018).

Mumford et al. (2000) advanced this work further to develop a skill-based model of leadership, which has also been widely adopted within management. The model examines the relationship between leadership performance and the individual leader's knowledge and skills and asserts that leadership qualities can be developed over time through education, training and experience.

The model is based on the belief that leadership is dependent upon the individual's ability to develop and implement appropriate solutions to complex problems. Mumford et al. (2000) propose that an individual's capacity to problem solve will depend upon:

- *complex problem solving skills,* which are concerned with identifying and understanding the problem and developing potential solutions;
- *social judgement skills,* which involve refining potential solutions and creating ways of implementing solutions within complex organisations;
- *social skills,* which relate to the ability to motivate and direct others during the implementation of solutions.

Application of complex problem-solving skills, social judgement skills and social skills is associated with various forms of knowledge, such as an understanding of the organisation and its processes and an understanding of people, particularly those who will be instrumental in implementing solutions. As with skills, knowledge is believed to develop with experience (Mumford et al. 2000). Mumford et al. (2000) argue that without knowledge, the skills outlined above are inadequate for effective leadership, as knowledge is essential to a leader's ability to define and solve complex organisational problems.

Effective communication is at the heart of effective management and effective leadership. Good communication skills can be broken down into the following:

- Three-level listening: internal listening to what the message means to you, listening to the words and phrases being said, and listening to non-verbal cues (an indication of intentions and feelings)
- Being able to ask powerful questions to achieve clarity
- Knowing the difference between accountability and responsibility. Responsibility (for objects, tasks or people) can be delegated but accountability can't!
- Providing high-quality feedback that can be used immediately
- Managing performance effectively and in a timely way
- Setting clear expectations regularly
- Delegating effectively by utilising the strengths and talents of their team
- Motivating others to achieve professional and organisational goals
- Feeling confident in having difficult conversations
- Coaching others to achieve their potential and overcome challenges (Stanley 2017).

The Need for Education

Whilst acknowledging the pivotal role of front-line leaders and clinical managers in healthcare, as we have acknowledged, the literature suggests that the role is characterised by particular challenges underpinned, largely, by its hybrid nature in that clinical managers are typically required to juggle patient care with leadership roles and vice versa. Consequently, these types of roles are largely part-time and highly demanding. These challenges are also frequently compounded by limited preparatory leadership and management education (Buchanan 2013). The skills- based approach to management and leadership aligns with the need for educational programmes that aim to support participants in developing their leadership and management skills. However, as Leech (2019) points out, in contrast to the clinical education that healthcare professionals receive to support them in their clinical roles, as they progress into leadership and management roles they are more likely to learn through experience, error and luck, due to a lack of availability of professional development opportunities available to staff *before* they take on leadership and management roles. We, therefore, advocate a cultural shift whereby leadership and management development programmes become an integral part of clinicians' continuing professional development.

Clinical Leader Stories: 5 Leaders in Midwifery

During my clinical placement in the post-natal ward, I was fortunate enough to experience a good clinical leader. I have seen many good and bad clinical leaders, but this person stood out as one of the better clinical leaders I have worked with. She was a clinical midwifery educator (CME) on the post-natal ward. She was knowledgeable, clinically competent, had vast experience and had previously worked as a senior RM. Her beliefs and values matched her midwifery practice as she advocated for the women in her care and the students who practiced on the ward. As well, she supported and empowered others, she was an effective communicator and skilled educator. She took her time to explain to me about certain skills I was unsure of and made sure that I knew the reason why each was important to perfect. She ensured staff were up to date with their professional development and ensured they could attend in-services when possible. She educated mothers and families on the ward about caring for newborns and looking for post-natal complications. Although very approachable, she was not always visible on the ward due to her busy schedule, but when she was, she would dedicate her time to help others. The leadership theory relevant to my personal experience with this CME aligns with congruent leadership. This clinical leader demonstrated a match between her values and beliefs of midwifery – with her actions. She believed in respecting, advocating, educating, and supporting others and her actions showed just that. Although she was in a senior position, her actions did not overrule anyone; they rather influenced not only me but other staff to provide safe and quality healthcare. She displayed many desirable attributes of a clinical leader, clinical competence, approachability, great communication skills and being supportive, but she also was a passionate and a committed leader. I am grateful I was able work alongside a great clinical leader in this ward. She enabled me to reflect on the necessary attributes and the importance of being a good clinical leader. I left this ward feeling inspired, well-educated and supported, just like other staff, to put my values and beliefs, respectfully and safely into my actions within practice. I learnt the importance of value-based leadership and practice, and patient, woman and family-centred care. Women and families were often left feeling reassured and confident and had trust in this clinician that many felt sure they could successfully look after their newborn. I learnt the necessary attributes of being an able and effective leader and I will take this knowledge into my future practice as a graduate RM. I also learned that clinical leaders are essential for change and innovation in healthcare to ensure healthcare professionals are consistently delivering safe and quality healthcare to improve patient outcomes.

Maggie: Student Midwife.

Reflection Point

Make an action plan, outlining how you could promote access to leadership and management development programmes for clinicians, as a continuing professional development opportunity, in your place of work.

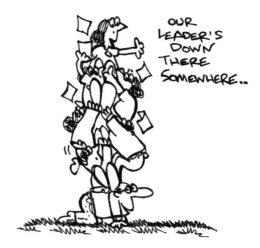

Toxic or Misunderstood?

Leech (2019) argues that '"Management" remains a toxic word for the NHS. Managers have long been associated with a bureaucracy that impedes, rather than improves patient care'. Likewise, The King's Fund (2021) outlines how management is often an unpopular concept across all political parties in the UK, with a desire to decrease the amount of 'management' in the NHS, yet effective management is central to maintaining performance and delivering change. The NHS Leadership Academy (2016) also describes an ill-ease among managers themselves, when taking on management roles or positions, but as they point out, effective management can profoundly impact upon how colleagues experience work and how patients experience healthcare organisations. Indeed, Veronesi et al. (2019) identified that hospitals with greater numbers of managers are characterised by better clinical and financial performance, more satisfied patients and lower infection rates than hospitals with fewer managers.

Kline and Lewis (2019), however, draw attention to how management and bullying can be perceived as synonymous for some employees, with 24% of NHS staff in England reporting having been bullied, harassed and abused by colleagues and managers. In a further paper, Kline (2019) argues that this is symptomatic of how the NHS is managed, with a constant stream of demands being imposed from the national level which, in turn, significantly influences workforce culture. Secondly, he cites cultural norms regarding the avoidance of 'difficult' conversations which illuminate such issues, meaning that staff are unable to share concerns and managers are reluctant to provide opportunities for frank discussions. The third reason that he proposes relates to decades of cut backs and staff shortages, which has led to managers being under immense pressure. A further reason, he argues, centres on flawed human resource systems that rely on individuals bringing bullying to the attention of the employer (Tarrant et al. 2017) rather than implementing proactive and preventative approaches that are underpinned by an evidence base. Finally, he argues that there has been a widespread failure across the NHS to use management and leadership to develop a culture in which staff, including managers themselves, feel valued and respected.

The power of effective management and leadership to positively affect patient outcomes is unquestionable (Kline 2018), but equally, there is no denying that hierarchical approaches to management that are characterised by a lack of openness are problematic and far too common (Kline 2019). Healthcare organisations should, therefore, be inclusive and employ compassionate leadership approaches in order to create a supportive culture for staff, which can reduce staff injuries, bullying, absenteeism and patient mortality (Carter et al. 2008; Kline 2018).

The Future

Reflection Point

What do you perceive as being the key challenges for leadership and management over the next 10 years?

Walker (2016) argues that the increasing complexity of healthcare systems requires a different style of leadership and management. She proposes that traditional hierarchical models should be replaced by an approach whereby accountability is distributed across the multiple stakeholders and that interdisciplinary collaboration is given priority. To bring the various nested systems, or subsystems, across healthcare together, Walker asserts that we need leaders who are able to:

- align purpose and practice
- create and nurture networks
- give up a degree of autonomy to foster interdependency

She also argues that leaders and managers will need to reorientate health services towards wellness and quality, which will create the need for buy-in through effective engagement with stakeholders as well as inspiring the workforce to want to achieve system goals through motivational communication.

Advanced clinical practice has gained momentum across the professions internationally, and this offers significant potential to influence healthcare reform (Rose 2015). Heinen et al. (2019) identified the leadership competencies expected of advanced practice nurses and clinical nurse leaders through a review of the international literature and identified the following themes:

- Clinical leadership
- Professional leadership
- Health system leadership
- Health policy leadership

Greater competence in the first three aspects of leadership are evident in the literature, with less prominence given to the health policy domain (Heinen et al. 2019), which may suggest that the potential of advanced clinical practitioners to shape healthcare reform is yet to be realised. It is time now for advanced clinical practitioners to seize this opportunity and develop the skills outlined by Walker (2016) above, so that their influence across the various facets of the healthcare system can be seen. Indeed, the same could be argued for all healthcare practitioners, but an important point to raise here us that 'all healthcare professionals' are not equal when it comes to leadership and management roles. As Chasma and Khonat (2021) demonstrate, significant racial and ethnic disparities exist in healthcare leadership and management, with Black, Asian and minority ethnic healthcare professionals consistently underrepresented in the NHS. In addition, gender inequalities exist in healthcare leadership, with Walden et al. (2018) highlighting the gender gap in healthcare leadership positions in the United States. For clinical leadership to be truly effective, equality and equity are imperative, so that all communities are represented and their voices heard. While these issues are complex and a full analysis is beyond the scope of this book, we echo Chasma and Khonat's (2021) recommendations that existing clinical leaders and managers should provide support for colleagues who have the potential to develop into leadership and management roles but lack support.

A Culture Shift

This chapter offers the view that leadership and management are different. It also provides evidence that management and leadership functions embodied in the same person, or within the same post, lead to values breach, confusion, conflict and diminished clinical and management effectiveness (Kippist and Fitzgerald 2009; Kerridge 2013; Cutcliffe and Cleary 2015; Nene et al. 2020).

Addressing this issue must surely be considered central to improving the efficiency of clinical areas and to developing sustainable improvements in the quality of patient/client care. The shift in culture to achieve this would be tremendous and has implications for the provision of appropriate continuing professional development and, indeed, maybe even a political shift in healthcare policy. However, the potential benefits in terms of improvements to patient care and staff retention could be tremendous too.

Since the 1970s (Zaleznik 1977), numerous authors have highlighted differences between leadership and management. The health industry is constantly dealing with change, and organisations need both effective and compassionate leaders and managers (Kline 2019). Sometimes it is the manager who fulfils a leadership role, while at other times others within the organisation lead. Indeed, one of the key criticisms of the Francis Inquiry (Francis 2013) was that confusion existed because a care culture had developed where management was separated from ward-level leadership, and where further confusion existed over who should be responsible for care. To suggest that only managers can lead would be a mistake. Maintaining the status quo requires considerable energy, and working as a manager in any health industry organisation demands resilience, commitment and dedication as well as recognition that leadership occurs on many levels. Managers therefore fulfil a vital role.

However, they may not be best placed to be effective clinical leaders. Managers are about stability, running the organisation and keeping things on an even keel. Some managers are able to lead and engage in both stable management tasks and creative risk-taking leadership – but only rarely (Anderson 2012).

Appointing and training people who are asked to function as managers, but with expectations that they will offer dynamic and risk-taking leadership, sets them up to fail or leads them to feel insecure in their role; a point identified by Vize (2015) in relation to medical practitioners' reluctance to take on 'senior managerial' roles in the NHS. Across all professional disciplines these practices are almost epidemic in proportion. No one wins and the health industry and patients suffer, as the Mid Staffordshire inquiry shows (Francis 2013). Clinical leaders with significant management responsibilities are potentially placed in positions of diminished clinical effectiveness (Vize 2015; Kline 2019). Ward managers, advanced clinical practitioners and a host of other senior clinical staff with managerial responsibilities find themselves climbing the managerial ladder, only to slide down the clinical snake. Advancing themselves or their organisation's objectives is too often at the cost of effective clinical leadership, often depriving some (neophyte healthcare professionals and unskilled or semi-trained carers at the bedside) of their guidance and clinical leadership that could significantly improve patient/client care.

For a genuine opportunity to develop more efficient clinical management and clearer, more effective clinical leadership, it may be time to accept that having leadership and management functions reside in one person or post is inefficient and counterproductive, both to the individual concerned and to the health service's future development and success.

Recognising the difference between leadership and management will also allow professional development to embrace education focused on leadership development that is based on clinical practice, and not simply management principles overlaid on clinical functions.

Case Study 5.1   Joan of Arc

Joan of Arc is one of France's national heroes. Born in 1412, she was a simple peasant girl who, at the age of 12 or 14, heard the 'voices of the saints', Michael, Catherine and Margaret, calling her to save France from the English. With this divine inspiration she rose to become a soldier, leader, martyr and finally a saint herself. She was convinced that God had called her to free France, and she showed remarkable moral courage and significant military leadership to inspire the demoralised, humiliated and discredited French army to fight on during the Hundred Years' War. Read this brief account of her life and consider the challenge that follows.

Joan defied convention and the obstructions of statesmen, churchmen and generals to follow her divine beliefs. She travelled across war-torn France to seek an audience with the Dauphin Charles, the uncrowned son of the previous king, Charles VI. Her quiet determination and religious devotion led to her gaining access to the Dauphin, and she persuaded him to allow her to lead his army to lift the siege of Orleans. Clad in white armour and wielding a battleaxe, Joan led the army to a stunning victory in only nine days and became known as the 'Maid of Orleans'. There is some debate about the contribution she made in actually planning or fighting during the battle, as her testimony

(Continued)

during her later trial implied that she preferred the standard to the sword. She may have been more influential on a motivational level, but she clearly had a dramatic impact on the reversal of the French army's fortunes. The English reviled her as a witch who must have had some sort of supernatural power. Other victories followed, and she witnessed the crowning of Charles VII at Rheims before convincing the new king to continue his offensive and liberate other parts of France.

In an attempt to lift the siege of Compiègne, Joan was captured by the Burgundians, sold to the English and tried as a heretic. She was so convinced of her divine mission that interrogators decided it would be useless to torture her, but when the church threatened to hand Joan over to the secular courts, she confessed to heresy and agreed to put on women's clothes again. She was sentenced to life in prison, but her 'voices' returned and she recanted. As a result, she was handed over to the secular authorities and at the age of 19 she was burnt at the stake as a witch. Charles VII, wishing to maintain the truce with Burgundy and not wanting to be seen to be associated with a witch, failed to intervene.

Joan's devotion and belief were unwavering, and as she died a priest shouted above the flames that she was assured of eternal salvation. The English were so concerned that no relic of her should remain that they burnt her body three times and scattered the dust from her ashes in the river Seine.

Twenty years later, Charles VII, now with a safe hold on the French throne, supported an inquiry into Joan's trial. Her conviction was overturned, and 500 years later, in 1920, the Roman Catholic Church made her a saint. Joan of Arc has remained a significant figure in Western culture, and in French politics the memory of Joan's devotion to the salvation of her country is often evoked.

As with the varied and vexing definitions of leadership, the story of Joan of Arc offers a contrary insight into leadership, when in an age of war and male dominance, a simple peasant girl rose to lead an army and conquer the English and their assumptions about strength and determination.

Challenge: Joan was able to lead the French Army into battle and stir the men to follow her and believe in her, in spite of their previous string of defeats. Was this leadership or management? To what extent are clinical leaders in positions of leading without managerial authority? How is it that leaders can motivate followers when they have little direct managerial authority or sometimes little awareness that they are even seen as leaders? When your values or beliefs are challenged, how strongly do you feel that you can hold on to them? Few female health professionals are threatened with being burnt alive; although this was not always the case, as Ehrenreich and English (1973) attest. To what extent does gender play a role in people's assessment of leadership potential today? (See Chapter 17 for more on this issue.)

Summary

- Leadership and management are different, but remain complementary.
- Misunderstanding the differences can lead to values conflict, confusion, a challenge to the clinician's values and beliefs, disassociation from the clinician's core clinical values, and ineffective leadership and management.

- There is considerable evidence that management and leadership functions, when embodied in the same person or within the same post, lead to confusion, conflict and diminished clinical and management effectiveness.
- Clinicians with managerial responsibilities find themselves climbing the managerial ladder at the expense of their clinical career, advancing themselves, or the employer's objectives, at the cost of effective clinical leadership.
- There may be other, more effective, productive and satisfying models for the facilitation of management and leadership approaches in clinical areas, such as the availability of continuing professional development opportunities being made available to staff *before* they embark on a leadership or management role.

Mind Press-Ups

Exercise 5.1

Think about your formative healthcare education. What did you learn about management? Was this adequate? Do you think that there are other matters or topics that health professionals should learn about to ensure that they are skilled managers (e.g. financial management, human resources management)? Did your formative healthcare education prepare you to function as an effective manager?

Exercise 5.2

Think about a leader (from your work, from history, politics, or any walk of life) whom you admire, look up to or have been inspired by. Write a short summary about what it is or was about them that you admire, respect or identify with. Look at the qualities and characteristics of leadership and management you have described. How do they match?

Now do the same, but this time think about a manager whom you admire, look up to or have been inspired by. Repeat the process. Again, how do the qualities and characteristics of leadership and management match?

Exercise 5.3

Are clinical leadership, management and profession-specific leadership different? Think for a moment about these three concepts and how they relate to your professional position. Is there something happening in the health service (wherever you work) that implies a shift in the way things are being done? Are we seeing the rise of leadership? If so, how is this manifest in practice? What do your colleagues think?

Exercise 5.4

In researching the difference between leadership and management in the health service, trying to undertake both roles (leadership and management in the one position) was found often to lead to considerable conflict. Have you ever experienced the types of values-based conflict suggested here?

References

Anderson, L. (2012). Difference between nurse leadership vs. management. http://Nursetogether.com, http://www.nursetogether.com/difference-between-nurse-leadership-(accessed 8 January 2016).

Bass, B. (2010). *The Bass Handbook of Leadership: Theory, Research, and Managerial Applications*. New York: Simon & Schuster.

Bennis, W.G. (1989). *On Becoming a Leader*. New York: Basic Books.

Bennis, W.G. and Nanus, B. (2005). *Leaders Strategies for Taking Charge*, 2e. New York: Harper Collins.

Bryman, A. (1986). *Leadership and Organizations*. London: Routledge.

Buchanan, D.A. (2013). How do they Manage? A Qualitative Study of the Realities of Middle and Front-line Management Work in Health Care. http://www.nets.nihr.ac.uk/projects/hsdr/081808238 (accessed 8 September 2021).

Carter, M., West, M., Dawson, J. et al. (2008) Developing team-based working in NHS trusts. Report prepared for the Department of Health. (accessed 8 September 2021).

Chasma, F. and Khonat, Z. (2021). How equal is access to senior management leadership roles in the NHS? *British Journal of Healthcare Management*, https://doi.org/10.12968/bjhc.2021.0057 (accessed 8 September 2021).

Cutcliffe, J. and Cleary, M. (2015). Nursing leadership, missing questions and the elephants in the room: problematizing the discourse on nursing leadership. *Issues in Mental Health Nursing* 36: 817–825.

Ehrenreich, B. and English, D. (1973). *Witches, Midwives, and Nurses: A History of Women Healers,* Issues 1–2. Feminist Press.

Francis, R. (2013). *Report of the Mid Staffordshire NHS Foundation Trust Public Inquiry*. London: HM Stationery Office.

Goleman, D. (1998). What makes a leader? *Harvard Business Review* 76 (6): 93–102.

GPOnline (2021). GPs told to stop non-essential blood tests amid shortage of tubes. https://www.gponline.com/gps-told-stop-non-essential-blood-tests-amid-shortage-tubes/article/1724562 (accessed 1 September 2021).

Gumbo, T. (2017). Unpacking the role of leadership and management styles in teaching and research output in South African higher education. Faculty of Engineering and the Built Environment, University of Johannesburg, Johannesburg.

Heinen, M., van Oostveen, C., Peters, J. et al. (2019). An integrative review of leadership competencies and attributes in advanced nursing practice. *Journal of Advanced Nursing* 75 (11): 2378–2392.

Hicks, H.G. and Gullett, C.R. (1975). *Organizations: Theory and Behavior*. New York: McGraw-Hill Book Company.

Jones, L. and Bennett, C.L. (2018). *Leadership for Nursing, Health and Social Care Students*. Banbury: Lantern Publishers.

Katz, R.L. (1955). Skills of an effective administrator. *Harvard Business Review* 33 (1): 33–42.

Kerridge, J. (2013). Why management skills are a priority for nurses. *Nursing Times* 109 (9): 16–17.

King, M.L. (1965). Excerpt from Rev. King's sermon on courage, delivered on March 8, 1965 in Selma, Alabama.

Kippist, L. and Fitzgerald, A. (2009). Organisational professional conflict and hybrid clinician managers: the effects of dual roles in Australian health care organisations. *Journal of Health Organizations and Management* 23 (6): 642.

Kline, R. (2018). Diversity and inclusion are not optional extras if the NHS wishes to improve. *Health Service Journal*, https://www.hsj.co.uk/equality-and-diversity/diversity-and-inclusion-are-notoptional-extras-if-the-nhs-wishes-to-improve/7023599 (accessed 8 September 2021).

Kline, R. (2019). Leadership in the NHS. *BMJ Leader* 3 (4): 129–132.

Kline, R. and Lewis, D. (2019). The price of fear: estimating the financial cost of bullying and harassment to the NHS in England. *Public Money and Management* 39 (3): 166–174.

Kotter, J.P. (1990a). What leaders really do. In: *Harvard Business Review on Leadership* (ed. M.A. Boston), 37–60. Harvard Business School Press.

Kotter, J.P. (1990b). *A Force for Change: How Leadership Differs from Management*. New York: Free Press.

Kotter, J.P. (2001). What leaders really do. *Harvard Business Review* 79 (11): 85–96.

Kotterman, J. (2006). Leadership versus management: what's the difference? *The Journal for Quality and Participation* 29 (2): 13–17.

Leech, D. (2019). Leadership and management are two different roles – what is your job, really?. *National Health Executive*. https://www.nationalhealthexecutive.com/Health-Service-Focus/leadership-and-management-are-two-different-roles--what-is-your-job-really (accessed 8 September 2021).

Morrison, M. (1993). *Professional Skills for Leadership: Foundations for a Successful Career*. St Louis: Mosby.

Mumford, M.D., Zaccaro, S.J., Harding, F.D. et al. (2000). Leadership skills for a changing world: solving complex social problems. *The Leadership Quarterly* 11 (1): 11–35.

Nene, S.E., Ally, H., and Nkosi, E. (2020). Nurse managers experiences of their leadership roles in a specific mining primary healthcare service in the West Rand. *Curationis* 43 (1): 1–8.

NHS Graduate Management Training Scheme (2021) NHS Graduate Management Training Scheme. https://graduates.nhs.uk (accessed 8 September 2021).

NHS Leadership Academy (2016). 8 ways to be a better manager. https://www.leadershipacademy.nhs.uk/8-ways-to-be-a-better-manager (accessed 8 September 2021).

NHS Leadership Academy (2021). Healthcare leadership model. https://www.leadershipacademy.nhs.uk/resources/healthcare-leadership-model (accessed 8 September 2021).

Orvik, A., Vagen, S.R., Axelsson, S.B., and Axelsson, R. (2015). Quality, efficiency and integrity: value squeezes in management of hospital wards. *Journal of Nursing Management* 23: 65–74.

Rose, L. (2015). Better Leadership for Tomorrow: NHS Leadership Review. https://www.gov. uk/government/publications/better-leadership-for-tomorrow-nhs-leadership-review (accessed 8 September 2021).

Scully, N.J. (2015). Leadership in nursing: the importance of recognising inherent values and attributes to secure a positive future for the profession. *Collegian* 22 (4): 439–444.

St George, A. (2012). *Royal Navy way of Leadership.* London: Preface.

Stanley, D. (2006). Role conflict: leaders and managers. *Nursing Management* 13 (5): 31–37.

Stanley, D. (2011). *Clinical Leadership. Innovation into action.* Palgrave: Macmillan.

Stanley, D. (2017). *Clinical Leadership in Nursing and Healthcare*, 2e. Chichester: Wiley Blackwell.

Tarrant, C., Leslie, M., Bion, J., and Dixon-Woods, M. (2017). A qualitative study of speaking out about patient safety concerns in intensive care units. *Social Science and Medicine* 193: 8–15.

The King's Fund (2021). The changing role of managers in the NHS. https://www.kingsfund. org.uk/publications/future-leadership-and-management-nhs/changing-role-of-NHS-managers (accessed 1 September 2021).

Veronesi, G., Kirkpatrick, I., and Altanlar, A. (2019). Are public sector managers a "bureaucratic burden"? The case of English public hospitals. *Journal of Public Administration and Research Theory* 29 (2): 193–209.

Vize, R. (2015). Why doctors don't dare go into management. *The BMJ* 350 (922): 16–18.

Walden, T., Snapp, H., Morgenstein, K., and Gregory, L. (2018). Starting the discussion about equality and equity in leadership. *Audiology Today* 30 (3): 37–47.

Walker, D. (2016). Managing moving pieces. In: *Talent Management*, 42–46.

Watson, C.M. (1983). Leadership, management and the seven keys. *Business Horizons* 26 (2): 8–13.

West, M., Armit, K., Loewenthal, L., Eckert, R. et al. (2015). Leadership and Leadership Development in Health Care: The Evidence Base, London: Faculty of Medical Leadership and Management/King's Fund/Center for Creative Leadership, http://www.kingsfund.org. uk/sites/files/kf/field/field_publication_file/leadership-leadership-development-health-care-feb-2015.pdf (accessed 1 September 2021).

Wood, C. (2021). Leadership and management for nurses working at an advanced level. *British Journal of Nursing* 30 (5): 282–286.

Wynendaele, H., Gemmel, P., Pattyn, E. et al. (2021). Systematic review: what is the impact of self-scheduling on the patient, nurse and organization? *Journal of Advanced Nursing* 77: 47–82.

Zaleznik, A. (1977). Managers and leaders: are they different? In: *Harvard Business Review on Leadership* (ed. M.A. Boston), 61–88. Harvard Business School Press.

Part II

Clinical Leadership Tools: How to Influence Quality, Innovation and Change

Man is a tool-using animal. Without tools he is nothing, with tools he is all.
Thomas Carlyle, Scottish philosopher, 1795–1881, from Sartor Resartus, 1834

The second part of this book deals with how clinical leaders who act in concert with their values can initiate change, enhance quality care, lead innovation and support their own development. Primarily, each chapter offers practical information about a range of 'tools' or topics that clinically focused health professional leaders can use to support a focus on values-based care and compassion-driven practice, as well as to lead innovation, quality initiatives and change practice through the employment of a congruent leadership style.

Chapter 6 discusses the relationship of organisational culture to congruent and values-based leadership and clinical leadership. Recognising that values are the primary driver for organisational culture change is central to this chapter's position. Chapter 7 offers a range of models for managing change. If the clinically focused leader's values are to be translated into action, a clear understanding is required of how to bring about innovation and change. Therefore, clinically focused health professionals need to understand models and processes that can be used to support the effective implementation of change. A range of models are offered in this chapter, including SWOT analysis, stakeholder analysis, Pettigrew's context/content/process model, the change management iceberg, the PEST model, Kotter's eight-stage change process model, the nominal group technique, process re-engineering and force-field analysis. Other approaches are mentioned and there is also a discussion of why health professionals may be resistant to change. Chapter 8 considers how clinical leaders make decisions and the relevance of that decision making. The core part of the chapter outlines potential strategies and refers to models, such as shared-decision making, that foster effective clinical decision making. Theories that support decision making are also outlined, along with a discussion of why decisions may go wrong, group decision making and the significance of decision making for clinical leaders. Chapter 9 explores the issue of creativity and why it is an important concept for clinical leaders seeking to initiate change, promote innovation and stand by their values. The chapter defines creativity, explores how

Clinical Leadership in Nursing and Healthcare, Third Edition.
Edited by David Stanley, Clare L. Bennett and Alison H. James.
© 2023 John Wiley & Sons Ltd. Published 2023 by John Wiley & Sons Ltd.

creative capacity can be built and considers what the barriers to creativity may be. It also elaborates on the significance of understanding creativity from a clinical leader's perspective. For clinical leaders to be effective they need a reasonable understanding of how teams function, why teams may sometimes fail to deliver and how they themselves can support the creation of powerful teams. Chapter 10 offers this information, as well as a discussion of the value of team working and the role of team members. The chapter also considers self-led teams and the impact of leadership on a team's ability to deliver. Chapter 11 focuses on networking and delegation, two essential skills for clinical leaders to acquire or hone. Networking is first explored in terms of the skills needed and strategies that can be used to enhance it. Then the skills of delegation are described so that clinical leaders can develop successful delegation attributes and strategies.

Conflict is recognised as a feature of most work environments and is central to the professional dichotomy between values-led care and other drivers for clinical practice. Chapter 12 offers information about how conflict is recognised, the different styles of dealing with it and how clinical leaders can more effectively manage conflict. Non-productive behaviour types are also outlined and approaches such as active listening, self-talk and I-messages are elaborated as strategies for coping with conflict. Chapter 13 offers information about motivation and inspiration, vital aspects of clinical leadership. The chapter considers approaches to motivating others and how people are inspired to follow and engage, with steps to improve patient care and the health service. In effecting change and initiating innovation, clinical leaders will benefit from an understanding of evidence-based practice. Chapter 14 provides an introduction to strategies to creating a spirit of enquiry and developing evidence-based research practice habits. The barriers to using evidence in practice, approaches to applying evidence-based practice and strategies for addressing the practice, research and education nexus are also discussed. Chapter 15 is about reflection and emotional intelligence. This chapter outlines what reflection is and how it can be used as a tool to support clinical leaders' development. It also describes what emotional intelligence is and how it can be applied in the clinical context. Moreover, the chapter considers how clinical leaders can employ emotional intelligence to focus on their own values and beliefs and use them in a productive and care-enhancing way. Finally, Chapter 16 explores the central place of quality initiatives and project management in helping clinical leaders express their values meaningfully and constructively. Learning where clinical leaders can direct their energies to greatest effect is central to magnifying the power of their values in the clinical domain.

6

Organisational Culture and Clinical Leadership

Sally Carvalho and David Stanley

> *Values aren't buses . . . they're not supposed to get you anywhere.*
> *They're supposed to define who you are.*
> > Jennifer Crusie, b.1949, author of *Maybe This Time* and many other novels

Introduction: Values First

This chapter addresses the relationship of organisational culture and leadership, and specifically the vital place that congruent leadership can play in helping leaders shape or influence an organisation's culture. In the introduction to the *Culture of Care Barometer* (Rafferty et al. 2015) it is made clear 'that quality and culture are not uniform within, let alone across organisations'. And as a result, the 'lack of consistency in care culture impedes the spread of good practice across organisations' (Rafferty et al. 2015, p. 6). The introduction goes on to suggest that in the main, 'failures are not usually brought to light by the systems . . . such as incidence reporting, mortality and morbidity reviews, inspections, accreditations clinical profiling and risk and claim management' (Rafferty et al. 2015, p. 6). This is because these approaches fail to capture the reality for most patients or clients and for health professional staff. Instead, it is only by understanding and influencing the 'culture of care' that genuine change and improvement can be made, with culture being seen as everybody's business and central to the way things are done within each organisation.

What Is Organisational Culture?

Organisational culture is not an easy concept to pin down, and it is vague and slippery at best, with many organisations unsure of what it is and how to change or guide it (Hall 2005). Schein defines culture as

Clinical Leadership in Nursing and Healthcare, Third Edition.
Edited by David Stanley, Clare L. Bennett and Alison H. James.
© 2023 John Wiley & Sons Ltd. Published 2023 by John Wiley & Sons Ltd.

a pattern of shared basic assumptions that the group learned as it solved its problems of external adaption and internal integration, that has worked well enough to be considered valid and, therefore, to be taught to new members as the correct way to perceive, think, and feel in relation to those problems. (Schein 2010, p. 17)

Hall (2005) aids in our understanding of organisational culture by suggesting that every organisation, regardless of its size, age or industry, has a culture. Hall adds that what separates leading organisations from each other is their ability to shape or direct the culture to bolster their business or support the organisation to better achieve its goals. In addition, organisations also find that they engage the 'hearts and minds' of their employees or create an environment where people are inspired to achieve extraordinary results (Hall 2005, p. 1).

Davies et al. (2000) suggest that there are two ways to conceptualise organisational culture. First, organisational culture can be seen as something that an organisation 'is'. Seen in this way, the social interaction of people within the culture makes the organisation and becomes the organisation. The second view of organisational culture is that an organisation has a culture of which it is part, but which is separate from the organisation and is described as one of its attributes (Davies et al. 2000; Scott et al. 2003). From this second perspective, it is possible to conceptualise organisational culture as something that can be modified, created or even managed (Davies et al. 2000).

The analogy of an iceberg is often used to represent the 'seen' and 'unseen' elements within an organisational culture. The 'seen' elements are described as the surface manifestations of the culture (rites and rituals) that are commonly thought to be more readily manipulated and open to change. The 'unseen' elements represent the deeper beliefs, feelings and values that are often below the surface, out of view and far more difficult to recognise or change. It is these deeper elements that are described as a reflection of the values of the organisation and point to its approach to key issues such as safety, quality and, in healthcare, compassion, patient care and a client-focused perspective (West et al. 2014).

However, there is far more to organisational culture than the definitions would suggest. An organisation's culture (in fact any culture) is deeply embedded, grown from shared emotional experiences, which are often unconscious and made up of mutual basic assumptions and beliefs that guide how people relate to each other. From this initial outline it can be seen that there are clear links between congruent leadership theory and shaping and developing an organisation's culture.

Culture also describes how things 'are done around here' (Fowke 1999, p. 1) and offers a source of stability, helping employees, customers, students or patients and clients recognise where their place is in the complex structures and systems of a large organisation. Culture is based on often unquestioned assumptions about values and beliefs, with each member of the organisation's culture commonly fitting in, or getting on, even if they do not realise that they are working towards shared basic assumptions and core beliefs. This may go some way to explaining why some congruent leaders do not recognise that it is their shared values and beliefs that mark them out as leaders.

Cultures are built from pivotal events (stories, myths and ceremonies) that form the bedrock of shared beliefs and values. As such, it is values and beliefs that are used to build an organisation's culture; again, this is why an appreciation of congruent leadership is so vital.

That said, an organisational culture can be built or made by design (or default), implying that if a culture is not consciously constructed or structured with intent, it will be grown from the power and influence of members of the organisation, or subcultures within a larger organisation, and become embedded of its own accord.

An organisational culture has a social energy built over time and it is something that can also change, over time. In fact, organisational cultures are always changing, as new staff, new employees, new managers, new circumstances and new politics or policies come into play on the goals, values, direction and actions of the organisation. Indeed, any organisation that does not embrace change will not survive (Handy 1999; Hall 2005). The message is, to be the master of the direction that the organisational culture takes so that the people with an investment in it can feel, at least in part, in charge of that direction.

Box 6.1   Why Did the *Titanic* Hit an Iceberg?

The story of how passenger liner RMS *Titanic* hit an iceberg in 1912 is well known and celebrated in film and literature. But why did it happen?

The answer is not a dark night, a still sea, minimal lookouts or the ship's swift passage through the sea, although they all played a part. The real reason is more central to organisational culture than you might think.

The captain, Edward Smith, knew about the presence of icebergs in the Atlantic Ocean, as the crew had been warned by at least one other vessel. He knew that speed put the ship at greater risk and he knew that the best course of action was to go slower. However, safety was not the driving value of the White Star Line, the company that owned the *Titanic*. What was of value to this organisation was speed and getting the record for crossing the Atlantic. The owner of the company, Joseph Ismay, was on board that night. He instructed the captain to ignore the iceberg warnings and to go as fast as possible.

Had the organisational culture valued safety, the ship would have gone more slowly, been designed with more lifeboats and put more value on the lives of the people on board than on the possibility of a record speed. The company's reputation and profits were based on speed and not safety, so it was this that drove the crew to ignore the warnings and go as fast as they could on the cold, still, dark night. Until they hit the iceberg.

Therefore, organisational culture is something that is constantly evolving and reacting to changes in the surrounding environment, such as the observation of Brooks (2009), who considers the NHS to be an organisation driven by the culture of the UK, noting that all four countries within the UK operate their healthcare systems individually, fostering their own subcultures. As such, organisational culture remains a matter of choice. It can be accepted, rejected or redesigned. However, even if it is not attended to, it is still there, invisible and all pervasive unless there is a move to try to change it.

An organisation's vision may assist in setting its direction and goals, and it may be these that help it see its way to the future. However, it is the organisation's culture that helps it get though day-to-day activities and thrive, survive or dive (see Box 6.1). It is the extent to which the managers and organisational 'brains trust' realise that culture is the key that enables an organisation to make it home, or hit an iceberg. The most recent evidence of this has been through the emergency responses worldwide to the healthcare needs resulting from the COVID -19 (SARS-CoV-2) pandemic; each country's response was driven by their individual healthcare organisation's culture.

Reflection Point

Talk to people in the area in which you work about what they think makes up or influences the organisational culture. How do their views link with or counter those in this chapter? And does it matter whether they do?

A Culture of Care and Compassion

It is clear that an organisation's culture is influenced by economic, political, legal and technological elements, and by the context within which the organisation operates (Rytterstrom et al. 2013). In addition, the culture is influenced by the dominant cultural views and behaviours of the majority of the organisation's members. These factors combined create the principal values, beliefs, norms and meanings that individuals infuse into the work they do. However, West (2021) recognised that those who work to inspire and support the health and well-being of all in health and social care settings are often affected by corroding cultures of compassion, which often harms their own health.

Therefore, the creation of an organisational culture of care and compassion is based on reinforcing the significance of care and compassion as key attributes, beliefs and values that build meaning and life into the organisation's culture. The central aspect of creating and maintaining a culture based on care and compassion relates to reinforcing and rewarding employees and members of the organisation who act on these values and beliefs and deliver performance consistent with the desired culture (Rytterstrom et al. 2013). Such a culture is known as 'supportive' (Luthans et al. 2008) and it is built on the practice of energising and fostering the activity of the organisation's members (in all positions) to value and behave in caring and supportive ways. However, Pink (2009) considers that it is through helping the individual within an organisation to understand what motivates them that a sense of purpose is fostered through intrinsic internal processes which will be reflected within the organisation as it evolves, resulting in an organisation of high-performing and satisfied members.

In 2015, the UK's Department of Health released a document entitled *Culture Change in the NHS: Applying the Lessons of the Francis Inquiry* (DoH 2015). In it, there is a recognition that while a culture change has begun, sustaining cultural change will only be possible if doctors, nurses and front-line staff feel free to speak out when they have concerns. This has led to a deliberate drive to ensure that the NHS is the 'most open and transparent (health) system in the world on key measures of patient safety and patient experiences' (DoH 2015, p. 7). To achieve this, a number of positive measures have been introduced, including the first national guardian for freedom to speak up in the NHS (Middleton 2016). This is in response to the new legal duty known as the duty of candour (DoH 2015), which places a responsibility on all NHS organisations to ensure that if anything does go wrong, patients and their relatives are informed immediately. It also makes clear that front-line clinicians, closest to patient care and the implications of poor judgements, need to have a voice in addressing problems with the healthcare culture (Middleton 2016). Another initiative is the introduction of a 'name above the bed' system, which will allow relatives and patients to know who is in charge of their care and who is accountable and responsible for their welfare. These few examples are evidence that change is taking place and, while only the beginning, that a series of initiatives aimed at making the NHS more open and transparent are being fostered. In addition, an unprecedented and bold effort has been made to capture feedback from patients, clients and their relatives using online and paper-based surveys, such as the Friends and Family Test (introduced in April 2013), to ask patients whether they would recommend their hospital to their friends and family (DoH 2015). Such is the value placed on NHS service users' and stakeholders' opinions that the Care Quality Commission (CQC 2015) conducted a national survey of patients who had received care in 154 acute and specialist NHS Trusts. The feedback is being used to bolster and support the positive steps that health professionals are taking to build a culture of care and compassion.

However, the NHS has also recognised that staff need a feedback mechanism too. Thus, in order to promote a positive emphasis on a transparent health service, NHS staff are supported and engaged to be confident about providing feedback on their own employing organisation's culture using the Staff Friends and Family Test (introduced in 2014), with results and case studies readily available on the NHS England website.

These changes and initiatives from the UK Department of Health and NHS Trust managers are essential, because where organisational members see a lack of care and compassion, for their welfare, for their skills or for the contribution they could or do make, or if feedback is used as a stick to beat staff, the message that is reinforced is that the organisation does not care for them, does not value them or their skills, and that employees are simply replaceable resources. This fosters a culture where suspicion, bullying, a lack of care and compassion and mistreatment are dominant (Francis 2013; Rytterstrom et al. 2013).

Where this style of culture develops there are inevitable consequences compromising patients, examples being the Public Inquiry related to children's heart surgery at the Bristol Royal Infirmary (Kennedy 2001) and the 33 patient deaths at Stoke Mandeville during an outbreak of *Clostridium Difficile* infection (Kennedy 2006), and more recently, the investigation into maternity and neonatal care services of the University Hospitals of Morecambe Bay NHS Foundation Trust between January 2004 and June 2013 (Kirkup 2015).

Moreover, all of the organisation's staff need to be trained and educated so that they can articulate their concerns when they do speak up. The training should include guidance and education about the pivotal place of values and beliefs when they are translated into actions (Stanley 2011; DoH 2015). While realising that the key staff of the health service are clinical staff, the Department of Health (2015) also recognises that leaders are central to shaping culture and that it is essential for leaders to be supported and educated to provide effective, culturally appropriate leadership based on an organisation's foundational values. This again points to the place of congruent leadership in helping foster education for leaders at all levels, but most significantly clinically focused leaders.

In the health arena (as in any industry/organisation), the powerful place of culture means that the dominant culture is fostered and infused into the organisation's product. If the product is healthcare, support and compassion, then it will be little surprise to find that quality healthcare, client support and compassion will fail to be consistently delivered if the dominant cultural narrative is negative, non-supportive or non-responsive. As Turkel (2006), Ranheim et al. (2011) and Rytterstrom et al. (2013) indicate, the mistreatment of staff can serve as an example of how poor care practices are influenced by a culture where care and compassion are not valued, as was identified by the Care Quality Commission's investigations related to poor patient care at Winterbourne View Hospital (DoH 2012).

Reflection Point

Access the NHS England website https://www.england.nhs.uk/fft/case-studies for case study reports where respondents to the 'Staff Friends and Family Test' have influenced cultural change. During your clinical practice experience, have you participated in providing your organisation with feedback about its performance, and did you experience any changes to the organisation's culture as a result?

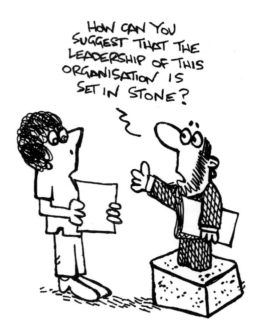

Culture and Leadership

For some time now, the health industry has recognised that to improve it has to develop or enact new cultural practices through new values and beliefs to initiate new ways of working (Mannion et al. 2008; Mannion et al. 2009). In the UK, the Department of Health has specifically identified the need for leadership education and training (DoH 2015, p. 16), because 'the right leaders are critical in shaping culture'. As such, it has recognised that with the right understanding of these leaders' values and the impact they have on how they lead, a greater effect on shaping organisational culture is likely. Reforms in government policy, organisational strategies and strategic documents across the globe have also called for improvements in organisational performance and better clinical care (Francis 2013; DoH 2015), with many focusing on how leaders can better support a value-based organisational culture.

The Francis Report (Francis 2013) offers the clearest example of such a document, with the dominant themes of its 290 recommendations indicating that at the core of the problems in Mid Staffordshire NHS Trust was a failure of organisational culture. This was followed in 2015 by a further report, *Sir Robert Francis' Freedom to Speak Up Review* (Francis 2015), which also highlighted the centrality of a culture of safety and learning becoming part of everyday practice. Even more recently, the CQC (2018) reported the strong link between the safety of services and the quality of the leadership, whilst NHS England and NHS Improvement (2019) published their strategy for maintaining patient safety with a clear focus upon developing safer cultures within the NHS.

What these and other reports and reviews have identified is that for organisations to address failures, they need to deal not with quality processes or quality assurance measures but with building or influencing their cultural practices and with how leaders within organisations do this in a positive way.

The key to this link lies in the actions of the organisation towards its employees. As congruent leadership theory indicates, leaders are followed because they put into practice their values and beliefs. These can be positive values as well as negative ones: staff follow the lead of people identified as 'leaders' and if they are treated in negative ways (not listened to, mistreated, bullied, ignored or not valued for their skills or efforts), then it will not be a surprise if they copy these behaviours or see them as central to the organisation. This is especially the case if the leaders they see behaving in this way are promoted, rewarded and even awarded. West et al. (2014) indicate that how staff talk to each other can help shape the organisation's culture, but significantly, these same staff reported that their behaviours were based on observations of how other staff were spoken to.

The role of the senior executive is vital in setting the tone for an organisation's culture. The King's Fund (2012) sought to elaborate the characteristics of an engaged form of leadership in response to research conducted by Storey et al. (2010) identifying the damage caused by over-dominant chief executives. As Hall (2005) and Storey and Holti (2013) indicate, most employees will see leaders at many levels, and in this regard, it is the actions and behaviours of mid- or lower level 'leaders' that are more likely to be dominant in setting an organisation's cultural tone. Rafferty et al. (2015) indicate that in health and clinically focused organisations, it will be clinically focused leaders who act to enrich the environment and deliver the key message about whether staff are valued or supported. Again, congruent leadership theory, which as already outlined has grown from attempts to understand clinical leadership, helps explain why clinical leaders are identified and followed and the significance of this theory in terms of linking leadership, actions, values and beliefs, all of which are central to setting, directing or modifying an organisation's culture.

> **Reflection Point**
>
> Read and reflect on the Winterbourne View hospital inquiry (DoH 2012) at https://www.gov.uk/government/publications/winterbourne-view-hospital-department-of-health-review-and-response
>
> The organisational culture at Winterbourne View was such that the senior nurse managers were exasperated at their powerlessness to challenge poor care, despite their qualifications and accountability, because they had less power than the front-line staff. This is an example of an organisational culture where the people perceived to have the least power actually had the most. What are some of the pivotal events that have built the culture of the ward, clinic or unit you work on? What does this mean in terms of creating or shaping culture? Can cultures be made or shaped by clinical leaders? If so, how might they go about it?
>
> Read how the report has since helped to shape the organisational culture at https://www.gov.uk/government/publications/winterbourne-view-2-years-on

How Congruent Leaders Shape Culture

It is possible to change an organisation's culture. However, this is not possible unless it is understood that organisations have more than just cultures – they have cultures, structures and systems. Each of these elements is vital and without all of them the organisation would crumble. The structure offers a skeleton for the organisation, helping link responsibilities, roles, frameworks, facilities and equipment. Systems deal with how processes work and how people interact. The culture is about 'people . . . not cash, equipment, facilities or even product and in a service focused organisation (e.g. the health industry) . . . culture is *the* critical variable' (Fitz-Enz 1997, p. 50).

Organisational cultures can change when the values and beliefs that constitute them are challenged. This point is supported by the NHS Leadership Academy, which asserts:

> Leaders create a shared purpose for diverse individuals doing work, inspiring them to believe in shared values so that they deliver benefits for patients, their families and the community. (NHS Leadership Academy 2013, p. 5)

Congruent leadership is not directly focused on change, but congruent leaders can influence change by acting in concert with their own values and beliefs, especially if these offer an alternative to the current, dominant or prevailing culture. Indeed, this is evident now in many organisations that are led by leaders who demonstrate their values and beliefs. However, these may be at odds with a culture of support, care and compassion, so that other values are on display and foster less productive, more negative cultures. Working to shape an organisation's culture becomes central to the facilitation of lasting and meaningful change, and therefore congruent leaders become significant agents for change (even if they do not know it). What is more, the change they institute can be very powerful and can be summed up in terms of vision and values:

- **Vision** is about where an organisation is going and what it is doing.
- **Values** are about how an organisation is doing what it is doing. Values drive decisions and become the foundation of the culture, contributing to the design and function of the operating system and organisational structure.

As such, establishing a values-based culture further underpins the organisation's vision. If the values and beliefs also link to people's emotional and relationship networks, congruent leaders are in a position to influence and build powerful and lasting organisational cultures.

Reflection Point

Access The King's Fund document about leadership culture and read about their position on NHS leadership and culture:
   www.kingsfund.org.uk/projects/positions/NHS-leadership-culture
   The factors identified can also be translated to organisational cultures outside of the healthcare.

Leaders are therefore required to shape culture by taking responsibility for where they sit within the organisation and recognising that their behaviours and actions will be seen, followed and role modelled. There are a number of ways in which leaders can foster organisational change. Hall (2005) suggested the following activities that I have developed further. Leaders need to do the following:

- Become models of the culture – 'champions of culture'. The research that forms the basis of the theory of congruent leadership identified that being a role model was central to how clinically focused leaders were recognised.
- Remain visible in their 'modelling role'. Being visible was another key attribute of clinical leaders and meant that congruent leaders were recognised as visible, approachable and present.
- Ensure other senior staff support and also model the desired culture (staff at all levels in an organisation see different people as 'senior leaders' depending on where they are placed and who they interact with). Mid-level and even lower-level leaders/managers are vital, and, in the healthcare arena, clinical leaders feature as pivotal leaders in this regard. This is reinforced in the research that underpins congruent leadership theory, with leaders recognised as clinical leaders seen at all levels of the organisation; significantly, they were less likely to be at a senior management level or in positions of control.
- Develop personal ownership and responsibility for their behaviour and how it will influence or be seen by other people. This suggests that leaders cannot just 'talk the talk', they need to be seen to 'live' their values and beliefs and put them into action.
- Employ personal communication approaches (avoid email where possible, speak with people, establish communication approaches that are personal). This supports the attributes of congruent leaders, who use excellent communication skills and lead by their actions rather than just what they say they will do.

- Repeat messages in multiple ways to ensure that the message is received consistently and effectively. This again rests on congruent leaders' ability to use excellent communication skills. The keys to establishing personal and meaningful communication and having others see leaders' values in action are to build respect and trustworthiness and to keep communication clear with open interpersonal skills.

Ask yourself:

- Can people believe what you are saying?
- Do you listen to others' concerns?
- Are your intentions clear?
- Are your actions consistent (congruent) with your values?
- Do you say and do what you mean?

In addition, Garvin and Roberto (2005) suggest that effective change leaders (congruent leaders) provide opportunities for employees to practise the desired behaviours repeatedly, while personally modelling new ways of working and providing coaching and support. In this way, effective congruent leaders explicitly reinforce organisational values on a consistent basis, using actions to back up their words.

In order to establish lasting cultural change, people need to be rewarded for actions that support and promote the new ways of operating. Appropriate rewards will send clear messages about the desired culture. How these behaviours are rewarded is also important, with more effective rewards producing more rapid and lasting change. There are a number of rewards that could be implemented, although Hall (2005) has suggested the following three as very effective:

- Individual team recognition at an organisational meeting or event
- Informal recognition by a manager
- Professional development opportunities

After interviewing a number of staff in the UK, Rafferty et al. (2015) report that NHS staff suggested that their commitment, productivity and engagement were strongly linked to four themes that were essential for them to feel part of a positive work culture. These were:

- The resources to deliver quality care
- The support to do a good job
- A worthwhile job that offers the chance to develop
- The opportunity to improve team working

There is considerable evidence to support the conclusion that monetary rewards or awards do not rate highly if the task calls for even rudimentary cognitive skills. Pink (2009) adds that there are three factors leading people to perform better and increase their personal satisfaction at work: mastery (the urge to get better at things), autonomy (a desire to be self-directed) and purpose (a desire to find meaning in the things we do). Pink (2009) is of the view that if the profit motive becomes unmoored from the purpose motive, bad things happen. This again links motivational forces based on values and beliefs to why leaders who demonstrate congruent leadership may be more effective in leading and changing organisational culture.

Reflection Point

Read the Executive Summary of Rafferty et al's (2015) *Culture of Care Barometer*. Does culture matter more than quality assurance measures in terms of gaining an insight into reality and meaning for patients and staff?

The Department of Health (2015) offers a raft of specific information in the report *Culture Change in the NHS* that can be used to guide organisational change. However, this can be distilled to the following broad areas:

- Prevent problems by employing transparency, acknowledging issues and responding to mistakes by recognising that more needs to be done. Report and respond to critical issues by monitoring patient safety and allowing and encouraging staff to speak up and speak freely.
- Detect problems quickly and do something about them. Handle patient complaints appropriately, seek relevant patient feedback and engage (connect) with a wider range of service users in the delivery of and consultation about the service.
- Take action promptly and maintain robust accountability, ensuring that what is meant to happen is happening, with inspections, ratings, clear lines of accountability and measures to ensure that clinical accountabilities are understood and acted on.
- Ensure that staff are trained and motivated. This involves developing leadership skills and practices in keeping with a culture based on values and beliefs. It also means that all members of the organisation need to be aware of the 'right values' and to focus on ensuring that clients and patients have better experiences of the service. Finally, it is incumbent on the organisation to support staff, because as Dixon-Woods et al. (2013) indicate, there is a close relationship between the well-being of staff and patient outcomes.

The key to changing culture lies in changing and reinforcing the desired behaviours and positive values. Leaders then need to encourage everyone to play their part in shaping the organisation's culture, and to model these behaviours and values themselves. Then leaders need to invite participation, ownership and commitment from colleagues and team members. It is often said that what people create, they cherish. Therefore, lasting change is based on using appropriate rewards to reinforce desired behaviours and values. From this standpoint, organisations can establish respect, grow trust and communicate more effectively (with staff, employees, students, clients, stakeholders, etc.). Then the organisation's vision, strategic plan and way forward can be planned.

If clinical leaders are recognised because their values and beliefs are on display and are acted on, then they are already in a position of being seen as leaders from a cultural perspective. Interestingly, however, they may not be demonstrating the culture that the organisation is hoping or wishing to promote, especially if the organisation's values clash or are in conflict with the clinical leaders' professional values.

Clinical Leader Stories: 6   Learning Leaders

The time that I definitely saw clinical leadership at its best was during an emergency department placement. The nurse unit manager (NUM) who ran the night shifts while I was there was an absolutely amazing leader. She shared the responsibilities of not only her own role but of everyone else's role. She was always willing to jump in and help people with even the simplest of tasks. She was involved with the care of patients and patient transfers, and she was willing to be a second pair of eyes for checking medications. She was great at education and always helped other people come in and learn new skills, and she was always hosting mini in-service sessions on a range of topics. She was a great leader because she showed that she was communicating with others on the floor, she was always asking 'what can I do?' 'Do you need a cup'a or a break?' and she was always willing to go out and get things for staff who were occupied in front-line care. She was great at delegating as well so that nurses were able to gain new or varied clinical experiences. She would always advocate for nursing staff too, pushing staff forward and helping to motivate them. She was inspirational and was able to look after patients and staff in equal measure. She was a great example of a congruent leader; she was driven by her values, helped others, including those in all health professions, she looked after her staff and she pitched in when needed. She led by example, she didn't look down on others and she helped push or support people around her to grow and develop.

Samuel: Student Nurse.

Clinical Leadership, Education and Training

Attempts to introduce clinically focused health professionals to leadership education are not new. For at least the past 20 years, professional bodies and health service providers have recognised that care, service quality and change are more likely to occur if health professionals at all levels are provided with access to appropriate education about leadership. Sadly, some of the clinical leadership education offered has been aimed at the wrong targets (managers), or focused on topics driven by 'management' and focused on 'management', with little on offer to genuinely promote an understanding of what clinical leadership is, or how and why clinical leaders are followed.

Many of the educational programmes are driven by an attachment to 'transformational leadership', even though there is little empirical evidence to support this leadership theory. Again, the organisational and management drivers were to the fore in plans for the training programmes. Some progress has been made, but I suggest that more could have been achieved if clinical leadership and an appropriate understanding of clinical leadership or leadership theories that support it were employed in leadership education.

Brown et al. (2016) and others (Scott and Miles 2013; Ailey et al. 2015) called (appropriately) for clinical leadership education to be infused into undergraduate nursing programmes and suggest that benefits would ensue if 'leadership' was recognised as an expectation of all registered nurses. This was to be the case for all clinically focused health professionals and was indeed a recommendation from a 2015 study into clinical leadership among allied health professionals in Western Australia (Stanley et al. 2015). Whereas the

UK undergraduate nursing programmes (NMC 2018) have since progressed to include the key element of leadership with the focus upon newly qualified nurses being the organisational culture influences of the future.

This is not the first time this call has been made. Rafferty (1993) also recommended that more attention needed to be paid to leadership training, management development and clinical leadership. The nursing profession, she declared, required more research into nursing leadership and an exploration of the role of research in leadership development. Leaders were required with 'verve and vision' who could support the development and creation of a healthcare system that allowed nurses to express their values and the value of nursing (Rafferty 1993, p. 27). However, she recognised that at the time of her report, nursing leadership development had been neglected and was in 'crisis'. She also saw the complexity, contradiction and confusion associated with leadership issues and recognised that immediate and vital action was needed if the nursing profession was to 'claim legitimacy in the leadership stakes' (Rafferty 1993, p. 26). The health professions have really made inroads into leadership education with a raft of leadership and clinical leadership programmes and other training programmes on offer all across the globe and in all health services. The Mid Staffordshire crisis refocused attention on leadership issues in the UK and ripple effects are being felt around the world. However, I believe that we are still a long way from realising Rafferty's recommendation and there remains much for us to learn about leadership from a clinically focused perspective.

In 1997, Malby indicated that the crisis persisted because there was a belief that nursing was incapable of promoting a leadership culture or consciousness. The 2010 Gallup Report from North America, *Nursing Leadership from Bedside to Boardroom: Opinion Leaders' Perceptions*, seems to suggest that little has changed and that nurses remain unable or poorly positioned to have any impact on health policy reform. This is in spite of the 2021 Gallup report suggesting that nurses earned a record 89% score for their honesty and ethics in the United States, four percentage points greater than their prior high, last recorded in 2019, and evidence that nurses are both respected and trusted professionals (Saad 2021).

In addition, in spite of Rafferty's (1993) call for more research into leadership, when compared with the academic, political and management domains the uniqueness of clinical leadership has remained largely unrecognised and undervalued (Lett 2002; Stanley 2008). It is certainly true that more and more research addressing clinical leadership is becoming evident and in the past five years more studies have appeared in the health-related literature. Even so, the realisation that clinically focused health professions can influence, change and improve quality care seems only slowly to be finding resonance with health service managers and educational program planners. Addressing this shortfall has been a powerful motivation behind the direction of my clinical leadership research and the approach taken in this book.

It is my contention, based on the research and literature that supports this book, that a new theory specifically related to clinical leadership would be more appropriate to gain an understanding of how to recognise and support the development of clinical leaders. As such, congruent leadership (Stanley 2006a, b, 2008, 2011, 2014; Stanley, Cuthbertson, & Latimer 2012; Stanley, Latimer & Atkinson, 2014; Stanley, Hutton, & McDonald, 2015) is proposed as a new theory to support the demonstration of qualities and characteristics attributable to clinical leaders (see Chapter 4).

Case Study 6.1   Marcus Rashford MBE

Marcus Rashford is an England and Manchester United footballer. In 2020, during the COVID -19 pandemic, aged just 22 years, he campaigned the British Conservative Government to reform their policy on the provision of free school meals outside of the school term-time.

Marcus raised millions of pounds with the help of charities and the Co-op to help both eligible families and those families where their income only just excluded them from free school meal provision and fuel bill aid. Had it not been for Marcus Rashford's campaign, there is every chance nothing would have been done to help these families. The free school meal scheme would have ended at the close of the school term, and millions of children would have gone hungry in the UK.

Marcus' campaigning was initially rejected by the government, but instead of giving up, Marcus conducted a high-profile campaign and pushed the Conservative government – who eventually relented under public pressure.

What is so impressive about what Marcus Rashford did is that he was just 22 years old, and yet he recognised his position, as well as the platform and influence it afforded him.

Marcus understood the plight of the most vulnerable in British society as he and his four siblings were raised by his single-parent mother who had to sometimes work three minimum pay jobs just to be able to buy a little food. Throughout his childhood Marcus often experienced the uncertainty of not knowing where the family's next meal was coming from. Marcus is widely quoted in the British media as being determined that he wants no child to ever experience the hunger and pain that he went through, and he wants no parent to experience what his own mother had to endure.

Unlike many people in more powerful positions, Marcus feels compelled to use his platform to help those less fortunate than himself. The relentlessness with which he has taken on these challenges has allowed him to transcend football and become a leader in British society.

At a time when he could easily and justifiably be using his platform to further his own profile and wealth, he is instead using it to shine a light on the areas which need improvement in British society and, as a result, hold the more powerful to account.

Challenge: If culture is people focused and if culture can be changed, how much power do we have as compassionate leaders to change negative or potentially disruptive/damaging influences so that we can be our best selves, be the best clinicians or do the best for our patients or clients?

Summary

- Culture is people focused.
- Culture is about how things are 'done around here'.
- Culture has some seen and unseen elements, making it a difficult issue for organisations to understand or deal with.
- The dominant culture will be infused into the product and atmosphere of an organisation.

- The key to changing culture lies in changing and reinforcing behaviour and values.
- Organisations can make or create their culture, or they can allow it to develop on its own.
- Congruent leadership theory strongly supports the links between culture, values and beliefs and leadership.
- Everyone in an organisation has an impact on the organisational culture, although leaders at all levels can have a dramatic effect on how an organisation develops and delivers its service.
- Clinical leaders may be the key leaders needed to secure solid organisational change that is genuinely focused on client/patient-centred care and compassion.

Mind Press-Ups

Exercise 6.1

If culture is people focused, what impact do you think technology is having on our relationships and our organisational culture? Talk to some of your senior colleagues and ask them how much impact changes in technology have had on their workplace culture

Exercise 6.2

Think about the 6Cs, discussed in Chapter 3. Bradshaw (2016) wrote a very interesting article about the hidden presence of M. Simone Roach's model of caring, which seems to have been the 'unwritten' precursor to the 6Cs. Bradshaw is of the view that the origins of the 6Cs should be acknowledged (I agree), but what do you think? Which matters more, what the 6Cs are based on or whether they are understood and enacted? Why might this matter?

References

Ailey, S., Lamb, K., Friese, T., and Christopher, B.-A. (2015). Educating nursing students in clinicalleadership. *Nursing Management* 21 (9): 23–28.

Bradshaw, A. (2016). 'An analysis of England's nursing policy on compassion and the 6Cs: the hidden presence of M. Simone Roach's model of caring. *Nursing Inquiry* 23 (1): 78–85.

Brooks, I. (2009). *Organisational Behaviour: Individual, Groups & Organisations*. Harlow: Prentice Hall.

Brown, A.M., Crookes, P., and Dewing, J. (2016). Clinical leadership development in a pre-registrationnursing curriculum: what the profession has to say about it. *Nurse Education Today* 36: 105–111.

Care Quality Commission (2015). *National NHS Patient Safety Survey Programme: National Results Fromthe 2014 Inpatient Survey*. London: Care Quality Commission.

Care Quality Commission (2018). *Opening the door to change: NHS safety culture and the need for transformation*. www.cqc.org.uk/sites/default/files/20181224_openingthedoor_report.pdf

Davies, H., Nutley, S.M., and Mannion, R. (2000). Organisational culture and quality in health care. *Quality in Health Care* 9 (1): 111–119.

Department of Health (2012). *A National Response to Winterbourne View: Department of Health Review: Final Report*. London: HM Stationery Office.

Department of Health (2015). *Culture Change in the NHS: Applying the Lessons of the Francis Inquiry*. London: Department of Health.

Dixon-Woods, M., Baker, R., Charles, K. et al. (2013). Culture and behaviour in the English National Health service: overview of lessons from a large multi-method study. *BMJ Quality & Safety* 23 (20): 106–115.

Fitz-Enz, J. (1997). *The 8 Practices of Exceptional Companies: How Great Organizations Make the Most of their Human Assets*. New York: AMACOM.

Fowke, D. (1999). Shaping corporate culture. *New Management Network* 12 (2): 1–4.

Francis, R. (2013). *Report of the Mid Staffordshire NHS Foundation Trust Public Inquiry*. London: H M Stationery Office.

Francis, R. (2015). *Sir Robert Francis' Freedom to Speak Up Review*. London: Department of Health http://webarchive.nationalarchives.gov.uk/20150218150343/http://freedomtospeakup.org.uk/the-report (accessed 1 July 2016).

Gallup Report (2010). *Nursing Leadership from Bedside to Boardroom: Opinion Leaders' Perceptions*. Princeton, NJ: Robert Wood Johnson Foundation http://www.rwjf.org/en/library/research/2010/01/nursing-leadership-from-bedside-to-boardroom.html (accessed 5 May 2016).

Garvin, D. and Roberto, M. (2005). Reinforcing values: A public dressing down. *HBS Working Knowledge*. 13 March, https://hbswk.hbs.edu/item/reinforcing-values-a-public-dressing-down (accessed 1 July 2016).

Hall, M.L. (2005). Shaping organisational culture: a practitioner's perspective. *Peak Development Consulting* 2 (1): 1–16.

Handy, C. (1999). *Understanding Organisations*, 4e. London: Penguin.

Kennedy, I. (2001). *Learning from Bristol: The Report of the Public Inquiry into Children's Heart Surgeryat the Bristol Royal Infirmary 1984–1995*, Command Paper CM5207, London: HM Stationery Office.

Kennedy, I. (2006). *Investigation into Outbreaks of Clostridium Difficile at Stoke Mandeville Hospital, Buckinghamshire Hospital NHS Trust, Commission of Healthcare Audit and Inspection*. London: HM Stationery Office.

King's Fund (2012). *Leadership and Engagement for Improvement in the NHS*. London: King's Fund www.kingsfund.org.uk/publications/leadership-engagement-for-improvement-nhs (accessed 5 May 2016).

Kirkup, B. (2015). *The Report of the Morcambe Bay Investogation*. London: H M Stationery Office.

Lett, M. (2002). The concept of clinical leadership. *Contemporary Nurse* 12 (1): 16–20.

Luthans, F., Norman, S.M., Avolio, B.M., and Avey, J. (2008). The mediating role of psychological capital inthe supportive organisational climate–employee performance relationship. *Journal of Organisational Behavior* 29: 219–238.

Malby, R. (1997). Developing the future leaders of nursing in the UK. *European Nurse* 2 (1): 27–36.

Mannion, R., Davies, H.T.O., Konteh, F. et al. (2008). *Measuring and Assessing Organisational Culture Inthe NHS*. London: National Coordinating Centre for the National Institute for Health Research Service.

Mannion, R., Konteh, F.H., and Davies, H.T.O. (2009). Assessing organisational culture for quality andsafety improvement: a national survey of tools and tool use. *Quality and Safety in Health Care* 180: 153–156.

Middleton, J. (2016). Nurses should lead the culture change. *Nursing Times*. Jan. http://www. nursingtimes.net/break-time/editors-comment/nurses-should-lead-the-culture-change/7001591.fullarticle (accessed 1 May 2016).

NHS England and NHS Improvement (2019) *Safer Culture, Safer Systems, Safer Patients*. https://www.england.nhs.uk/wp-content/ uploads/2020/08/190708_Patient_Safety_Strategy_for_website_v4.pdf

NHS Leadership Academy (2013). *Healthcare Leadership Model: The Nine Dimensions of Leadership Behaviour*. Leeds: NHS Leadership Academy http://www.leadershipacademy. nhs.uk/wp-content/uploads/dlm_uploads/2014/10/NHSLeadership-LeadershipModel-colour.pdf (accessed 2 May 2016).

Nursing and Midwifery Council (2018). *Future Nurse: Standards of practice for registered nurses*. www.nmc.org.uk/globalassets/sitedocuments/standards-of-proficiency/nurses/ future-nurse-proficiencies.pdf

Pink, D. (2009). *Drive: The Surprising Truth about What Motivates us*. New York: Riverhead.

Rafferty, A.M. (1993). *Leading Questions: A Discussion Paper on the Issues of Nurse Leadership*. London: King's Fund.

Rafferty, A.M., Philippou, J., Fitzpatrick, J.M., and Ball, J. (2015). *Culture of Care Barometer*. London: National Nursing Research Unit, King's College London.

Ranheim, E.A., Karner, A., and Bertero, C. (2011). Eliciting reflections on caring theory in elderly caringpractice. *International Journal of Qualitative Studies on Health and Well-Being* 6 (3): https://doi.org/10.3402/qhw.v6i3.7296.

Rytterstrom, P., Unosson, M., and Arman, M. (2013). Care culture as a meaning-making process: a study ofa mistreatment investigation. *Qualitative Health Research* 23 (9): 1179–1187.

Saad, L. (2021). U.S. Ethics Ratings Rise for Medical Workers and Teachers. https://news. gallup.com/poll/328136/ethics-ratings-rise-medical-workers-teachers.aspx

Schein, E.H. (2010). *Organizational Culture and Leadership*, 4e. San Francisco, CA: Jossey-Bass.

Scott, E.S. and Miles, J. (2013). Advancing leadership capacity in nursing. *Nursing Administration Quarterly* 37 (1): 7–82.

Scott, J.T., Mannion, R., Davies, H.T.O. et al. (2003). The quantitative measurement of organizationalculture in health care: what instruments are available? *Health Service Research* 38: 923–945.

Stanley, D. (2006a). In command of care: clinical nurse leadership explored. *Journal of Research in Nursing* 11 (1): 20–39.

Stanley, D. (2006b). In command of care: towards the theory of congruent leadership. *Journal of Research in Nursing* 11 (2): 134–144.

Stanley, D. (2008). Congruent leadership: values in action. *Journal of Nursing Management* 16: 519–524.

Stanley, D. (2011). *Clinical Leadership: Innovation into Action*. South Yarra, VIC: Palgrave Macmillan.

Stanley, D. (2014). Clinical leadership characteristics confirmed. *Journal of Research in Nursing* 19 (2): 118–128.

Stanley, D., Cuthbertson, J., and Latimer, K. (2012). Perceptions of clinical leadership in the St. John ambulance service in WA. *Response* 39 (1): 31–37.

Stanley, D., Latimer, K., and Atkinson, J. (2014). Perceptions of clinical leadership in an aged care residential facility in Perth, Western Australia. *Health Care: Current Reviews* 2 (2): http://www.esciencecentral.org/journals/perceptions-of-clinical-leadership-in-an-aged-care-residential-facility-in-perth-western-australia.hccr.1000122.php?aid=24341 (accessed 1 May 2016).

Stanley, D., Hutton, M. and McDonald, A. (2015). *Western Australian Allied Health Professionals'Perceptions of Clinical Leadership: A Research Report*, http://www.ochpo.health.wa.gov.au/docs/WA_Allied_Health_Prof_Perceptions_of_Clinical_Leadership_Research_Report.pdf (accessed 1 July 2016).

Storey, J. and Holti, R. (2013). *Towards a New Model of Leadership for the NHS*. Leeds: NHS Leadership Academy.

Storey, J., Holti, R., Bate, P. et al. (2010). *The Intended and Unintended Outcomes of New Governance Arrangements within the NHS*, Final Report for the National Coordinating Centre for NHS Service Delivery and Organisation R&D (NCCSDO) SDOResearch Project, 08/1618/129, http://www.nets.nihr.ac.uk/__data/assets/pdf_file/0006/82338/ES-08-1618-129.pdf (accessed 1 July 2016).

Turkel, M.C. (2006). Applications of Marilyn Ray's theory of bureaucratic caring. In: *Nursing Theories and Nursing Practice*, 2e (ed. M.E. Parker), 369. F. A. Davis: Philadelphia, PA.

West, M. (2021). *Compassionate leadership: Sustaining wisdom, humanity and presence in health and social care*. www.SwirlingLeafPress.com

West, M., Steward, K., Eckert, R., and Pasmore, B. (2014). *Developing Collective Leadership for Health Care*. London: King's Fund.

7

Leading Change

Clare L. Bennett and Alison H. James

> *Be the change that you wish to see in the world*
>
> Mahatma Gandhi

Introduction: Tools for Change

In many ways this chapter sits at the heart of what clinical leadership is about – change. If health services are to improve, healthcare professionals need to be able to recognise what is not working well and develop strategies and solutions to change practices, attitudes and processes. This is especially so because service improvement is based on effective change and, in turn, leadership is central to bringing about and facilitating change (Nadler and Tushman 1990; Kotter 1996; Burke 2017).

Effectively dealing with change implies that clinical leaders require a tool kit of skills and techniques (Ford et al. 2021) and the courage to champion change (Hendy 2012). Clinical leaders are also in the ideal position to initiate innovative change, focused on service improvement and quality and on patients/clients/services, that has the potential to be ongoing, practice driven and clinically relevant (Dougall et al. 2018). This chapter aims to outline why change is a key clinical leadership issue and offers healthcare professionals the tools to deal with or lead change successfully. It also offers insights into recognising resistance to change and managing it. Michael Leunig explores the issue of change in his poem 'A Common Prayer' (2003, HarperCollins Australia):

> We struggle, we grow weary, we grow tired.
> We are exhausted, we are distressed, we despair.
> We give up, we fall down, we let go.
> We cry. We are empty, we grow calm, we are ready.
> We wait quietly.

Clinical Leadership in Nursing and Healthcare, Third Edition.
Edited by David Stanley, Clare L. Bennett and Alison H. James.
© 2023 John Wiley & Sons Ltd. Published 2023 by John Wiley & Sons Ltd.

A small, shy truth arrives. Arrives from within and without.
Arrives and is born.
Simple, steady, clear. Like a mirror, like a bell, like a flame.
Like rain in summer.
A precious truth arrives and is born within us.
Within our emptiness.

We accept it, we observe it, we absorb it.
We surrender to our bare truth. We are nourished.
We are changed. We are blessed.
We rise up.

All Change

Many healthcare professionals will recognise the undulations of the change process described in Leunig's poem in their working lives. Change seems to be an almost unrelenting feature of the health service industry (Jones and Bennett 2018), with staff having to consistently adapt to new ways of working, often following little or no consultation or involvement.

Reflection Point

Consider your own feelings about change, in your work life and personal life. How well do you adapt to change when it's enforced? Talk to your colleagues about how change makes them feel – is it something they view positively or negatively? What was the dominant emotion?

In healthcare, as in the wider community, there are those who want to change but do not know how to effect it, those who want to change and think they know what is best and try to impose it on others, and those who do not want to change at all and would willingly settle for a quiet life. As part of a teaching exercise, one of the authors asked a cohort of 53 healthcare professionals to list words commonly associated with change. The words are outlined in Table 7.1. Interestingly, these are almost identical to a list that was compiled almost a decade earlier (Jones and Bennett 2012), although the healthcare professionals differed

Table 7.1 Words associated with change.

Apathy	Threatening	Exhaustion	Resistant	Fearful
Anxiety	Scared	Uncomfortable	Distrust	Unwilling
Worrying	Concerned	Apprehensive	Uneasy	Fretful
Nervousness	Exciting	Positive	An opportunity	Cynical

across the two groups, with the former comprising only nurses employed in England and the latter comprising physiotherapists, podiatrists, occupational therapists, dietitians and nurses employed largely in Wales, with a small number employed in the Middle East. It is also important to note that the second cohort discussed this question mid-pandemic.

As you may have noticed, only 3 of the 20 words listed by the healthcare professionals were positive, with reasons largely centring on change fatigue, underpinned by the sheer amount of change that practitioners were required to adapt to during the pandemic. Kubler-Ross's (1973) grief and loss model can be useful in understanding people's responses to change. Originally, the model was developed to describe common emotional responses to death, outlining sequential stages of denial, followed by anger, bargaining, depression and finally, with appropriate support, acceptance. Today, the model is widely accepted as being applicable to any significant life change, including workplace change, which demonstrates the challenging nature of change for some people and the need for effective leadership approaches to support people in adapting positively to change.

Change is not necessarily always perceived negatively, however, with many individuals actively seeking it out. Communication skills, preparation and the mode of implementation, as well as factors that are unique to the individual such as confidence and prior experiences, will significantly shape how people feel about change. Rogers and Shoemaker (1971) classify six different categories of people who are involved in change:

- Innovators: individual team members who are excited by new ideas and are eager to implement them
- Early adopters: individuals within the team who take a few days to think about the change and then go on to adopt the change
- Early majority: several team members adopt the idea
- Later majority: a number of the team accept and take up the idea
- Laggards: individual team members who have a tendency to lag behind in accepting and adopting change
- Rejecters: individuals who usually oppose new ideas and are against change

Change is a necessary condition of survival whether for individuals, communities or organisations. Differences are a necessary ingredient of change and a never-ending search for improvement. Improving quality in healthcare involves changing the way things are done, changing processes and the behaviour of people and teams of people. The challenge for any one of us is to harness the energy and thrust of differences so that the individual, community or organisation does not disintegrate during the process of change but instead, develops and grows.

Transformational Change

Transformational change leads to the emergence of an entirely new way of doing things, which is often prompted by a shift in perceptions of what is considered possible or necessary and profoundly impacts the workplace culture and levels of performance (Dougall et al. 2018). An example of transformational change is how COVID-19 revolutionised the conduct of clinical trials, as seen in the Randomised Evaluation of COVID-19 Therapy

(RECOVERY) trial, with Park et al. (2021) asserting that COVID-19 has fundamentally changed the conduct of clinical research in global health. Transformational change differs from incremental change, which focuses on improving existing processes, and is the more 'usual' approach to change in health services internationally. The King's Fund has been giving prominence to the need for transformational change since 2012 (Ham et al. 2012), arguing that transformation is at its most effective when it is brought about 'from within' (Ham 2014). Furthermore, in contrast to traditional discussions about the 'management' of change, Ham et al. (2016) and Hulks et al. (2017) contend that transformational change is most effective when supported by collaborative leadership.

Reflection Point

Make a mind map of all the changes you would like to make in your area of clinical practice. Then think about what these changes might entail – are the changes required 'incremental' or 'transformational'? In other words, would 'tweaks' to existing processes be enough or are the changes required more fundamental? Next, think about how different leadership styles may affect the success or otherwise of your proposals.

Dougall et al.'s (2018) research into transformational change shows that it is emergent and, therefore, messy and fluid, involving multiple layers of healthcare systems. They emphasise that this kind of change isn't just about changing how part of a service is delivered, instead it involves new ways of thinking, relationships and a redistribution of power. Rather than the traditional 'command and control' approach which has characterised 'change management' in healthcare historically, this approach to change prioritises 'curiosity and invitation' (priority 1) and employs organic approaches that centre on one central priority – improving people's lives. To achieve this, Dougall et al. (2018) argue that three things are key:

- Learning from each other, joining up understandings and connecting efforts
- Collaborative and distributed leadership that brings diverse groups of people together and allows them to harness their shared potential
- Transformational leadership

The next part of this chapter outlines a number of models that can be used to facilitate change when used in partnership with transformational leadership styles that foster collaboration and a re-distribution of power.

Approaches to Change

A variety of tools can be used to support change, and some will be explored in this section. However, before these are explained, a note of caution: tools for change do not mean that the intended change will result. The models will help, but the outcomes are dependent upon the leadership styles employed. Effective communication, a good relationship and mutual trust are key to eliciting a positive response to new ways of thinking and working (Jones and Bennett 2018). As Scholtes (1998) argued, trust comes from a combination of competency and caring. Competency on its own within a leader will bring about respect, but not trust. Equally, if an individual feels cared for by a leader but does not consider the leader to be competent or capable, it is likely that the individual will have affection for that person but may not trust them. So remember, regardless of how good the following tools may appear to be, your success in bringing about change will be contingent on *how* you use the tools, your leadership styles and the culture of the organisation in which you work (see Chapter 6).

SWOT Analysis

A SWOT analysis can facilitate an individual, team or organisation to examine the Strengths, Weaknesses, Opportunities and Threats that are relevant to them in a particular context. For example, many healthcare practitioners find that a SWOT analysis can be very useful in relation to developing their proficiency as a leader. However, in relation to leading change, a SWOT analysis can help to analyse the current direction of an organisation (ward/clinical area/workplace), to formulate future goals and objectives, or to analyse specific situations, ideas, groups or activities. Then, once the assessment is made, it is good practice to question whether it is possible to change or challenge the threats so that they become opportunities and, likewise, question whether any weaknesses can become strengths.

By looking at these areas we have found that practitioners are better able to identify potential obstacles to change. To be effective, a SWOT analysis requires scrupulous honesty and the capacity to be open in reflecting on the threats and to consider whether they may actually be weaknesses. The exercise can often be very difficult and it may require uncomfortable realisations and difficult admissions. Indeed, in some cases, a SWOT analysis might be more useful in identifying reasons *not* to change (Box 7.1).

Box 7.1   SWOT

The four parts to a SWOT analysis applied to an organisation or team are:

- **Strengths**: What are the strengths of your organisation? In what areas does it function well?
- **Weaknesses**: What are the weak points in your organisation?
- **Opportunities**: Are there circumstances present that create openings and the potential for positive change?
- **Threats**: Are there other circumstances that could threaten or jeopardise your organisation?

Use a SWOT analysis to consider your unit's/team's position in relation to making one of the changes that you outlined in the reflection point above. Identify your strengths and weaknesses, and consider the opportunities that present themselves and the potential threats.

Strengths	Weaknesses
Opportunities	Threats

By considering these four areas, you may be able to identify where you need to target resources or energy to bolster the strengths or reduce the weaknesses of a situation or problem. The task also encourages you to reflect on the opportunities evident and what threats there could be. It is a simple approach, but it relies on you having access to significant insight and information to ensure that all the relevant details are taken into account.

Stakeholder Analysis

NHS England and NHS Improvement (2021) advocate the use of a stakeholder analysis in the early stages of a change project, to ensure that everyone who needs to be involved is identified and to realistically establish the amount of time and resource required to maintain their commitment. The approach involves five sequential steps (NHS England and NHS Improvement 2021):

1) Identify your stakeholders
Brainstorm the individuals and groups who are most likely to be affected by the intended change. This may involve you talking to other people who have wide networks and who are well informed of both the project and its broadest implications.

2) Prioritise your stakeholders
Next, analyse how powerful the people you have identified are, in terms of influence and the degree to which they are affected by the change. People who have high levels of power and high impact on the project need to be fully engaged through good communication and consultation. Individuals who have high power and low impact tend to be opinion formers and should be kept abreast of the project's progress. People who have low levels of power but high impact (for example, patients) should be encouraged to contribute their thoughts and ideas to the programme of change. Next, identify which parties support, oppose or are neutral about the proposals. This will enable you to identify any influencing activities that may be required. You may also wish to evaluate individuals' levels of commitment to the project at this stage.

3) Understand your key stakeholders
It is also advisable to give some thought to how stakeholders might react to your project and what the best way to communicate with them might be. You may wish to consider:

- What interests they have in the outcome of the project
- What motivates their involvement
- What information they want from you
- The best way to communicate your message to them
- Whether their opinions are grounded in accurate information
- Who influences their opinions
- If they are opposed to the project, how you might convince them to support it
- How you will manage opposition

4) Building trust

Trying to understand stakeholders' expectations for the proposed change can help build trusting relationships and shared values. Trust can be developed by:

- demonstrating empathy
- being straightforward
- owning-up to mistakes
- keeping promises
- moving on from grievances
- being consistent in thought and action

5) Working with your stakeholders

Finally, it is advisable to communicate in advance how you intend to work with your stakeholders, for example the nature and frequency of meetings, an appropriate Chair, modes of communication and progress monitoring.

Pettigrew's Model

Andrew Pettigrew is one of the foremost writers on change in the UK health service, and he formulated a model with which to analyse change. The core of the model emphasises the importance of a broad, contextual approach to change. Pettigrew felt that an analysis of change should not just look at the processes of change, but also at the political features of the organisation, and the history and cultural context in which the change might take place (Pettigrew and Whipp 1998). Pettigrew et al. (2001) suggest that the model offers a continuous interplay between ideas about the context of change, the process of change and the content of change. You can see these three components in Figure 7.1.

Pettigrew defined the context as the 'why and when' of change. He also differentiated between the inner and outer aspects of the context (outer might be the prevailing economic circumstances and the social and political climate at the time; inner might refer to the resources, structure, culture and local politics). Content is described as the 'what' of change and is concerned with areas of transformation (what is to be changed). The process covers the 'how' of change and refers to how the change will be made to come about, what actions are needed, who will do what and how things will get done.

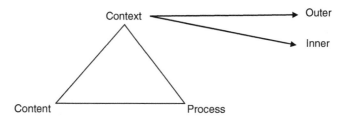

Figure 7.1 Pettigrew's change model.

The usefulness of this model is that it reminds the change agent that it is important to consider and keep in mind the complexities of the organisation, and that change is commonly influenced by characteristics in the internal and external environment.

The Change Management Iceberg

The change management iceberg was developed by Wilfried Kruger and is based on the concept that dealing with change means dealing with barriers. Kruger's view (Ackerman-Anderson and Anderson 2001) is that many managers or change agents only consider the tip of the iceberg – cost, quality and time – as significant issues. However, a number of other issues are below the surface, waiting to influence the proposed change (Figure 7.2). These are the management of perceptions and beliefs about the proposed change, and issues of power and politics. Such factors imply that more needs to be understood about the proposed change for it to be implemented successfully.

Dealing with the types of barriers that arise and how the change can be implemented is dependent on the kind or type of change and the strategy for change that is followed or applied.

Change may be 'hard' (information systems/processes/policies), which can be difficult enough to implement but only scratches the surface in terms of impact on the iceberg. It can also be 'soft' (e.g. values/mindsets/capabilities), which can result in more profound change, and be more difficult to initiate or suffer from more ingrained barriers.

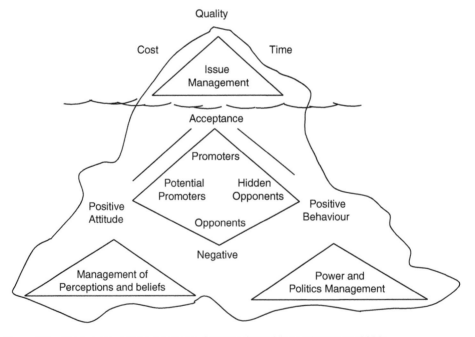

Figure 7.2 Change management iceberg. *Source:* Adapted from 12manage (2009).

The iceberg model also offers insight into the types of people who might be involved in the change, and, like stakeholder analysis, Kruger asks that the people involved in the change are incorporated in the assessment. They are described as one of the following:

- **Opponents** have a generally negative attitude to the change and behave negatively towards it. Their minds need to be changed by managing their perceptions and beliefs (as far as this is possible).
- **Promoters** have a positive attitude to the change, seeing it as an advantage and offering their support.
- **Hidden opponents** appear to be supporting the change on a superficial level but have a negative attitude to it. They need more information or involvement so that their attitude can be swayed to one of support.
- **Potential promoters** remain unconvinced or sceptical. They are open to the change and generally positive but may need further influencing to gain their full support.

In the change management iceberg model, it is recognised that change is a constant feature of a manager's (leader's) task, but that superficial (tip of the iceberg) issue management can only achieve results on a limited level (structural change). For greater impact and control of the change, the interpersonal and behavioural dimensions, cultural dimensions, power and politics, perceptions and beliefs all need to be addressed and considered when the change is planned and implemented. The model supports the concept of a complete and thorough assessment of the barriers that may have impacts on change, so that it is likely to be implemented with a greater chance of success.

PEST or STEP

PEST (Political, Economic, Social and Technological) analysis (sometimes called STEP by changing the letters or words around) performs an overall environmental scan of an organisation. It is not generally as beneficial as some of the other change tools at a local or ward/unit-based level. However, it is very useful to gain an overview of the 'health', sustainability or resilience of an organisation as a whole.

The factors assessed are the following:

- **Political** factors including tax policy, employment laws, environmental regulations, trade restrictions and tariffs, and political stability.
- **Economic** factors including economic growth, interest rates, exchange rates and inflation rate.
- **Social** factors including health consciousness, population growth rate, age distribution, career attitudes, emphasis on safety and generational make-up of the workforce.
- **Technological** factors including research and development (R&D) activity, automation, technological incentives and rate of technological change.

This tool may take a considerable amount of time to use and may also be undertaken by a range of individuals with specialist skills in the various areas suggested. It may also be employed in conjunction with a range of other change management tools, for example, SWOT analysis.

Kotter's Eight-Stage Change Process

John Kotter (1996) offers an eight-stage process for progressing change. The model is quite simplistic, although it offers a pattern or map that can support and direct clinical leaders and others when initiating or planning change (Jones and Bennett 2018). The steps are as follows:

1) Establish a sense of urgency.
2) Create a guiding coalition (involve people at all levels to construct a shared vision and address specific needs).
3) Develop a vision and strategy (this needs to work towards the planned change).
4) Communicate the change/vision to others.
5) Empower employees for action (let people know that their opinions matter).
6) Strive for short-term wins (good leadership is essential for short-term achievements).
7) Consolidate gains and produce more change (address resistance and strengthen leadership approaches).
8) Anchor new approaches in the culture (which is frequently overlooked and requires as much energy as the earlier stages).

Nominal Group Technique

The nominal group technique is an excellent change tool for helping groups solve problems or propose changes. It may not be as useful for driving change through, but it is very handy for identifying where scarce resources and personnel with limited time can focus their energies. It is also an excellent approach for helping to engage wide numbers of people in the change process.

The technique establishes what problems exist and what priority is placed on these various problems. Significantly, it employs the stakeholders in the process of decision making, so that the priority problems or change issues have been identified from within the stakeholder group. The process for the nominal group technique is relatively simple, but it takes time to set up and requires the majority of the stakeholders to engage in it for it to be successful.

Have all the stakeholders gather together and follow these steps:

- Ask the group to split into smaller groups and discuss the first question: 'What are the problems with ...?' or 'What are the bad aspects of ...?' (you can add the relevant problem/ issue). Have them write their problems clearly on flip-chart paper, because it will need to be put up on a wall for all the other groups to see. Make it clear that each group has a certain time frame (you will need to decide this based on the total time available or the nature of the problem being discussed). Once the groups are finished, ask them to put up their lists for all the other groups to read. Make sure that the group's discussion sticks to the one question asked: 'What are the problems with ...?' or 'What are the bad aspects of ...?'
- Ask the same small groups to discuss the second question: 'What are the good things about ...?' Again, give them flip-chart paper to record their lists and a suitable time frame, and once they have finished once again put up the 'good things' list on a wall for all the

groups to read. We have used this method many times and it is worth noting that just to get to this point can take between one and two-and-a-half hours.

- Have the whole group review the smaller groups' problems and good points. Ask them to read and possibly discuss these informally as they review what the other groups have written.
- Now ask everyone to vote for their top three problems. To do this, offer a large number of felt-tip pens and have each person vote for the three main problems by ranking them 3, 2, and 1. After everyone has voted, calculate the results, with the highest number being the issue of most concern to the majority of participants (stakeholders).

In this way, the whole group has considered all the issues and decided for themselves what the three primary issues are. This can be very empowering for stakeholders. Identifying the good aspects as well is important to retain a fair perspective on the issues being discussed. The process is not over, though: the final step is to ask stakeholders to focus only on the three main problems identified. In their smaller groups again, ask them to propose potential solutions.

Of course, the problems will still need to be addressed, but using this approach means that implementing change (which is often suggested by the stakeholders) has a greater chance of success, as the people involved have had a significant hand in identifying the issues and the possible solutions. They have also had a public and detailed opportunity to express their feelings among people who are often in a position to support or direct resources for change.

Process Re-Engineering

Process re-engineering can be a very complicated process to implement, but it is also a clear and practical response to certain problems. It is all about sticky notes (small, usually yellow, low-adhesive notes that can be removed and repositioned easily).

The process is to decide on an issue or process that you would like to change, such as how patients are moved through a busy Emergency Department (ED). Meet with all the relevant stakeholders, in one place. Give out a stack of different-coloured sticky notes for each participant. Depending on the process under review, it may be wise to break the large group into smaller groups. Usually, the group needs to have representation from all areas involved in the process under review for it to be successfully assessed and replanned. For example, it would be foolish to plan process re-engineering in an ED department without including the clerical staff who are central to the patient's journey through the department.

The next step is to brainstorm what the issues/problems/current processes are. These are then written on a separate sticky note. Thus, everything is broken down into its smallest part. Then with everyone's input, put the issue/problem/process back together using the sticky notes to manipulate the process, make changes or suggest new aspects.

It is helpful to foster discussion by physically moving the sticky notes around to see if a new process evolves. This requires a great deal of creativity and may also need people to suspend established ideas about 'how things get done around here'. This approach has the potential to offer a whole new set of solutions to significant problems or issues. It may imply restructuring (in terms of job activities and physical environments) and could need to be used in tandem with some of the other change tools, for example, stakeholder analysis or SWOT.

Process re-engineering can also be an empowering tool and often brings all the stakeholders together by valuing everyone's input. As such, a key to its success is skillful facilitation of the sticky note activity.

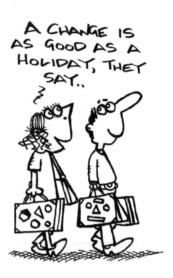

Force-Field Analysis

Force-field analysis (FFA) has a clear advantage over the other models in relation to its use in the health arena; that is, it allows the change agent to place themselves clearly in the picture and see their part in the process of change. The other advantage of FFA is that it is very easy to follow and use. Brager and Holloway (1992) describe it as a tool for assessing the prospects of organisational change, and Egan (1990) sums it up by describing FFA as an analysis of the major obstacles to, and resources for, the implementation of strategies and plans for change.

The 'field' theory was developed by Kurt Lewin as early as 1947, but subsequent developments in the late 1960s led to the development of FFA. By 1969, what we now know as Lewin's FFA model of change management was developed. It was born from the realisation that stability within a social system is a dynamic rather than static condition, and is therefore the result of opposing and constraining forces. Lewin (1951) speculated that these operate to produce what we see or sense as stability. Changes occur when the forces shift, thus causing a disruption in the system's equilibrium, as depicted in Figure 7.3.

Lewin's model is therefore a way of listing, discussing and dealing with the forces that make change possible or obstruct it (Jones and Bennett 2018). An analysis of these forces helps generate options that can help achieve or work against the objectives:

- **Restraining forces** work against the change
- **Driving forces** or **facilitating forces** work for the change

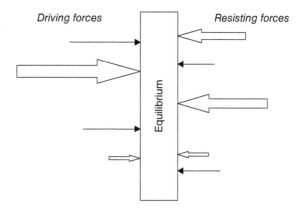

Figure 7.3 Driving and resisting forces. *Source:* Adapted from Lewin (1947).

Analysing these forces can determine whether a solution can get the support needed, identify obstacles to successful solutions, suggest actions to reduce the strength of the obstacles and determine where the change agent's part in the change process might be.

Egan (1990) also indicated that there are four reasons why FFA may be useful:

- By focusing on the potential or real environmental influences, the nature of these perceptions becomes open to scrutiny, revision and test. In effect, there is an opportunity to test out what you feel the situation or 'lay of the land' is.
- A complete account of the obstacles and resources decreases the likelihood that pitfalls or potential opportunities will be overlooked. This will prevent any surprises when the change process begins.
- Using knowledge of the influences in the environment (ward/unit/workplace) helps to capitalise on opportunities. These may even be extended to go beyond the resources under your direct control.
- Alternative strategies to implement an action plan can be created and assessed in the context of the force field.

In effect, an FFA is a judicious look at the potential future and can lead to meaningful insights. The various forces involved are discussed in what follows.

Restraining Forces

These are the potential and actual obstacles in the external or internal environment and can include a self-analysis. They represent a census of the probable pitfalls (rather than a self-defeating search for every possible thing that could go wrong). Once the pitfalls are identified, then ways of coping with them can be identified too. Sometimes being aware of a pitfall is enough; sometimes you may need to take more explicit action.

Driving or Facilitating Forces

These can be the resources or things you have to hand, other people who can help or those with power or influence and evidence to support the change proposal. The aim, though, is not so much to list every possible factor but to capture an insight into the force or strength of the features that will support, drive, facilitate or restrain the planned change.

How Do You Find Either Restraining or Facilitating Forces?

There are many approaches to discovering or realising the restraining or driving forces. They can be discovered alone, or it may be useful to employ a collaborative approach to identifying the relevant factors. Approaches can include:

- Brainstorming
- Mind maps
- Considering what is in it for you, for colleagues and for others
- Asking what the key issues are and whether you have thought of everything
- Check or think steps, used as a bridge between planning and action. Stop, question what you have done, consider it again. Is a re-plan required?
- Social support and challenge (clinical supervision)
- Seeking advice from others, experts, people who may have more experience or insight than you. Ensure that you have the support you need to take on the challenge of a change
- Feedback on performance: get confirmation that you are on the right track
- Education and training: can these provide the information you are looking for? Will they give you more information to place you in a stronger position?
- Research and development: has someone else done it before you?

To be clear, FFA is all about the 'force'. It is not a pros and cons list. Once the analysis is complete, consider how you can address the restraining forces or bolster the driving forces to bring about the change. While the driving forces matter and should be supported, the gift of the FFA model is that it allows you to take stock of the restraining forces and plan ways to limit or minimise them.

Reflection Point

The change models offered in this chapter may also be applied to other aspects of your life. Choose SWOT analysis and apply it to a professional or personal issue that you are facing at the moment. What are the advantages and disadvantages of the SWOT analysis? Would other models be more or less useful for the issues you have considered?

Clinical Leaders Stories 7: Change

Reflections on Congruent leadership and change: Congruent leaders are not focused solely on initiating change, although they can be significantly influential in the change process. Nurses who display congruent, clinical leadership are those that hold a strong value for high-quality care for patients and are subsequently visible role models that initiate change strategies. They are receptive and positive towards change and innovation and actively implement change that proposes maximum potential to support their strong values for optimising patient care. In contributing to and demonstrating an

(Continued)

openness towards change and innovation in the workplace, graduate nurses grow professionally and personally as they nurture the development of their leadership attributes, and their personal ability to be change agents in the workplace, which as emphasised, is a fundamental skill in contemporary nursing. All nurses, as pivotal front-line healthcare workers, are placed in a critical position to identify and implement change and be change agents. Change agents 'are people with either formal or informal legislative power, to lead change and influence other people's responses to change'. Compared to other healthcare professionals, nurses, being the front-line utilisers of policies and skills and those that spend the most time in contact with patients, are more likely to identify opportunities to optimise patient care. Moreover, innovation and change are not new concepts in the nursing profession. Nurses, on a daily basis, problem solve new ideas and methods of performing tasks in order to improve and implement patient-centred care and meet the unique needs of individual patients. All nurses are critically positioned to provide creative and innovative solutions that make a real difference to the day-to-day lives of our patients, organisations, communities and the health professions.

It is evident that in order to deliver a high-quality standard of nursing care, that is safe and effective, nurses must demonstrate the foundations of clinical leadership. Embedding the leadership styles of authentic and congruent leadership, fostering and developing attributes including being highly visible in practice, clinically competent, supportive and holding a high value for patient safety and quality care are imperative to becoming a competent nurse. In achieving this standard consistently, positive attitudes and support for change and innovation in the workplace must be employed. Graduate nurses and experienced registered nurses alike, both have an undeniably significant role to play in enhancing, maintaining or recovering a patient's health, with change, innovation and clinical leadership in all forms being fundamental to the attainment of this goal.

Kat - Student Nurse

Initiating, Envisioning, Playing, Sustaining: A Theoretical Synthesis for Change

This model offers a cyclical approach to change with four stages. The first is for the change to be **initiated**. In effect, goals are set and the problem is stated. The second stage is **envisioning**, where a vision for the future is outlined. In the third stage, **playing**, the vision and goals are tested throughout the organisation. The implication is that the 'leader' observes how the vision and goals are being implemented and makes appropriate adjustments to lead followers to success. The final stage, **sustaining**, implies that the change has taken root and with evaluation can be seen to be sustained change. It is concluded that the process never really stops, since evaluation and initiation are ongoing, so that as new problems arise and new goals are set the stages renew and develop (Edgehouse et al. 2007).

Beckhard and Harris's Change Equation

Beckhard and Harris's (1987) model places staff engagement at its heart, with the equation offering a solution to resistance encompassing dissatisfaction (D) with the present situation, a vision (V) for what can be achieved and the first steps (F) taken towards the vision (Jones and Bennett 2018). All of these lead to a path to overcoming resistance (R). The model is expressed as:

$$D \times V \times F > R$$

In keeping with sound mathematical principles, if any one of the variables is not addressed, the net result will be zero or an inability to negate the resistance to change.

People-Mover Change Model: Effectively Transforming an Organisation

This model has four parts: reflective motivation, team-based preparation, strategy implementation and evaluation. It begins with the change agent asking themselves vital or key questions about the planned change. The aim is to identify their passion for the proposed change. The next step is to select partners (team members) who will work with the change agent to support the change. In the third stage, strategy implementation, the change is communicated to others, and finally the impact of the change is evaluated. The process is about moving people along by motivating them and winning them over to the proposed change (Edgehouse et al. 2007).

Instituting Organisational Change: An Examination of Environmental Influences

In this model it is suggested that sustainable change is best achieved if the environment is most suitable for change to occur. In this regard, organisations need to have a high value placed on change, a safe environment for change to occur and open dialogue with those affected by change. This implies that a change-willing organisation will be prepared to assess its strengths, weaknesses and resources; plan for future development; and then apply itself to effective change (Edgehouse et al. 2007).

Change Is Never Simple, Even with a Model

Thus, there are many change models and many approaches overlap or encroach on the methods and theories of others. In this regard, choosing a model or set of change models is crucial if clinical leaders are to make effective plans for change. However, change is not an easy thing to effect and it is never just a matter of selecting or applying a model. As we argued at the beginning of this chapter, leadership styles that are collaborative, distributive and transformational are vital in initiating, implementing and sustaining change (Dougall et al. 2018). None of the models that we have presented in this chapter will facilitate change unless they are implemented by clinical leaders who are able to influence others to work together to accomplish a common goal (Smith 2015; Bender 2016; Kitson 2016) and create a culture that is supportive of change (Mannion and Davies 2018).

Resistance to Change

Resistance to change has been defined as 'a tridimensional (negative) attitude towards change, which includes affective, behavioural, and cognitive component' (Oreg 2006, p. 74). In the health arena, change is often difficult to implement and frequently faces stiff resistance. Kouri et al. (2020) estimate that 70% of intended changes fail. It is often assumed that resistance to change relates directly to how complex the intended change is. However, Kouri et al. (2020) argue that this is far from the truth because change is not only a technical process, it has a social side too, and it is this social aspect of change that is most likely to give rise to resistance (Lawrence 1954). In healthcare, this may be a phenomenon of the culture that seems to dominate, where hierarchical structures and constant rounds of change produce scepticism on unprecedented levels. Therefore, if clinical leaders are to facilitate or lead change, they need to acknowledge that resistance is common and they should be aware of both its likely cause and strategies for combating or acknowledging resistance.

There are a number of reasons why people may resist change, and these are discussed in what follows.

Self-Interest and Conflicting Agendas

Some health professionals resist change because they do not see it as in their best interests (Jones and Bennett 2018). They may fear a loss of power, influence, status, money or position. Weihrich and Koontz (1993), Griffin (1993) and Daft (2000) suggest that fear of loss may be the greatest obstacle to change within organisations. Such a fear may stem from professional rivalry, issues of low self-esteem or a lack of personal resources for dealing with change. Healthcare professionals with low self-esteem may react to change negatively, feeling that change will undermine them, whereas professionals with high self-esteem will generally see change as an opportunity, confident in their capacity to exploit the change or find benefits for themselves within it. It is suggested that clinical leaders will find themselves more commonly in the latter group, but they will need to be aware that reactions which are labelled self-interest may come from deeper feelings of insecurity or fear. Failing to recognise these deeper feelings or deal effectively with them may stall or affect the success of a change proposal.

Increased Stress

Dent and Galloway-Goldberg (1999) propose that resistance may in fact be a result of the perceived consequences of change. Any change requires a readjustment, and this, good or bad, implies an increase in stress. If it is combined with fear or feelings of loss (of position, power or status), increased stress in itself will lead to growing resentment and resistance to the change. Again, this should be acknowledged and addressed along with the actual change proposed.

Uncertainty

Being aware that change is planned and that it will affect them may create a level of uncertainty that can push people into rejecting the change, even before they understand it (Jones and Bennett 2018). Announcing a change and then expecting people to follow the organisation on a journey into the unknown, without providing information or insight, remains a main reason for people offering resistance to planned change. Fear and uncertainty are again the net result (Griffin 1993; Weihrich and Koontz 1993; Daft 2000). Uncertainty often produces the sense that people are not in control of their destiny, and this can have significant negative consequences for any planned change. Knowing what is coming allows people to make a decision to support the change, or at least to make decisions about any action that they feel is appropriate for them. Uncertainty again produces fear and increases stress. Organisations keen to hold on to power over their employees may favour uncertainty, but this approach is seldom successful, as staff who are fearful, destabilised, uninformed and anxious are seldom productive and useful within any organisation.

Diverging Points of View

Festinger (1957) labelled this issue 'cognitive dissonance'. What the managers see as an appropriate change may not be change that employees or staff consider appropriate. Such a situation commonly leads to conflict, as management and staff's goals, values or beliefs are at odds. The battle lines are about core beliefs, and if new systems or models of practice are being introduced, only behavioural change on the part of one side or the other will lead to effective progress. However, behavioural change will only result if there is a change in thinking about the new system or model. Some people will refuse to modify their thinking, believing that the planned change is inappropriate, unhelpful or unnecessary. The fight goes on in their mind as much as it does in the open as they struggle to accommodate the new values that the change will herald (Jones and Bennett 2018).

Cognitive dissonance may continue even after the change has taken hold, with resistance in the form of non-compliance with all aspects of the change, or a form of cognitive rebellion as individuals seek to superimpose some of their values back onto the change without being seen to oppose it overall. In order to combat this form of pernicious rebellion, clinical leaders need to effectively 'sell' any change that may challenge cultural ideals or long-held practices. The main reason clinical leaders are followed is because of their values and beliefs, and in this regard, bringing followers along with a change in values or beliefs may require considerable preparation and role modelling.

Ownership

Resistance may also follow if participants in the change do not feel connected to it or have ownership of it. Understanding the purpose of the change is a key factor in bringing participants along. Introducing change 'because you can', because you have authority over others, or doing so in an insensitive way will result in resentment, uncertainty, distrust and dissociation of participants from the planned change. Simply not allowing participants significant participation in the change process will ensure a negative result and resistance. A word of caution here: participation is not what the change instigator thinks it is, but what the participants think it is. This may be a confronting concept, but many a useful change proposal has come unstuck when resentment at a lack of inclusion was increased by management's insistence that collaboration was achieved when the vast majority of participants were convinced that they remained in the dark and were under-valued.

Recognising the Drivers

People may resist change simply because they see it as a threat to their self-worth or personal integrity. People like being in control or consulted; they do not feel comfortable if their values and beliefs are under threat or at risk of assault. Therefore, initiating change successfully may involve assessing the motivational forces that sit behind the people the change will affect. This implies a need for being compassionate to them and working in a collaborative relationship or partnership. However, the planned change will have a better rate of success and be less prone to attracting resistance if those who will be affected by the change are involved, consulted and respected.

Some People Just Do Not Like Change

It needs to be acknowledged that some people with specific personality types are more inclined to be resistant to change than others. Individuals bring with them their own beliefs, values, support systems, cognitive levels, personality types, languages, behaviours, cultural influences, maturity levels, emotional intelligence levels, emotions and emotional needs, and in the end some people have a low tolerance for change (Jones and Bennett 2018). Planning for these individual variances is impossible, so it could be expected that with every change, on some level, there will always be individuals within a group who will feel compelled to rebel or resist. These issues can be anticipated, but it is hardly an exact science, so even with personality type indicators, determining where resistance will come from may be impossible to predict. The best a change agent can hope for is to be aware that resistance is likely on some level and to be prepared with inclusive approaches, easy access to information about the change, and effective communication and information.

Recognising Denial and Allowing Time for Reflection

When faced with change, people commonly go into an initial period of denial. This is normal, as adjusting to the concept and reality of change takes time, and denial offers a period of reflection and thought. It is during this time that information should be provided, explanations offered and time given for the proposal(s) to take form in people's minds. Those planning change need to recognise that denial will occur and remember to have information about the planned change ready, respect the time this process of assimilation will take, and not rush participants into accepting the change without sufficient reflection time. Forcing participants to accept change without allowing them some time to grasp its consequences may force them into a pattern of resistance based on many of the reasons cited in this chapter.

> **Reflection Point**
>
> Why do you think some people are resistant to change? Speak with some colleagues about changes that have occurred in the past. How did your colleagues cope? How were these changes viewed then, and what impact do they have now?

Successfully Dealing with Change

Marquis and Hudson (2012) and Curtis and White (2002) suggest that managers, leaders and change agents should not only expect resistance but also be prepared to deal with it when it occurs. They also recommend consideration of the following points for change to be successful:

- Introduce change slowly, allowing time for thinking about and assimilating the change proposal.
- Participation of those involved or affected is essential, allowing all to take an active part in the change.
- Participants need to be able to take ownership of the proposed change at a cognitive level; that is, they need to feel that as individuals they are invested in the process of change.
- Information about the proposed change needs to be accessible and put forward as early as possible to allow people to adjust and accept or take part in it.
- Open and honest communication needs to be established. This will facilitate trust and limit misunderstanding. It will also promote two-way communication, questioning and feedback.
- It is important to offer support (psychological/emotional/informational) for people struggling with the proposed change.

Dignam et al. (2012), writing from an educational perspective, further suggest that collaboration is essential for change to be successful. It may also be helpful to employ an external change agent, an objective outsider who may be able to facilitate the change. However, this outsider may also be viewed with cynicism or mistrust if they do not follow the recommendations given here.

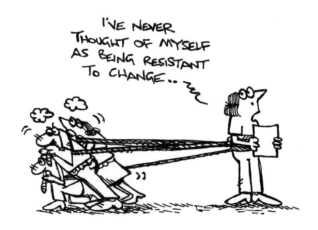

Organisations reflect the dynamics of small (and sometimes large) communities, and working within them requires considerable skill. There are champions and heroes, cynics and nay-sayers. Change, no matter how positive, has the power to promote feelings of stress, anxiety, anger, hope, liberation and indifference, and whatever the change being proposed, managing it and dealing with the inevitable resistance will be central to the clinical leader's role and function.

Recognising that resistance may be prevalent and acknowledging the complexities of planning and implementing a programme of change is essential. Robbins et al. (2001) claim that to bring about change successfully there needs to be a clearly defined action plan, adequate resources to facilitate the planned change, the incentive to change, the skills to push through what is required, and a vision of what is to be achieved that is shared with all stakeholders. If confusion, anxiety and frustration are to be avoided and if resistance is to be addressed or minimised, planning the change process requires the application of a suitable change model and the steps that Robbins et al. (2001) suggest.

It is clear that for the health service and care practices to improve, health professionals need to be able to recognise what does not work well and develop strategies and solutions to change care practices, attitudes, systems and processes.

This is relevant to clinical leadership practices because service improvement and developing the health service are based on effective change and innovation, which leadership is central to bringing about and facilitating, with clinical leaders often in the role of 'change champion' (Hendy 2012).

A range of tools for effectively managing change have been considered in this chapter. Learning to employ these change management models avoids a haphazard approach to change and innovation and offers health professionals an opportunity to make a genuine impact on change in a planned, measured and strategic way.

Case Study 7.1 Marie Curie

Marie Curie was born at a time when women were seen as secondary to men, in a poor family and in an area of Europe were women had few rights and limited access to education. Yet she was able to contribute significantly to our knowledge in the realm of science. Read the outline of her story and consider the challenge that follows.

Marie was born in Warsaw (then part of the Russian Empire) in 1867. Her early years were spent in and around the city, where she was supported and instructed by her father. At the age of 10 she attended her mother's boarding school, but her mother died from tuberculosis when Marie was 12, and after this she attended a gymnasium (school) for girls.

She came from a relatively poor family, and in order to support herself (and her older sister Bronislawa) Marie did some tutoring and then took a number of positions as a governess, first in Krakow, then with a prominent family in Ciechanow who were relatives of her father. Here she fell in love with a son of the family, Kazimierz Zorawski, and although it was reciprocated, the match was considered inappropriate by the head of the family and Marie lost her position as governess. Her sister asked Marie to join her

(Continued)

Case Study 7.1   (Continued)

in Paris, but Marie was still hoping to marry Kazimierz and remained with her father, where she did some further tutoring and began practical scientific training at a laboratory at the Museum of Industry and Agriculture. In 1891, at the age of 24, when it was clear that any relationship with Kazimierz Zorawski was impossible, Marie moved to Paris.

She studied at the Sorbonne during the day and tutored at night. She quickly earned a degree in physics and then mathematics. In 1894 she met Pierre Curie. Marie was studying the magnetic properties of various metals, and it is ironic that they were drawn together by their mutual interest in magnetism. Marie returned to Warsaw, but was denied a place at Krakow University because she was a woman. She returned to Paris – and Pierre. They were married in 1895, and after this the two physicists hardly left the laboratory, although they shared two hobbies, long bicycle rides and journeys abroad.

In 1896 Marie and her husband began to explore uranium. Their systematic research led to many discoveries, including the radioactive properties of the element thorium, the element polonium and radium. Radium was an incredibly difficult element to isolate and a tonne of the base metal pitchblende produced only one-tenth of a gram of radium chloride. The idea to look for an element with greater radioactive properties than uranium was Marie's, and her biography makes it clear that there was no ambiguity about who made the discoveries.

In 1903, Marie Curie and Henri Becquerel were awarded the Nobel Prize in physics, making her the first woman to be awarded a Nobel Prize. In 1897 and 1904 Marie gave birth to daughters (Irene and Eve, respectively) and in 1911 she was awarded a second Nobel Prize for services to chemistry. Marie was also the first person to share or win two Nobel Prizes, and she is one of only two people to have been awarded a Nobel Prize in two different fields. In spite of these achievements, the French Academy of Science refused her admission on the grounds that she was a woman. It would be one of Marie's students (Marguerite Perey) who would be the first woman admitted to the Academy, over 50 years later in 1962.

In 1906, Pierre Curie was killed in an accident. Marie was left devastated, but she focused on her work to regain some meaning in her life. This was facilitated by her appointment as a professor at the Sorbonne, the first woman to hold this type of post. In 1910, Marie began an affair with a former student of her husband's, creating a degree of scandal, but her hard work, the second Nobel Prize in 1911 and her determination persuaded the French government to overlook her personal life and provide funding for the establishment of what is now the Curie Institute. The building, a research centre, was completed in 1914 and became a hotbed of Nobel Prize winners, including Marie's daughter Irene and her son-in-law.

During World War I, Marie donated both her own and her husband's gold Nobel Prize medals to the war effort and worked to provide mobile radiography units, known popularly as 'little Curies', which were used to treat wounded soldiers.

(Continued)

Following the war, Marie travelled to the United States twice to raise research funds to establish a research institute in Poland. She died in 1934 from aplastic anaemia, almost certainly contracted as a consequence of her exposure to radioactive substances in her research work. Due to their radioactivity, her research papers from the 1890s – and even her cookbook – are still considered too dangerous to handle and are stored in lead-lined boxes.

During her life, Marie Curie had to overcome many societal and equality barriers. The fact that she was a woman and from a poor Eastern European country presented many obstacles to her progress in the field of science, and she is regarded as a genuine pioneer, emancipated and independent. Albert Einstein suggested that she was the only scientist not corrupted by the fame she had achieved.

Challenge: Change is seldom achieved without great courage and conviction. Models of change are therefore only a small part of the process, for without courage and determination even the best laid plans for change are likely to fail. Marie Curie faced numerous obstacles and was still able to achieve much. What sorts of obstacles do you face in your workplace, and how can you overcome them? Consider the change management tools in this chapter. Can these be used to address or support any plans you have for change? And how can you deal with or find the courage and determination to hold on to the ideas you have to improve your work or the experience of your clients/patients?

Summary

- Clinical leaders need to recognise and develop strategies and solutions to address what is not working in their clinical area.
- Workplaces are not machines, they are communities, and as such dealing with change involves recognising and dealing effectively with the people affected by it.
- There are a number of tools that will facilitate a measured and strategic approach to change. Choosing an appropriate tool to support the planned change is crucial for health professionals to effect positive and genuine change, but these tools will only be effective if they are used in partnership with collaborative, distributive and transformational leadership styles.
- When choosing a change management tool, remember to consider your own place within the change process and model of change to avoid bias and an ill-considered evaluation.
- For change to be introduced successfully, clinical leaders need to appreciate that often what is really required is for culture to be shaped, modelled and remodelled.
- For lasting cultural change to be effective, people need to be rewarded for actions that support and promote the culture or new culture being proposed.
- There are a number of reasons why people are resistant to change: self-interest and conflict, perceived stress from the proposed change, uncertainty, cognitive dissonance, issues of ownership, conflict over values and denial that things need to change. Dealing with resistance to change sensitively will help support both the change proposal and those involved in or affected by the change.

Mind Press-Ups

Exercise 7.1

Listen to the songs 'The times they are a-changin' by Bob Dylan (1967), 'Changes' (1971) by David Bowie and 'Revolution' by the Beatles (1968). Are the times always 'a-changin' or was it just that the 1960s and early 1970s were key times of change? Why do some people want change to be quicker and more revolutionary? Which approach do you think will best support the future of healthcare? Is David Bowie's struggle with change common?

Exercise 7.2

Draw up your own version of the FFA model. Think of a problem you want to address. It can be personal or work related. Begin by listing the driving then restraining forces that have an impact on the problem or issue you want to change. Look at your lists. What power does each element bring to bear on the force for or against the change? Represent the forces with thick or thin arrows on your diagram or with numbers showing the strength of each factor. Use the structure in Box 7.2 to support this exercise.

Box 7.2 Force-Field Analysis	
State the issues or problem here:	
Driving forces (Indicate the strength of each force)	Restraining forces (Indicate the strength of each force)

Exercise 7.3

Return to your mind map of the various changes you would like to make in your area of practice and apply the various models presented in this chapter to two of these proposed changes. Next, think through the leadership styles you would employ throughout the change process.

References

12Manage (The Executive Fast Track) (2009) *Change Management Iceberg.* http://www.12manage.com/methods_change_management_iceberg.html (accessed 4 October 2021).

Ackerman-Anderson, L. and Anderson, D. (2001). *The Change Leader's Roadmap: How to Navigate Your Organization's Transformation.* San Francisco, CA: Pfeiffer.

Beckhard, R. and Harris, R. (1987). *Organizational Transitions: Managing Complex Change*, 2e. Boston: Addison-Wesley.

Bender, M. (2016). Clinical nurse leader integration into practice: developing theory to guide best practice. *Journal of Professional Nursing* 32 (1): 32–40.

Brager, G. and Holloway, S. (1992). *Assessing Prospects for Organizational Change: The Uses of Force Field Analysis*. New York: Haworth Press.

Burke, W.W. (2017). *Organization Change: Theory and Practice*. London: Sage.

Curtis, E. and White, P. (2002). Resistance to change. *Nursing Management* 8 (10): 15–20.

Daft, R.L. (2000). *Management*, 5e. Fort Worth, TX: Dryden Press.

Dent, E.R. and Galloway-Goldberg, S. (1999). Challenging resistance to change. *Journal of Applied Behavioural Sciences* 35 (1): 25–41.

Dignam, D., Duffield, C., Stasa, H. et al. (2012). Management and leadership innursing: an Australian educational perspective. *Journal of Nursing Management* 20: 65–71.

Dougall, D., Lewis, M. and Ross, S. (2018) Transformational change in health and care: reports from the field. *The Kings Fund*. www.kingsfund.org.uk/publications/transformational-change-health-care (accessed 4 October 2021).

Edgehouse, M.A., Edwards, A., Gore, S. et al. (2007). Initiating and leading change: a consideration of four new models. *The Catalyst* 36 (2): 3–12.

Egan, G. (1990). *The Skilled Helper: A Systematic Approach to Effective Helping*, 4e. Pacific Grove, CA: Brooks/Cole.

Festinger, L. (1957). *A Theory of Cognitive Dissonance*. Stanford, CA: Stanford University Press.

Ford, J., Ford, L., and Polin, B. (2021). Leadership in the implementation of change: functions, sources, and requisite rariety. *Journal of Change Management* 21 (1): 87–119.

Griffin, R.W. (1993). *Management*, 4e. Boston, MA: Houghton Mifflin.

Ham, C. (2014). *Reforming the NHS from within: Beyond Hierarchy, Inspection and Markets*. London: The King's Fund. Available at: www.kingsfund.org.uk/publications/reforming-nhs-within (accessed 4 October 2021).

Ham, C., Dixon, A., and Brooke, B. (2012). *Transforming the Delivery of Health and Social Care: The Case for Fundamental Change*. London: The King's Fund www.kingsfund.org.uk/publications/transforming-delivery-health-and-social-care (accessed 4 October 2021).

Ham, C., Berwick, D., and Dixon, J. (2016). *Improving Quality in the English NHS*. London: The King's.

Hendy, J. (2012). The role of the organisational champion in achieving health system change. *Social Science and Medicine* 74 (3): 348–355.

Hulks, S., Walsh, N., Powell, M. et al. (2017). *Leading Across the Health and Care System: Lessons from Experience*. London: The King's Fund www.kingsfund.org.uk/publications/leading-across-health-and-care-system (accessed 4 October 2021).

Jones, L. and Bennett, C. (2012). *Leadership and Social Care: An Introduction for Emerging Leaders*. Banbury: Lantern.

Jones, L. and Bennett, C.L. (2018). *Leadership for Nursing, Health and Social Care Students*. Banbury: Lantern Publishers.

Kitson, H.G. (2016). PARIHS revisited: from heuristic to integrated framework for the successful implementation of knowledge into practice. *Implementation Science* 11 (33): https://doi.org/10.1186/s13012-016-0398-2.

Kotter, J. (1996). *Leading Change*. Cambridge, MA: Harvard Business School Press.

Kouri, G., Stamatopoulou, M., Tzavella, F., and Prezerakos, P. (2020). The Greek resistance to change scale: a further validation. *International Journal of Caring Sciences* 13 (1): 294–306.

Kubler-Ross, E. (1973). *On Death and Dying*. London: Routledge.

Lawrence, P. (1954). How to deal with resistance to change. *Harvard Business Review* 32: 49–57.

Leunig, M. (2003). *A Common Prayer: A Cartoonist Talks to God*. Sydney, NSW: HarperCollins.

Lewin, K. (1947). Frontiers in group dynamics: concept, methods and reality in social science; socialequilibrium and social change. *Human Relations* 1: 5–41.

Lewin, K. (1951). *Field Theory in Social Science*. New York: Harper & Row.

Mannion, R. and Davies, H. (2018). Understanding organisational culture for healthcare quality improvement. *BMJ* 363: k4907.

Marquis, B.L. and Hudson, C.J. (2012). *Leadership Roles and Management Functions in Nursing: Theoryand Application*, 6e. Sydney, NSW: Lippincott Williams & Wilkins.

Nadler, D.A. and Tushman, M.L. (1990). Beyond the charismatic leader: leadership and organizational change. *California Management Review* 32 (2): 77–97.

NHS England and NHS Improvement (2021) *Stakeholder Analysis*. https://www.england.nhs.uk/wp-content/uploads/2021/03/qsir-stakeholder-analysis.pdf (accessed 4 October 2021).

Oreg, S. (2006). Personality, context, and resistance to organizational change. *European Journal of Work and Organizational Psychology* 15: 73–101.

Park, J.H., Mogg, R., Smith, G.E. et al. (2021). How COVID-19 has fundamentally changed clinical research in global health. *Lancet Global Health* 9: e711–e720.

Pettigrew, A.M. and Whipp, R. (1998). *Managing Change for Competitive Success*. Oxford: Blackwell.

Pettigrew, A.M., Woodman, R.W., and Cameron, K.S. (2001). Studying organizational change and development: challenges for future research. *Academy of Management Journal* 44 (4): 697–713.

Robbins, S.P., Millet, B., Cacioppe, R., and Waters-Marsh, T. (2001). *Organisational Behaviour : Leading and Managing in Australia and New Zealand*, 3e. Frenchs Forest, NSW: Prentice Hall.

Rogers, E.M. and Shoemaker, F.F. (1971). *Communication of Innovations: A Cross Cultural Approach*, 2e. New York: Free Press.

Scholtes, P. (1998). *The Leader's Handbook: Making Things Happen, Getting Things Done*. New York: McGraw Hill.

Smith, P. (2015). Leadership in academic health centers: transactional and transformational leadership. *Journal of Clinical Psychology in Medical Settings* 22: 228–231.

Weihrich, H. and Koontz, H. (1993). *Management at a Global Perspective*, 10e. New York: McGraw-Hill.

8

Patient Safety and Clinical Decision Making

Clare L. Bennett and Alison H. James

'We are not here to curse the darkness, but to light the candle that can guide us through that darkness to a safe and sane future'.

John F Kennedy, 1960

Introduction: A Choice

This chapter will focus on how clinical practitioners and leaders make decisions and the relevance and significance of decision making for clinical leaders, for care and service delivery and, ultimately, patient safety. It is impossible to deliver healthcare without making decisions, and poor decision making can have devastating consequences for patient safety and care. This chapter introduces the field of patient safety, outlines the theoretical background underpinning clear, effective decision making, explores why decisions sometimes go wrong and considers how clinical leaders use more than technical rational approaches when they make decisions.

Patient Harm

Here are some key statistics regarding patient safety/patient harm:

- Unsafe care is one of the 10 leading causes of death and disability internationally (Jha 2018).
- Approximately 1 in 10 patients in high-income countries experience harm in inpatient settings (Slawomirski et al. 2018) and nearly half of these incidents are preventable (de Vries et al. 2008).
- 134 million adverse events related to unsafe care occur in hospitals in low- and middle-income countries annually, leading to 2.6 million deaths (National Academies of Sciences, Engineering, and Medicine 2018).

Clinical Leadership in Nursing and Healthcare, Third Edition.
Edited by David Stanley, Clare L. Bennett and Alison H. James.
© 2023 John Wiley & Sons Ltd. Published 2023 by John Wiley & Sons Ltd.

- Internationally, up to 40% of patients experience harmful incidents in primary and out-patient healthcare, with up to 80% of incidents being preventable (Slawomirski et al. 2018).
- 15% of expenditure and activity in hospitals relates to adverse incidents (Slawomirski et al. 2018).

Perrow's (1984) normal accident theory explains that failures are inevitable in complex systems such as healthcare because a failure in just a few areas of the system can impact significantly on other areas. This is particularly the case when these failures are unexpected (Plsek and Greenhalgh 2001). Reason (2000) contributes further by asserting that human error and adverse events can be understood in terms of latent conditions (weaknesses within the system) which can lay dormant in the system but can also be triggered by, or induce, active failures (unsafe acts of individuals), leading to an adverse event.

Reason (2000) also introduced the Swiss cheese model (Figure 8.1), which demonstrates that within a system there are many levels of defence; however, each level of defence has latent conditions which are depicted as holes. If these holes become aligned because of a breach in defences, it increases the likelihood of a safety incident and harm occurring.

Reflection Point

Consider how safe you think healthcare is, whether patients ever experience avoidable harm and if they do, what do you think are the main contributors to harm?

What Is Patient Safety?

The World Health Organisation (WHO 2019) describes patient safety as a healthcare discipline that aims to prevent and reduce risks, errors and, subsequently, harm to patients. They argue that to achieve this goal leadership capacity is key, along with other areas that clinical leaders can influence such as the availability of clear evidence-based policies, data that identifies where improvements are required, competent healthcare professionals and the involvement of patients in their care.

Reflection Point

Consider the following scenario:

A surgical patient receives the wrong anaesthesia because of a mix-up that occurs due to similar packaging. The anaesthetist verbally requested the drug by the correct name but the operating department practitioner passed the wrong drug to her. The correct drug had been dispensed by pharmacy but had been placed next to a drug of a very similar name in the same colour packaging. The operating department practitioner was rushing and had picked up the drug which was next to the correct one in error and the anaesthetist did not spot the error when she checked it.

   Who should be held accountable for this error?

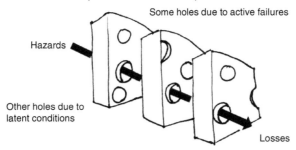

Reason's model helps us understand the complexities of an accident's pathology.

Some holes due to active failures

Hazards

Other holes due to latent conditions

Losses

Successive layers of defences, barriers and safeguards.

Figure 8.1 The Swiss Cheese Model (Adapted from Reason 2000).

In the example above, Reason's (2000) account of latent (weaknesses within the system) and active (unsafe acts of individuals) failures is relevant because both led to this adverse event. This is a classic example of Reason's (2000) Swiss cheese model in practice. Because of a lack of adherence to safety processes at various levels in this (real) scenario, such as standard procedures for the storage of medications that look alike, poor communication between team members and a lack of checking prior to drug administration, this error occurred. Even if just one of these strategies had been present the error would have been detected and corrected. Historically in this kind of scenario, the individual who actively made the mistake (active error) by giving the wrong drug would be blamed for the incident, but this overlooks the factors in the system that contributed to the occurrence of error (latent errors).

Mature healthcare systems, therefore, seek to reduce both active and latent errors by focusing on reducing the risk of error due to system factors (WHO 2019). However, this can only be achieved through clinical leadership that facilitates an open and transparent environment, which leads to a culture which prioritises patient safety (Workplace Health and Safety Queensland 2013).

Reflection Point

Identify 'near-miss' patient safety events that you are aware of in your clinical area, for example, a patient 'nearly' falling in a bathroom, incorrect manual handling that could compromise a patient's skin integrity, unsafe pre-operative checks, etc. Consider both latent (weaknesses within the system) and active (unsafe acts of individuals) errors that have contributed to the near misses.

Leadership and Patient Safety

Clinical leaders can contribute to patient safety by promoting an open culture underpinned by trust which, in turn, supports the workforce in communicating openly about errors and, importantly, learning from errors (Auer et al. 2014; Zaheer et al. 2021).

With regard to leadership styles, the literature suggests a positive relationship between transformational leadership and patient safety (Wong et al. 2013; McFadden et al. 2015; Merrill 2015; Weng et al. 2015; Farag et al. 2017; Fischer et al. 2017; Lappalainen et al. 2020). Motivational theory informs transformational leadership (Bass 1990) with its focus on empowering others to achieve excellence. In relation to patient safety, the transformational leader's authenticity regarding congruence between their values and ethical conduct is key, since this, in turn, facilitates trust among colleagues and positive role modelling in promoting behaviours that enhance patient safety (Lappalainen et al. 2020). In contrast, laissez-faire leadership styles are associated with a culture of blame (Merrill 2015; Farag et al. 2017), which negatively impacts patient safety.

Reflection Point

The WHO 2019 identified the following as the most common preventable adverse patient safety events internationally:

- Medication errors
- Healthcare-associated infections
- Unsafe surgical care procedures
- Unsafe injections practices
- Diagnostic errors
- Unsafe transfusion practices
- Radiation errors
- Sepsis
- Venous thromboembolism (blood clots)

Consider how your personal leadership style could contribute to reducing the risk of two of these events occurring among the patients in your care.

Clinical Decision Making and Patient Safety

Clinical decision making may involve decisions at the patient (micro) level regarding clinical procedures, the organisational (meso) level such as decisions regarding patient flow or at the national and international (macro) level such as the approval of and investment in vaccines and medications. As such, healthcare professionals' clinical decision making can lead to or negate both active and latent patient safety failures.

The provision of healthcare invariably requires patients and/or carers to make treatment choices, and health professionals to make clinical care decisions. The Latin root of the word 'decision', *decisio*, means 'to cut away'. So decision making should cut away the surrounding clutter to enable one to see a path to an objective, which one can follow with all of its implications (Russell-Jones 2015, p. 4). Rider-Ellis and Love-Hartley (2009) define a decision as a systematic cognitive process in which healthcare professionals need to identify alternatives, evaluate those alternatives and come to a conclusion. More recently, decision making has been described as the crux of patient-centred care, with shared decision making (SDM) being the process by which a patient and the healthcare professional make health-related decisions together based on the best available evidence. However, there has been a tendency to consider SDM primarily in terms of making treatment decisions.

A broader conceptualisation of SDM, whereby patients and health professionals jointly take an active role in decisions concerning the patient's health, can be applied to a range of decision-making activities such as the patient's contribution to identifying and articulating the nature of their problem, treatment monitoring and the way care is delivered. SDM presents new opportunities to improve health outcomes and healthcare services (Couët et al. 2015). Marquis and Huston (2009) view decision making as a complex, cognitive process related to choosing a particular course of action, and Carroll (2006, p. 93) supports this, indicating that decision making is the 'process of establishing criteria by which a nurse leader can develop and select a course of action from a group of alternatives'. Therefore, a decision may lead to a specific action or refraining from action, depending on the situation in which individuals find themselves.

The delivery of safe, high-quality patient care is dependent on the skills, judgement and decisions of health professionals, often working in teams (Mannion and Thompson 2014). Increasingly, healthcare professionals are leading and taking responsibility for making clinical decisions. All healthcare practitioners are accountable for their actions, and actions are based on decisions, whether those decisions are made consciously or otherwise. However, digital developments and new technologies, such as clinical decision support systems, have been shown to enhance diagnostic reliability and reduce variation (NHS England and NHS Improvement 2019). Likewise, prescribing tools such as electronic prescribing and medicines administration (EPMA) reduce medication errors (NHS England and NHS Improvement 2019). Equally, strategies such as SDM, where patients are empowered to become a part of the decision-making process (NHS England and NHS Improvement 2019) along with wider members of the healthcare team (Montague et al. 2019), can reduce the risk of patient harm.

Reflection Point

Consider whether the decision-making improvements described above are aimed at decreasing active or latent errors.

The above interventions aim to reduce human error in clinical decision making. Another successful intervention which aims to achieve the same is the patient safety huddle (PSH) (Montague et al. 2019; Burr et al. 2021). PSHs are brief multidisciplinary meetings which focus on patient safety and support decision making with the aim of mitigating identified risks and reducing adverse events (Montague et al. 2019; Burr et al. 2021). Beyond reducing patient harm, PSHs have been instrumental in enhancing the patient safety culture in organisations (Glymph et al. 2015; Burr et al. 2021).

Terminology

There are many terms used in healthcare that relate to decision making. These are often used interchangeably and should not be confused. The list includes:

- Making judgements: reaching a considered choice
- Clinical judgement: reaching a considered choice in clinical practice based on reflection, previous knowledge, data and client preference
- Clinical inference: an educated guess about a clinical issue, often based on heuristic insight
- Clinical reasoning: the process of applying logic to the clinical decision-making process
- Diagnostic reasoning: using the decision-making process to reach a diagnostic decision
- Problem solving: a systematic approach to analysing a difficult situation

Judgement, inference and reasoning are commonly employed to make decisions. However, decision making can occur without the complete analysis that is commonly seen in problem solving. A useful distinction between judgements and decisions is offered by Dowie (1993), in that a judgement is about assessing the alternatives, whereas a decision is about choosing between alternatives.

Decision-Making Approaches

If it is the case that decision making is a central part of healthcare, then it is important to explore how health professionals come to make decisions. Being able to make decisions in a considered, consistent and judicious way is vital, particularly so in the dynamic, changeable and ethics-laden environment of healthcare.

In healthcare, where quality and safety issues dominate, decision-making models can aid the decision-making process. Internationally, professional bodies are increasingly offering support for health professionals to assist them with making planned, considered choices and to minimise the 'ad hoc' nature of decision making.

Reflection Point

Explore decision-making models in your particular profession and specialism.

Relevant guidance also includes advice from the National Institute for Health and Care Excellence (NICE) (2021), which advocates SDM as a process in which patients and their carers, when they reach a decision crossroads in their healthcare, can review all treatment options available to them and participate actively in making that decision. In this model, patients and their carers are helped to work through any questions they may have, explore the options available and take a treatment route that best suits their needs and preferences. To achieve this, NICE (2021) encourages the development of new relationships among patients, carers and clinicians, where they work together, in an equal partnership, to make decisions and agree a care plan.

In clinical practice, a growing number of clinical decision-making models are emerging, with the aim of reducing human error. For example, there are algorithms that guide telephone healthcare triage and advice services, pressure sore development risk calculators which guide interventions, and vital sign monitoring packages that calculate and trigger early warning scores and systems. However, all clinical decision-making models require clinical judgement as there may be deviations to normal parameters that need to be understood and acted upon. For example, Early Warning Systems are often programmed to trigger based on a pulse oximetry reading that is less than 95–90%, but for some people their normal measurement is less than this.

Reflection Point

Consider the advantages and disadvantages of decision-making models.

Russell-Jones (2015) offers an example of a decision-making framework, suggesting that in any decisions there are potentially seven steps:

1) Define (the real issues to be decided on)
2) Understand (the context within which the decision is needed)
3) Identify (the options)
4) Evaluate (the consequences of each option)
5) Prioritise (the options from one choice)
6) Review (the decision taken)
7) Take action (to effect the decision)

A useful starting point when considering options is to begin by framing the decision and thinking about how the process should be implemented. Should the choice be made alone? Would it be better made in a group and, if so, who should be involved? Health professionals are becoming increasingly aware that many decisions that we have taken ourselves in the past are now better left in the hands of appropriately informed clients, patients or their relatives in some cases. What urgency is placed on the decision? Does it need to be taken at all? Finally, has this type of choice been made before and what was the outcome? Is there something that can be learnt from past decision-making episodes that were similar to the one being considered?

The characteristics of an effective model are essentially a representation of a traditional problem-solving process. While they are robust, there is some weakness in the time it takes to solve problems using these approaches when often, especially in clinical practice, problems require a speedy solution. It is clear that a systematic approach is required and that health practitioners already employ some sort of systematic approach on a daily basis in the clinical area, and indeed everywhere, when decisions need to be made. The real value of frameworks is that they make explicit the decision-making process and can at times be employed very quickly when faced with critical clinical decisions.

In order to make an appropriate clinical decision, practitioners should first consider the knowledge they already have regarding the following:

- the client/patient about whose care you are about to make a decision
- the personal impact your decision may have (on your patient, on you, on others)
- the decision-making process in use
- the impact of the decision on the quality of care
- the external factors that will influence the decision
- whether the decision is within the scope of professional practice (for your professional role)
- whether you have the appropriate skills, knowledge and attitudes to make the decision

There are also other issues that should be considered when applying a systematic approach to decision making:

- Can the patient make a choice or contribute to the decision?
- What are the patient's wishes?
- Are you the most appropriate person to make a decision in this circumstance?
- What information is available?
- Are there other options?
- Which option would be best for this patient at this time?
- What will be the implications of the decision?
- What evidence is available to support the decision?

Theories of Clinical Decision Making

A range of theory-based models attempt to explain how health professionals make judgements about patient care and reach clinical decisions. It has been suggested that the process of decision making is influenced by professional roles and socialisation processes (Hamers et al. 1994). Theoretical perspectives on decision making draw on information processing theory (IPT), cognitive continuum theory (CCT) and the intuitive approach (Goransen et al. 2008). IPT suggests that problem solving reflects how well people are able to adapt and that it is influenced by how good their short-term memory is (Newell and Simon 1972). CCT asserts that effective decision making is dependent upon the individual's ability to adapt to complexity, ambiguity and variations in how the task is presented. It also suggests that decision making is both analytical and intuitive (Hamm 1988; Thompson 1999). Intuitive theory emphasises the role of experience in decision making, with novices being described as reliant on context-free rules whereas experts use intuition (Benner 1984; Benner et al. 1996). In relation to healthcare, the literature suggests that the skills required for clinical decision making and the role of contextual factors in influencing decision making are not fully understood. However, although our understandings are incomplete, there are some useful nuggets of information in the literature that can help enhance the quality of clinical decision making and, thus, patient safety. These are summarised below.

Knowledge and Information

When considering theories of clinical decision making, it is important to reflect on where our knowledge and information come from, as being conscious of this can help practitioners avoid making decisions based on misinformation. Knowledge and information may stem from:

- tradition (knowledge that is passed down within cultures and subcultures)
- trial and error (from experience, but not very reliable)
- intuition (from experience, built up over time)
- personal experience (based on a person's individual clinical or life experiences)
- authority figures (advice, guidance, coaching and leadership from those whose experience we value)
- education (what we have learnt, what professional development or life experiences have supported our learning)
- logical reasoning (our capacity to apply logic and reasoning to the events in our life)
- reflection (our capacity to draw on past experiences and build a frame of reference to the past)
- research (our capacity to ask searching questions or analyse others' ability to ask and then answer questions)

Tradition, trial and error, intuition and personal experience all have their place and help in the development of knowledge and skills and, therefore, the decision-making process. However, caution is required, as these are not necessarily based on evidence or critical thinking. We often make decisions unconsciously, without the use of a systematic approach, which may lead to quick decisions. It is proposed that people such as healthcare professionals who are confronted with time-sensitive or life-threatening situations apply modified decision-making strategies that are less formal or less structured (Sinha 2005; Wolgast 2005). This unconscious process, known as heuristics (Marquis and Huston 2009), allows professionals to maximise what is already known, recognise patterns and, as a result, make a decision or solve a problem quickly and efficiently (Pritchard 2006). This type of decision making can work a great deal of the time, but not always, and is therefore not foolproof.

We also learn from authority figures and, of course, education, in whatever form that may take. Logical reasoning or using a technical rational approach (Fish and Coles 1998) is useful in the problem-solving or decision-making process, and through reflection we can learn much from decisions that were made in the past. In the health arena it could be argued that the most important facet of knowledge generation in the decision-making process is research or evidence-based practice, which provides the facts or knowledge on which to base our decisions. All these points are considered when established theories of decision making are employed. These include the following examples.

Intuitive-Humanistic Model

This approach to decision making accepts expert intuition in the reasoning process, but is rarely given any real credence (Hansten and Washburn 2000). Intuition does, however, appear to be a legitimate and essential aspect of clinical judgement and decision making so long as it is remembered that intuition can be overruled by a person's emotions, thus weakening it as a tool for systematic, rational decision making (Benner and Tanner 1987). The characteristics of intuitive decision making are that the context within which the decision is taken is usually quite specific (e.g. an occupational therapist could employ it in their area of specialism, say hand rehabilitation, but not in an area outside this, say paediatric spinal cord rehabilitation). The outcome of the decision is usually unknown, since the decision is based on frameworks and theories rather than formal, scientific rules. This remains a valuable decision-making approach, nevertheless, and sits at the heart of the debate in the healthcare literature (and common rooms) about whether healthcare is an art or a science.

Weber (2007) undertook a qualitative analysis of how advanced practice nurses (APNs) used clinical decision-support systems in the US Midwest and found implications for decision making based on how art and science are seen. What Weber (2007) demonstrated was that APNs were most comfortable with the capacity of an electronic clinical decision-making system's ability to forecast patient outcomes when the predictions that the software presented were consistent with the practitioner's personal judgements about the potential patient outcomes. Therefore, if the clinical decision-making system 'failed to support, confirm, or substantiate the APN's professional clinical judgment, it was disregarded' (Weber 2007, p. 667).

The fact that the nurses involved in Weber's study were 'advanced' clearly had an impact on their confidence to 'override' the predictors of the system's software, but it also highlighted the application of the artistry that healthcare practitioners employ in relation to decision making. Weber's results are supported by Andrews (2009), who proposed that the implementation of intuition in decision making is one of the critical skills that separates good from great leaders, with lesser leaders relying on traditional (technical rational) approaches when making decisions. Chen et al. (2016) also found similar results in a later study with nurse practitioners where they were discovered to use an intuitive-analytical model in clinical decision making.

Systematic-Positivist, Hypothetico-Deductive and Technical Rational Models

The systematic-positivist, hypothetico-deductive and technical rational approaches are all very similar. They rely on hypothesis generation, formal scientific rules, deconstruction and outcome prediction, and use schedules or protocols to interpret problems and make decisions. These would seem highly appropriate, but in fact they leave little room for heuristics, intuition, creativity or, indeed, what the patient may want. Fish and Coles (1998) also offer a view on how professionals make decisions, outlining a combined technical rational (scientific) view and a professional artistry view of how clinicians act in terms of decision making. This supports Andrews (2009) and Chen et al. (2016) in their findings, in that clinical leaders who combine their expertise with technical rational approaches achieve greater success in decision making.

Integrated Patient-Centred Model

The integrated patient-centred approach involves a process in which the clinician, interacting with the client or their significant others, structures meaningful goals and health management strategies based on clinical data, client choice, professional judgement and knowledge. This offers a combined approach to decision making that specifically focuses on the patient or client when framing goals.

IDEALS Model

This is similar to other models for supporting decision making. Its primary advantage is that it offers the mnemonic 'IDEALS' to help practitioners recall the relevant steps (Facione 2010):

- **I**dentify the problem
- **D**efine the context
- **E**numerate the choices
- **A**nalyse the options
- **L**ist the reasons for change explicitly
- **S**elf-correct

Managerial Decision-Making Process

There are a number of different managerial decision-making models. Most offer a modification of the traditional decision-making model with the addition of goal setting or objectives into the process. The steps involved may include the following:

- Determine the context of the decision
- Set objectives or goals
- Search for alternatives
- Evaluate alternatives
- Choose
- Implement
- Follow up and control

The model selected should preferably be one the clinical leader is comfortable and familiar with, and should be appropriate to the decision being considered. Using a specific model consistently is likely to increase the user's critical thinking skills and development of intuition (artistry) within the rational structure of the model (Marquis and Huston 2009).

Clinical Leaders Story 8: Bars

A physiotherapist on a cardiac rehabilitation ward noted that patients were usually assisted to the ward toilet and then left there. They were given a bell and told to ring it when they had finished. Then a nurse or physiotherapist would help them off the toilet and walk them back to their bed. Apart from taking considerable time on the busy ward, this whole process did not seem to be supporting the features of effective cardiac rehabilitation and helped foster greater client dependence on nursing and therapy staff. This practice had been in place for many years and was described as part of the 'ward culture'.

(Continued)

Clinical Leaders Story 8   (Continued)

The physiotherapist and a registered nurse suggested to the ward manager that if bars were placed in front of the toilet, patients could hold onto these and help themselves to stand, before walking slowly back to their bed unaided. The bell would only be used for emergencies, and busy clinical staff could focus on more pressing client needs. True rehabilitation and a focus on patient independence could also be encouraged. When they took the idea to the ward manager, she had no idea about the practice of ringing the bell, the clinical time being wasted or the missed opportunity for rehabilitation on her ward – as it was not her job, she had never answered the bell or helped anyone off the toilet and back to their bed.

Ironically, there were bars in the toilet area, but they had been attached to the wall behind the toilet, well out of anyone's reach. Indeed, it looked as though they had always been there and yet were never used. It cost nothing to ask a hospital maintenance employee to remove and reattach the bars where they could be reached, in front of the toilet.

The net result of this clinically driven initiative was that patients engaged in more positive cardiac rehabilitation activities and developed a greater sense of their role in their rehabilitation journey. The toilet bell was only used in emergencies, nurses and the physiotherapist were less distracted by frequent calls to answer the bell, and other patients benefited from greater attention to their needs afforded by the time saved. The physiotherapist and nurse were in our view clinical leaders, and this quality initiative, which cost nothing to initiate, is an example of the value of engaging and fostering clinical leaders in addressing client-focused change.

Jane – Physiotherapist

Clinical Leadership and Decisions

Leadership is commonly seen in terms of the leader's capacity to take decisions, to make the big call, to choose a course of action or a strategy (Marquis and Huston 2009). The big decisions that politicians or CEOs take are significant in the course of a country's progress or a corporation's success. However, in the scheme of people's lives, the choices that healthcare professionals make each day, each hour or each minute are as big for the individuals they affect. The point here is that health professionals who are in any doubt about their leadership capacity need only tally the number and impact of the myriad decisions they make each day to gain an insight into their leadership role.

Barriers to health professionals' participation in decision making should be explored and interventions developed so that clinically focused healthcare professionals may be able to participate fully in decision making that affects both patients and the work environment (Bacon et al. 2015). Globally, there is a growing emphasis on the importance of transforming the education of healthcare professionals to develop a shared vision and common strategy that reach beyond the confines of national borders and the silos of individual professions. Transformative learning involves a fundamental shift from fact memorisation to searching, analysis and synthesis of information for decision making (Frenk et al. 2015).

Why Decisions Go Wrong

It would be foolish to suggest that health professionals always make the right choice or decision, in spite of the existence of decision-making frameworks. There are a number of reasons for this.

Not Using the Decision-Making Framework

Not using a decision-making model or critically applying a decision-making framework is the surest way to an ill-informed decision in clinical practice. These tools and models have been designed to support clinicians and help develop a culture of informed decision making that employs critical thinking and a technical rational approach to care choices.

Flawed Data

If we have the wrong information, we make mistakes in our choices through lack of knowledge. Thus, it is incumbent on all health practitioners to gather the most relevant and up-to-date information from all available sources before effecting a decision.

Bias

Called 'filtering' by Russell-Jones (2015, p. 10), this implies that we do not believe the data or evidence because we have a personal bias (prejudice) against the method used to collect the data or the person who collected it. Furthermore, if the results contradict long-standing views, then our capacity to make effective decisions is compromised. Florence Nightingale's slow awakening to the possibility of germ theory can be used as an example of this type of bias (Bostridge 2008). She had for some time been engaged in an argument with William Farr, a scientifically minded member of her 'circle', and in a letter in 1859 he asked her to be more 'scientific in her arguments'. She replied that she did 'not venture to argue with' him and added:

> I only modestly and really humbly say, I never saw a fact adduced in favour of contagion [disease passed from person to person by germs] which would bear scientific enquiry. And I could name to you men whom you would acknowledge as scientific who would place 'contagion' on the same footing as witch-craft and other superstitions.

Nightingale was not the only doubter in her day, but her faith in sanitation, and in the idea that 'filth' was the cause of disease, meant that she was particularly slow to recognise the evidence building from the scientific work of Louis Pasteur, Joseph Lister, Robert Koch and others.

Seeking to Avoid Conflict or Change

Decision making is not easy and may not always be fair on everyone affected by the decision. This means that sometimes choices are made to avoid conflict or to negate change rather than solving the problem at hand.

Ignorance

If we do not have all of the available information, or worse, if we just do not bother to get the data or find the relevant information, the result is what is commonly called a guess. Patient care and a quality health service would be poorly served if health professionals routinely employed guesswork in their clinical decision making.

Hindsight Bias

Mistakes can be made because of second-guessing or poor or biased reflection. In effect, this means using new decisions to justify previously made decisions, especially if the previous decisions were incorrect or inadequate (Carroll 2006).

Availability Heuristics

Going by a 'rule of thumb' (Russell-Jones 2015, p. 10) or hoping that 'close enough is good enough' is essentially a failure to recognise that everyone is different and that a decision made for client 'A', even if the intervention worked, may not be relevant for client 'B', even if they have the same condition, wound, illness and so on.

Over-Confidence in Knowledge

Trusting that what we know is correct every time is where practitioners may jump to conclusions that are in fact wrong (Russell-Jones 2015).

Haste

This is not about speed; it is about poor decisions because they are made before all the facts are gathered (Russell-Jones 2015).

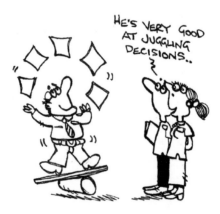

How about Emotion?

Given the nature of clinical decision making, it is interesting that the role of emotion is less evident in the literature. This reflects the dominant traditional discourse in the field, which assumes that clinical decision making is a purely rational process, requiring cognition and objectivity. However, recent research by Kozlowski et al. (2017) has linked emotional intelligence with clinical decision making. The findings of an integrative literature review (Kozlowski et al. 2017) have identified that the healthcare professionals' emotions do affect clinical decision making, although this acknowledgement is largely lacking in the literature as is educational preparation concerning emotional competence in the context of clinical decision making.

Group Decision Making

Depending on the decision, it may be appropriate to employ group decision making. This has some advantages and some disadvantages over individual decision making (outlined shortly), but when groups are encouraged to participate it is important that group members feel they are free to express themselves and state their opinions and ideas without duress or pressure to conform. Group decision making has real advantages when the impact of the decision will be felt by the group; therefore, they may prefer to be actively involved in the process of making that decision. Because group decision making takes longer, it is also important to recognise that more time will need to be assigned to the data collection and reflection stages of the decision-making process.

When supporting groups in making decisions, it is important to aim for a consensus decision and as such it may be useful to employ a nominal group technique (see Chapter 7) or, if the group cannot meet, the Delphi technique (see Box 8.1).

The Delphi technique allows many people to contribute to the decision-making process, and it may reduce the dialogue and chatter or even conflict between members of a larger group. However, it may be a very protracted process. Choosing the best approach to engage the group will depend on the group size, as small groups tend not to generate as many options and large groups may lack structure and consensus (Yoder-Wise 2015).

There is also evidence to suggest that groups take more risks when they engage in decision making (Russell-Jones 2015). This may be because a group has a shared feeling of

---

Box 8.1   Delphi Technique

The Delphi technique has the following steps:

- Send out a questionnaire addressing the issues to be decided.
- When the results are returned, summarise them and send out another questionnaire influenced by the summary data.
- Continue this process of questionnaire and summary results until the group feedback demonstrates a consensus.

responsibility and, as such, the risks are either explored in greater detail or the collective responsibility makes groups less cautious in general.

Advantages of Group Decisions

Groups bring more complete information and knowledge, as it is generally considered that two (or three or 10) heads are better than one. Groups tend to have more diverse views and thus group decisions are more likely to be accepted. There is also the issue of 'safety in numbers', since one person will not be held responsible for the decision. Group decisions tend to be more accurate and more creative than those made by individuals.

Disadvantages of Group Decisions

It can take a great deal of time to organise a group, ensure that appropriate personnel are among its members and find a convenient time for them to meet. Consensus may not be reached within the group, so potential actions may be delayed. Quick action is rarely the result of group decisions. There can be arguments and difficulties among the members, but a group can also lead to conformity, as some members can dominate, influencing their less assertive colleagues and potentially skewing the group view, making any decisions less effective. Moreover, Mannion and Thompson (2014) draw on theories from organisation studies and decision science to explore the ways in which patient safety may be threatened as a result of four systematic biases arising from group decision making: groupthink, social loafing, group polarisation and escalation of commitment.

Challenges

Effective decision makers take a 'step approach' to finding the root cause of an issue before acting and do not jump to conclusions. They employ an analysis and problem-solving approach and are wise enough to understand when they have reached their limitations. Effective decision makers avoid 'paralysis of analysis' (Russell-Jones 2015, p. 93) and learn from each decision-making experience.

Considered decision making can significantly contribute to patient safety and the avoidance of harm. Decision making models in the form of digital technologies and algorithms can reduce human error, but clinical judgement is still required. Latent errors caused by flaws in healthcare systems can also contribute to the risk of human error and require as much consideration as the prevention of active errors. With the increasing complexity of patients and healthcare systems, it is paramount that work environments are conducive to safe decision making and that staff have sufficient breaks and rest periods, quiet space to think and support from colleagues in exploring alternative decisions and coming to considered shared decisions with patients and their carers.

Case Study 8.1   Jo Brand

Jo Brand is a popular and respected comic and television personality. She was also a mental health professional and offers some unique insights into nursing. Consider her story and the challenge that follows.

Josephine Grace 'Jo' Brand was born in 1957 and has established a career as a notable English comedian, writer and actor. After working in a number of service jobs, she took a joint social science degree with a registered mental nurse qualification at Brunel University. She then worked as a psychiatric nurse for 10 years, at Cefn Coed Hospital in Swansea and the Bethlem Royal Hospital and Maudsley Hospital in London.

Jo's personal life and career as a comedian have been consistently linked to healthcare; she proactively uses her high public profile and popularity to promote the wellbeing of people with health problems, in particular but not exclusively those with mental health problems. As a staunch advocate for and campaigner on behalf of people with mental health problems, in 2007 she was awarded an honorary doctorate by the University of Glamorgan for her work as a psychiatric nurse. Professor Donna Mead, Dean of the School of Health, Sport and Science, commented 'Jo incorporates much of her experience working in the field of mental health into her current work as a comedienne. This has increased awareness of the work done by nurses in the mental health field. She has also used her experiences of working with individuals with conditions such as Alzheimer's to promote awareness of and raise funds for the Alzheimer's Society'.

In 2014, Jo was awarded a second honorary doctorate by Canterbury Christ Church University, for her work in raising awareness of mental health issues and challenging the stigma surrounding such illnesses.

In her entertainment career, Jo has appeared on various television shows, including being a regular guest on *QI*, *Have I Got News for You* and *Would I Lie to You?* In 2003, she was listed in *The Observer* as one of the 50 funniest acts in British comedy.

During her first gig as a comedian, she was scheduled to perform last in front of 'an audience from hell' and drank seven pints of lager while waiting. She humorously described how she therefore faced her first live audience with a 'bursting bladder'. As she climbed onto the stage, a male heckler started shouting 'Fuck off, you fat cow' and kept up the abuse until her performance finished. There was no applause at the end of her act. However, she persevered and her early comedy style involved her delivering jokes in a bored monotone, one line at a time, with pauses in between. She drew heavily from pop culture and the media, with many jokes containing references to well-known celebrities and public figures.

Jo delivered a guest lecture on the subject of psychiatric nursing to the University of Derby Psychology Society in 1997 in return for a donation to Derby Rape Crisis. Also in 1997, at Lambeth Hospital in South London, she opened the first major exhibition of the Adamson Collection since the death of Edward Adamson, the pioneer of art therapy, in 1996.

Jo co-created, co-wrote and co-starred in the BBC Four sitcom *Getting On*, for which she won the 2011 Best TV Comedy Actress BAFTA. The series, set in a geriatric ward, is a funny and realistic satire on the UK National Health Service.

(Continued)

Case Study 8.1   (Continued)

In 2010, Jo took part in *Channel 4's Comedy Gala*, a benefit show in aid of Great Ormond Street Children's Hospital. She is a supporter of a number of charities, and she was one of the celebrities, along with Tom Hiddleston, Benedict Cumberbatch, E. L. James and Rachel Riley, to design and sign her own card for the UK-based charity Thomas Coram Foundation for Children. In 2014, Jo was a part of the *All Star Choir*, who released a cover version of 'Wake Me Up' to raise money for BBC's *Children in Need*, which entered the UK Singles Chart at number one. She is the president of the Ectopic Pregnancy Trust and is a patron of the National Self Harm Network, the Prader-Willi Syndrome Association and London Nightline. In 2016, Jo Brand completed a highly publicised 150-mile walk across Britain in aid of Sport Relief.

Challenge: This chapter on patient safety and clinical decision making focuses on the relevance and significance of decision making for clinical leaders and for care and services delivery. Jo Brand never forgot her education and experience as a mental health nurse. On the contrary, she used the opportunities presented by her 'second career' as a comedian to advocate for and champion the causes of those in society who need support due to their health conditions. She campaigns for national and international charities and draws on her experience of clinical decision making when she was a practising nurse to highlight to national and international decision makers the challenges for those living with the consequences of health problems. She puts herself under considerable pressure in order to raise much-needed charity funds and help develop and promote healthcare services so that current healthcare professionals can work with patients to participate in SDM to enhance patient safety. Do you use your privileged knowledge and understanding within your area of healthcare to help ensure that SDM is a reality? Think about how you promote SDM in healthcare and whether there are areas of your personal life in which you could advocate for the wider political and societal needs of those in your care. Are there ways in which you use your professional education and experience to help others understand the needs of the groups or individuals you involve in decision making around their health problems?

Summary

- Too many patients are harmed each year internationally.
- Transformational leadership can actively contribute to patient safety.
- Consideration of both active and latent failures is essential when reducing the risk of adverse events.
- Health professionals are accountable for their decisions, actions and failures to act.
- Effective decision making can contribute positively to patient safety.
- Clinically focused health professionals need to ask how and why we do things, constantly challenge decisions and therefore practice, to ensure that we do the best for patients.
- Decisions should be based on the best available evidence at all times.
- The application of a range of approaches, including intuitive-analytical decision making, can help us make better decisions.

Mind Press-Ups

Exercise 8.1

Identify five potential adverse incidents that could occur in your clinical area and develop strategies that you could implement to minimise the risk of the incident occurring. Share these with your team.

Exercise 8.2

Reflect on the predominant leadership styles used in your clinical area. What impact do they have on the safety culture of the clinical area?

Exercise 8.3

Undertake a small survey where you work. Ask a number of colleagues if they have ever made a mistake with a clinical decision. Do not focus on what they did wrong or the outcome, but ask about why they think they made a poor decision and how they think they could avoid doing so in the future.

Exercise 8.4

Access the internet and see if you can find references to the decision-making approaches detailed in this chapter. Once you have found the information, try the techniques out. Consider decisions you have made and see if you can use these models or if they help with a particular problem.

References

Andrews, J. (2009). Intuitive decision-making profile. In: *Leadership Roles and Management Functions in Nursing: Theory and Application*, 6e (ed. B.L. Marquis and C.J. Huston). Philadelphia, PA: Wolters Kluwer/Lippincott, Williams & Wilkins.

Auer, C., Schwendimann, R., Koch, R. et al. (2014). How hospital leaders contribute to patient safety through the development of trust. *Journal of Nursing Administration* 44: 23–29.

Bacon, C.T., Lee, S.-Y., and Mark, B. (2015). The relationship between work complexity and nurses' participation in decision making in hospitals. *Journal of Nursing Administration* 45: 200–205.

Bass, B.M. (1990). *Bass & Stogdill's Handbook of Leadership: Theory, Research & Managerial Applications*, 3e. New York: Free Press.

Benner, P. (1984). *From Novice to Expert. Excellence and Power in Clinical Nursing Practice*. New York: Addison-Wesley Publishing Company.

Benner, P. and Tanner, C. (1987). Clinical judgement: how expert nurses use intuition. *American Journal of Nursing* 87 (1): 23–34.

Benner, P., Tanner, C.A., and Chesla, C.A. (1996). *Expertise in Nursing Practice. Caring, Clinical Judgment and Ethics.* New York: Springer Publishing Company.

Bostridge, M. (2008). *Florence Nightingale: The Woman and Her Legend.* London: Viking.

Burr, K.L., Stump, A.A., Bladen, R.C. et al. (2021). Twice-daily huddles improve collaborative problem solving in the respiratory care department. *Respiratory Care* 66 (5): 822–828.

Carroll, P. (2006). *Nurse Leadership and Management: A Practical Guide.* Sydney, NSW: Thomson/Delmar Learning.

Chen, S.-L., Hsu, H.-Y., Chang, C.-F., and Chang-Lan-Lin, E. (2016). An exploration of the correlates of nurse practitioners' clinical decision-making abilities. *Journal of Clinical Nursing* 25: 1016–1024. https://doi.org/10.1111/jocn.13136.

Couët, N., Desroches, S., Robitaille, H. et al. (2015). 'Assessments of the extent to which health-care providers involve patients in decision making: a systematic review of studies using the OPTION instrument. *Health Expectations* 18 (4): 542–561.

Dowie, J. (1993). Clinical decision analysis: background and introduction. In: *Analysing How We Reach Clinical Decisions* (ed. H. Llewelyn and A. Hopkins), 7–26. London: Royal College of Physicians.

Facione, P.A. (2010). *2010 Update: Critical Thinking, What It Is and Why It Counts.* Milibree, CA: Measured Reasons/California Academic Press.

Farag, A., Tullai-McGuinness, S., Anthony, M.K., and Burant, C. (2017). Do leadership style, unit climate, and safety climate contribute to safe medication practices? *Journal of Nursing Administration* 47: 8–15.

Fischer, S.A., Jones, J., and Verran, J.A. (2017). Consensus achievement of leadership, organisational and individual factors that influence safety climate: implications for nursing management. *Journal of Nursing Management* 26: 50–58.

Fish, D. and Coles, C. (1998). *Developing Professional Judgment in Health Care: Learning through the Critical Appreciation of Practice.* Oxford: Butterworth Heinemann.

Frenk, J., Chen, L., Bhutta, Z.A. et al. (2015). Health professionals for a new century: transforming education to strengthen health systems in an interdependent world. *The Lancet* 376: 1923–1958.

Glymph, D.C., Olenick, M., Salvatore, B. et al. (2015). Healthcare utilizing deliberate discussion linking events (HUDDLE): a systematic review. *American Association of Nurse Anesthetists Journal* 83 (3): 183–188.

Goransen, K.E., Ehnfors, M., Fonteyn, M.E., and Ehrenberg, A. (2008). Thinking strategies used by registered nurses during emergency department triage. *Journal of Advanced Nursing* 61 (2): 163–172.

Hamers, J.P.H., Abu-Saad, H.H., and Halfens, R.J.G. (1994). Diagnostic process and decision making in nursing. *Journal of Professional Nursing* 10 (3): 154–163.

Hamm, R.M. (1988). Clinical intuition and clinical analysis: expertise and the cognitive continuum. In: *Professional Judgment a Reader in Clinical Decision-Making* (ed. J. Dowie and A. Elstein), 78–102. New York: Press Syndicate of the University of Cambridge.

Hansten, R. and Washburn, M. (2000). Intuition in professional practice. *Journal of Nursing Administration* 30 (4): 185–189.

Jha, A. K. (2018). Presentation at the "Patient Safety – A Grand Challenge for Healthcare Professionals and Policymakers Alike," A Roundtable at the Grand Challenges Meeting of the Bill & Melinda Gates Foundation (18 October 2018).

Kozlowski, D., Hutchinson, M., Hurley, J. et al. (2017). The role of emotion in clinical decision making: an integrative literature review. *BMC Medical Education* 17 (255): https://doi.org/10.1186/s12909-017-1089-7.

Lappalainen, M., Harkanen, M., and Kvist, T. (2020). The relationship between nurse manager's transformational leadership style and medication safety. *Scandinavian Journal of Caring Studies* 34: 357–369.

Mannion, R. and Thompson, C. (2014). Systematic biases in group decision-making: implications for patient safety. *International Journal of Quality Health Care* 26: 606–612.

Marquis, B.L. and Huston, C.J. (2009). *Leadership Roles and Management Functions in Nursing: Theory and Application*, 6e. Philadelphia, PA: Wolters Kluwer/Lippincott, Williams & Wilkins.

McFadden, K., Stock, G., and Goween, C. (2015). Leadership, safety climate and continuous quality improvement: impact on process quality and patient safety. *Health Care Management Review* 40: 24–34.

Merrill, K. (2015). Leadership style and patient safety. *Journal of Nursing Administration* 45: 319–324.

Montague, J., Crosswaite, K., Lamming, L. et al. (2019). Sustaining the commitment to patient safety huddles: insights from eight acute hospital ward teams. *British Journal of Nursing* 28 (20): 1316–1324.

National Academies of Sciences, Engineering, and Medicine (2018) *Crossing the global quality chasm: Improving health care worldwide*. Washington (DC): The National Academies Press. https://www.nap.edu/catalog/25152/crossing-the-global-quality-chasm-improving-health-care-worldwide

Newell, A. and Simon, H.A. (1972). *Human Problem-Solving*. Englewood Cliffs, NJ: Prentice Hall, Inc.

NHS England and NHS Improvement (2019). *Shared Decision Making*, Redditch: NHS England, https://www.england.nhs.uk/ourwork/pe/sdm (accessed 4 March 2016).

NHS England and NHS Improvement (2019) *The NHS Patient Safety Strategy. Safer culture, safer systems, safer patients*. https://www.england.nhs.uk/patient-safety/the-nhs-patient-safety-strategy (accessed 23 October 2021).

NICE (2021). Shared decision making. www.nice.org.uk/about/what-we-do/our-programmes/nice-guidance/nice-guidelines/shared-decision-making (accessed 23 October 2021).

Papers of John F. Kennedy Pre-Presidential Papers. Senate Files, Box 910, "'The New Frontier,' acceptance speech of Senator John F. Kennedy, Democratic National Convention, 15 July 1960." John F. Kennedy Presidential Library.

Perrow, C. (1984). Normal accidents: living with high-risk technologies. *Administrative Science Quarterly* 29 (4): 630–632.

Plsek, P.E. and Greenhalgh, T. (2001). Complexity science: the challenge of complexity in health care. *BMJ* 323 (7313): 625–628.

Pritchard, M.J. (2006). Professional development. Making effective clinical decisions: a framework for nurse practitioners. *British Journal of Nursing* 15 (3): 128–130.

Reason, J. (2000). Human error: models and management. *BMJ* 320 (768): 768–770.

Rider-Ellis, J. and Love-Hartley, C. (2009). *Managing and Coordinating Nursing Care.* Philadelphia, PA: Lippincott, Williams & Wilkins.

Russell-Jones, N. (2015). *Decision-Making Pocketbook.* Alresford: Management Pocketbooks.

Sinha, R. (2005). *Impact of experiences on decision making in emergency situations.* Psychology C/D extended essay, Engineering Psychology, Lulea University of Technology, Sweden, http://epubl.ltu.se/1402-1781/2005/15/LTU-CDUPP-0515-SE.pdf (accessed 1 July 2016).

Slawomirski, L., Auraaen, A. and Klazinga, N. (2018). The Economics of Patient Safety in Primary and Ambulatory Care: Flying blind. Paris: OECD http://www.oecd.org/health/health-systems/The-Economics-of-Patient-Safety-in-Primary-and-Ambulatory-Care-April2018.pdf (accessed 22 October 2021).

Thompson, C. (1999). A conceptual treadmill: the need for 'middle ground' in clinical decision-making theory in nursing. *Journal of Advanced Nursing* 30 (5): 1222–1229.

Thompson, C. and Dowding, D. (2002). Clinical decision making and judgement in nursing: an introduction. In: *Decision Making and Judgement in Nursing* (ed. C. Thompson and D. Dowding), 47–65. Edinburgh: Churchill Livingstone.

de Vries, E.N., Ramrattan, M.A., Smorenburg, S.M. et al. (2008). The incidence and nature of in-hospital adverse events: a systematic review. *Quality and Safety in Health Care* 17 (3): 216–223.

Weber, S. (2007). A qualitative analysis of how advanced practice nurses use clinical decision making support systems. *Journal of the American Academy of Nurse Practitioners* 19 (12): 652–667.

Weng, R.H., Huang, C.Y., Chen, L.M., and Chang, L.Y. (2015). Exploring the impact of transformational leadership on nurse innovation behaviour: a cross-sectional study. *Journal of Nursing Management* 23: 427–439.

Wolgast, K. (2005). *'Command decision-making: Experience counts', USAWC strategy research project, Master of Strategic Studies degree*, USA Army War College, Pennsylvania, www.au.af.mil/au/awc/awcgate/army-usawc/cmd-decis-mkg.pdf (accessed 1 July 2016).

Wong, C., Cummings, G., and Ducharme, L. (2013). The relationship between nursing leadership and patient outcomes: a systematic review update. *Journal of Nursing Management* 21: 709–724.

Workplace Health and Safety Queensland (2013). *Understanding Safety Culture.* Brisbane: The State of Queensland.

World Health Organization (2019). Patient Safety. https://www.who.int/news-room/fact-sheets/detail/patient-safety (accessed 22 October 2021).

Yoder-Wise, P.S. (2015). *Leading and Management in Nursing*, 6e. St Louis, MO: Mosby.

Zaheer, S., Ginsburg, L., Wong, H.J. et al. (2021). 'Acute care nurses' perceptions of leadership, teamwork, turnover intention and patient safety – a mixed methods study. *BMC Nursing* 20 (134): https://doi.org/10.1186/s12912-021-00652-w.

9

Creativity

David Stanley

> *Come with me and you'll be*
> *In a world of pure imagination*
> *Take a look and you'll see*
> *Into your imagination.*

Anthony Newley/Leslie Bricusse, songwriters from the
Charly and the Chocolate Factory film – Pure Imagination, 1971

Introduction: A New Way Forward

This chapter looks at the issue of creativity: what it is, why it is important for nurses and other health professionals to develop creativity skills, and how to develop creativity. The chapter also addresses the barriers that hinder creative development and how creativity and leadership are linked. There is very little formal training in undergraduate or even postgraduate health education that deals with the issue of creativity. It is implied perhaps in learning goals for critical thinking and problem solving, but creativity and idea generation are seldom the focus of specific learning goals. And yet, being creative and bringing new ways of working and practice into being are the fundamental building blocks of clinical progression. Everything we do in healthcare had to start from a creative idea, a new thought or the courage to try something new. In some areas of practice, such as occupational therapy, finding creative solutions to complex clinical needs is clearly a key part of the role. This is less evident (perhaps) in other areas of practice, although recognising that clinically focused leaders commonly act to initiate and propose new ideas and solutions for often complex problems means that it is important to consider creativity in terms of the catalogue of tools to support innovation and implement values and beliefs in practice.

Clinical Leadership in Nursing and Healthcare, Third Edition.
Edited by David Stanley, Clare L. Bennett and Alison H. James.
© 2023 John Wiley & Sons Ltd. Published 2023 by John Wiley & Sons Ltd.

What Is Creativity?

Like leadership, creativity can be a difficult concept to pin down and define (de Bono 2015). Doyle (1993) and Rickards et al. (2008) suggest that creativity is much easier to detect than define. However, Barez-Brown (2006, p. 30) sees creativity as 'simply doing something new and differently that creates some benefit'. de Bono (2016) explains this with a new term or tool; 'bonting', which means the adding of value to something which is already good but not good enough. He argued that thinking to create value is not normally included as an aspect of thinking, but that if one starts with 'a value dream', which is like a hypothesis, then thinks creatively, down to a concept, then to an idea and then to a practical idea, creativity can be engaged. Edward de Bono (who, sadly, died in 2021) said at a book launch in 2016, that 'just as creativity can be taught, with the formal tools of lateral thinking, so thinking to create value can be taught' (de Bono 2016). Barez-Brown (2006, p. 31) adds that 'creativity gives us choices, gives us hope that in some way we can be special, we can be ourselves, we can create our own futures'. The *Oxford Dictionary* (Tulloch 1997, p. 336) suggests that to be creative is to be 'inventive and imaginative' or to 'originate', be 'artistic, original, ingenious or resourceful'. A broad view of creativity is that it is the ability to generate new, novel or useful ideas, solutions and propositions to everyday problems and challenges. De Bono (2015, p. 16) describes it as 'bringing into being something that was not there before'. Rickards et al. (2008) suggest that a definition of creativity needs to satisfy two requirements. First, an idea needs to be original, surprising, and novel; and second, it needs to be adaptive, effective and functional.

Sharma (2010, p. 231) states that the essence of creativity is original thought, offering the phrase 'see what all see, think what none think' to describe creativity in practice. Sharma (2010) adds that to foster innovation in organisations it is vital to create a workplace that rewards curiosity and recognises new ideas.

Thinking creatively is a highly desirable human trait, as it enables and supports us to keep up with or drive change. In this regard, most (if not all) people may be considered to be creative; it might be that some people just do not act on their ideas to the same extent as people consciously identified as 'creative', such as artists, painters, musicians or architects. However, if creativity is understood to be a basic human ability, then we all have the capacity to become creative or express our creativity (Klemm 1990). Creativity can be learnt and therefore it may be that some people are simply encouraged to do so more than others.

Creativity is rarely identified as a desirable skill for nurses or health professionals, so maybe its expression within nursing and the health professions is simply not encouraged, or it may even be suppressed in favour of processes, procedures and techniques or organisational structures that – hopefully unwittingly – discourage innovative thinking. Although I am sure this is less so for health professions, where creativity is an essential aspect of the role, such as in occupational health or physiotherapy. However, nursing and other health professions are commonly described as both an art and a science, and other health professionals are likewise supported to develop 'artistry' in the expression of their professional skills. The extraordinary talents of people whom we consider 'creative' or who work within creative fields (the arts, advertising or music) are commonly recognised when they combine their talents with determination and persistence to achieve mastery in their field. However, there may be a tendency not to recognise the 'creativity' expressed by others in areas not traditionally seen as creative, such as healthcare or business. Each person can be creative in their own domain by recognising their own skills and talents and developing mastery of them. Creativity is described as the ability to develop unique ideas and solutions to problems and challenges, and, in the health arena, health professionals are constantly employed in thinking about problems and searching for solutions to often complex and demanding issues.

Nevertheless, creativity is not a talent in the sense that it is inherited. Creativity is not a gift, even though some very creative people are often described as 'gifted'. Creativity is more a state of being, and being creative is about accepting that someone has new ideas and novel solutions and is prepared to act on them to help solve a problem. In this way, it can be seen that creative ability can be studied, learned, developed, improved on or increased over time (de Bono 2015, 2016).

In the 1920s, Graham Wallas (Doyle 1993) described the creative process as having four parts, which he called preparation, incubation, illumination and verification. They are still relevant today, and each is thought to set out how the creative process may be explained and offers an understanding of creativity so that we may learn how to develop creative skills and evaluate the effectiveness of the creative process.

- *Preparation:* This can only come from a solid grasp of the area or a degree of specialist knowledge. Writers, in order to become great writers, must have developed their craft, practised their art and understand the principles that underpin the writing process. They also need to know their subject and maintain an open, inquisitive and confident attitude to their endeavours. Following a formula or established practice may result in a new novel, but its potential creative impact is likely to be diminished. Preparation is about getting ready to build ideas and creative opportunities.
- *Incubation:* Wallas felt that while the conscious mind may help develop the ideas, it is in the subconscious that ideas and creative thoughts germinate (Doyle 1993). Solutions are therefore commonly described as being 'revealed' rather than arrived at consciously.
- *Illumination:* Wallas describes eureka moments as the issues being illuminated (Doyle 1993). As an extension of incubation, the idea may arrive without warning and may be accompanied by the feeling that a solution has been found.
- *Verification:* This involves critical analysis and assessment, evaluating the idea for its practical application and verifying its suitability to solve the problem or address the issues at hand.

Barez-Brown (2006) describes the creative process more simply, suggesting that it involves three steps: **insight**, which is about becoming clear about what your opportunities may be; **ideas**, which are about how to make the opportunities work for you; and finally **impact**, which is about doing something with the ideas. He indicates that because the process is so straightforward it can work on anything and lead to inspiring opportunities. Barez-Brown (2006) is also clear that ideas and thoughts are different, in that ideas change the world while thoughts do not. The difference he proposes is that you can 'do' ideas.

Creativity, therefore, may be more than simply having a thought about an issue or even just discussing a concern (say in the tearoom at morning coffee). Creativity implies a capacity or willingness to act on an idea and follow it through. This does not mean you have to be a genius, just that you need to apply yourself to an issue or problem and spend conscious or even unconscious or subconscious time ruminating positively on a solution. In the health service, nurses and other health professionals do this constantly, often with problems that they or their colleagues have encountered before. The application of creativity is why we are not still using scarification or blood-letting techniques for the treatment of, well, practically everything, and why new and enlightened approaches are being suggested for how we deliver health services across the globe.

De Bono (2015) suggests that the sources of creativity are the following:

- **Innocence**–like that of a child, so that if you do not know the usual approach, or the way things are 'normally' done, then you might have the advantage of 'fresh' eyes on the problem.
- **Experience**–the opposite of innocence and dependent on some people knowing because they have been there before, so they know what might work and what might not.
- **Motivation**–having the willingness to focus and look for novel solutions.
- **Tuned judgement**–recognising the potential of an idea at an early stage.
- **Chance, accident, mistake and madness**–history is full of advances that were not planned or even imagined, but happened because luck or misadventure played a part.
- **Style**–while not always generating new ideas, styles lead to creativity within existing approaches.
- **Release**–where the brain or person is freed to engage their creative options.
- **Lateral thinking**–the use of creative thinking techniques specifically and deliberately to focus the mind on being creative.
- **Values** (de Bono 2016) – the use of a belief system and values set to imagine the world into being.

Here is a selection of statements that people have made about creativity to elaborate on these concepts further:

> We are what we repeatedly do. Excellence then, is not an act, but a habit.
>
> *(Aristotle)*

> An idea can turn to dust or magic, depending on the talent that rubs against it.
>
> *(Bill Bernbach)*

> Imagination rules the world.
>
> *(Napoleon Bonaparte)*

> Blessed are the flexible, for they shall not be bent out of shape.
>
> *(Anonymous)*

> This telephone has too many shortcomings to be seriously considered as a means of communication. The device is inherently of no value to us.
>
> *(Western Union internal memo, 1876)*

There is no failure, except in no longer trying: no defeat, except from within; no insurmountable barrier, except our own inherent weakness of purpose.

(Elbert Green Hubbard)

The analysis of data will not by itself produce new ideas.

(Edward de Bono)

Live and work, but do not forget to play, to have fun in life and really enjoy it.

(Eileen Caddy)

We have to understand that the world can only be grasped by action, not by contemplation. The hand is more important than the eye . . . the hand is the cutting edge of the mind.

(Jacob Bronowski)

The essential conditions of everything you do must be choice, love, and passion.

(Nadia Boulanger)

Building Creative Capacity

Nurses and health professionals are commonly not perceived as possessing creative thinking skills or as being creative, although I suspect some aspects of healthcare lend themselves to a greater expression of creativity than others. Zuber and Moody (2018) are clear that there is an increasing push in healthcare for creativity and innovation to tackle key healthcare challenges, address issues of access and quality, and reduce harm or costs. In the past, as a nurse educator, I have had occasion to express myself creatively, and the most frequent response to these occasions has been: 'Why are you still a nurse, why not do something that allows for fuller creative expression?' I have always been satisfied with the capacity of nursing to allow me to be creative, and I believe that nurses and other health professionals are indeed creative, expressing their creativity every day in each and every healthcare environment. For example, the occupational therapist who employs a new moulding technique to make a physical aid or the physiotherapist who develops a new patient record system are both acts of creativity. Or it could be a play therapist who notices that a toy can be creatively used to encourage a child to develop strength in their upper body as they play. All these types of interaction offer evidence that creativity and innovation have a place in clinical practice in the hands of clinical leaders.

However, I accept that many health professionals and nurses may not see how creativity can be developed or applied to their work environment. Yet innovation (and creativity) is the cornerstone of a responsive and developing health service (Weintraub and McKee 2019). Enhancing your creative, innovative or critical thinking skills is not a one-off activity, and it requires attention over the course of your career.

Clinical Leader Stories: Nine Physiotherapy Challenge

At a workshop exploring clinical leadership in Western Australia, two physiotherapists offered some feedback. Two months earlier, at the first part of the workshop, the participants had been given the task of identifying areas in their practice where they might be able to bring about some measure of change. The physiotherapists outlined the change they had initiated on return to their clinical area, a medical rehabilitation ward in a busy city hospital. They had for some years been following a practice by which cardiac patients, prior to discharge, had to demonstrate that they could climb a set of stairs. This had become a pre-discharge prerequisite and no cardiac patient could be discharged until success in this task had been demonstrated and recorded. The issue the physiotherapists identified was that often this meant that a patient's discharge was delayed until a physiotherapist could undertake the activity. They set out to identify where the practice had originated and what clinical evidence sat behind it. They met with all the cardiac medical officers in the hospital and consulted a wide range of literature. The literature proved of limited value and the medical staff even less so, as none of them suggested that it was their idea to have the test undertaken prior to discharge.

Faced with a practice that seemed to have no basis in clinical evidence or medical practice, the two physiotherapists applied some creative thinking and suggested that it served no sound clinical purpose and that it should be stopped. While such a change clearly offered several benefits to the hospital, in terms of reducing the length of stay and speeding up the discharge process, the hospital and ward managers were at first not keen to change the practice. They were not sure that a change like this, initiated as it was by two physiotherapists, was worthy of consideration. They were concerned that not all medical practitioners were in favour of the change, and they were less convinced of the lack of literature to support this practice, given that 'it had been going on for so long'.

The physiotherapists persisted and recruited key medical staff to argue their position. They knew that the change to a less specific and more individualised cardiac assessment was a better outcome for the patients, the assessment process and the discharge issues, and because of these factors they were resolute and determined.

These physiotherapists were also congruent leaders. They had been motivated to look for change issues through their participation in the workshop, but it was their values and beliefs that a better outcome could be had by changing the cardiac patient assessment process that kept them focused on their values and determined in their belief that the practice should change. They used creativity, excellent communication skills and were seen as collaborative and collegial by their medical partners. The eventual outcome was a better, more flexible and appropriate assessment strategy that allowed many more patients access to a speedier and safe discharge.

Techniques for Developing Creativity

The following activities or suggestions offer practical advice and a range of skills that can be used to foster greater creative capacity. They are not all for everyone and it may be that only a few suit the type or range of creativity you intend to apply. The aim here is to offer a smörgåsbord of options to enhance your choice.

Relax

Listen to music (I find the classics particularly relaxing). Sit on the lawn in the sunshine. Take a walk, do some meditation, ride a bike, swim or have a spa. These activities allow you to take time for yourself and unwind, enabling your subconscious to take you out of yourself. Establish a 'work/life' balance that you are happy with.

Keep a Notebook or Journal

I have a small notebook with me all the time. In it, I write ideas and notes about significant events. Some I transfer into more elaborate reflections in my professional portfolio. Most remain just notes made from day to day. I don't keep a diary, although this might do as well. I record thoughts, ideas, observations and wonderful quotes I come across or I write affirmations. Some authors recommend that you use different colours to emphasise parts of your notes and make the notebook or journal your constant companion. I use underlines or bold print to highlight different parts of my notes.

Journaling

This is more specific than just keeping a journal. Here you need to wake up each morning and write a few pages about anything. Typically, it will be about the events of the previous day, but it could include dreams, ideas, thoughts, problems, solutions, needs or things to be thankful for. You may have to get up earlier than usual, but you will develop a deep insight into many areas of your thoughts and creative talents.

Record Your Ideas

Your brain is always working. The trick is to keep up with it and capture what it is thinking about. As well as a notebook or a journal, you can use cartoons, drawings, mind maps, index cards, a range of coloured pens or pencils, whiteboards, jotter pads or even a tape recorder. A laptop or tablet computer (particularly if marketed for audio and visual media such as books) now offers all these tools in a portable and readily accessible format, boosting the capacity to record ideas and thoughts easily. Take care with online social networking websites, though. You can record these thoughts on one of these, but everyone can see what you write, and someone might either react negatively or take your idea further without your consent.

Do or Learn Something New Each Day

Maybe there is no need to do one new thing absolutely every day, but the idea is to stimulate your creativity by learning or doing something different, something you might not have ever considered before or something you have wanted to do for a long time. Learn a new language, learn to parachute, learn new clinical skills. Take a course in history. Develop an interest in gardening or cooking or massage.

Learn to Draw

There are courses and books about drawing skills, and what is wonderful about drawing is that it uses the right side of your brain (the creative side). Learning to draw helps you grow your creative brain. It also helps you learn about perspective, light and shade and might help you meet new people.

Become a Cartoonist

Cartoonists see the world from a unique perspective, yet they can encapsulate simple humour, satire, political commentary and a wide range of other perspectives in their work. Cartoons appeal to the right side of the brain and Mukerjea (1997) refers to them as 'ideavisuals', where the imagery used bolsters the viewers' understanding because our eyes take in more detail than our other senses. Like drawing, cartooning can allow creative expression that ranges from doodling to carefully crafted and detailed images.

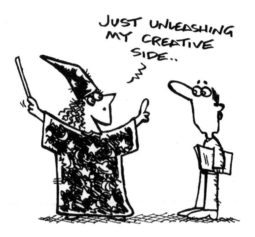

Learn to Map Your Mind

Mind maps are great tools to help you capture a concept or develop an idea. Use coloured pens, large sheets of paper or online programs, and even as you start the process you are being creative. You can develop your own style with icons, symbols, lines, links and space supporting your developing insights into a particular topic.

Try Associational Thinking

This is like mind mapping. You can use stories (your own and other people's) to compare your thoughts on a particular topic. Again, the technique uses a large sheet of paper, a trigger word and links that join your thoughts about the word. You can ask others (friends or colleagues) to do the same and then compare how each person thought about the same topic.

Go for a Walk

If you are stuck with a problem, take it for a walk, work in the garden, wash the dishes or go for a drive in the country. Change your space, and ideas sometimes flow. Even if they do not, the fresh air and exercise are good for you and your brain.

Adopt a Genius

There are people we recognise as having been gifted and creative, such as Leonardo da Vinci, Abraham Lincoln, T. S. Eliot, Andrew Lloyd Webber or Albert Einstein. Why not read about them, or look into their lives for clues about creative thinking?

Open a Dictionary

Sometimes if you are stuck for an idea, just open a dictionary and random words may stimulate some creative thoughts. In a way, the point is to restrict or direct your thinking, and while some people may feel that it is 'freedom' that stimulates creativity, a disciplined mind may also embrace restrictions to guide the creative process and help it to flow.

Study Books about Creative Thinking

Do not stop at this chapter. There is a fascinating range of books and web pages about creativity that will be a great support in developing your creative abilities. Edward de Bono's books are especially wonderful.

Flood Yourself with Information

Choose an area of interest and immerse yourself in it. Attend to this new interest fully so that you become completely respectful of the new topic or subject. Respond to your own needs to learn and feed yourself with knowledge. The internet makes this task much more accessible.

Attend Courses

You could do a course in anything you want to learn, but I am specifically recommending developing your creative potential. Creativity needs feeding, and the best food is the diversity of human life. If all you do is work, you will become dulled and blunt. Attending a course is an extension of the idea that you should be active and involved, opening doors for your mind.

Listen to Baroque Music

Wolff (2009) suggests that baroque music synchronises brain waves to about 60 cycles per second, and it produces a relaxed alpha state, which is frequently associated with creativity.

Face a New Fear Every Day

This is about being challenged. It may not be every day, but facing challenges is a great way to help create solutions. If you are worried about riding a motorbike, is it because you are afraid, you have seen the consequences of accidents in A&E or because your mother, husband or partner said you cannot? Maybe there are other solutions to facing this fear. Perhaps your fear is of swimming, or rock climbing or spiders. If fear is stopping you having a full and happy life, then finding a creative solution to it would be an excellent approach to developing more creative skills.

Develop Your Imagination

A great way to enhance your creative capacity is to foster a deep and active imagination. There are a number of ways to do this in a positive and healthy way. Here is a list of a few recommendations:

- Travel is a fabulous way to refresh your outlook and widen your tolerance and horizons. Travel also fosters greater self-reliance, so that you become more dependent on your own capacity to think, solve problems and generate new ideas.

- Develop personal contacts and associate yourself with creative people, fun people with a sense of humour and interesting views and those who stimulate your mind.
- Learn from children. A child's world is full of fun, games, fantasy and play and interacting with children is a great way to get in touch with your own imagination.
- Play games and do puzzles to get to grips with your creative side. Not everyone likes games and often you need to find a partner to play one. Puzzles are better if you can only try these activities alone. Both challenge your strategic skills, communication skills and creative talents. Sport can offer the same rewards but is not everyone's cup of tea.
- Take up a new hobby of the hundreds you could consider. Any hobby will help get your creative juices flowing. Many new hobbies can be undertaken from home and on the computer, so that expense, or time, or having to stand on a train platform for hours can no longer be offered as a valid excuse for not having a go.
- Read more, of anything. I find time to get through a book or so a week, and while there are some genres I do not enjoy reading, I do like to have a go at a range of different books to see what I can learn, or just to escape for a while. If you are time poor, listen to a 'talking' or audio book.
- Write something. This is not for everyone, but putting pen to paper or fingers to keyboard can be a very creative and stimulating activity and a wonderful outlet for your imagination.
- Learn to recognise your own abilities. Understand and acknowledge that you are a creative person. Remember that your imagination is there to be activated and developed. While you may need to nurture these skills, they exist, and you do not need permission, just opportunity.

Leave Things Alone for a While

It may be that the best thing to do is just put the problem down and walk away for a while. Getting away can offer a fresh perspective or allow you to 'sleep on it' – as long as you remember to come back!

Find a Creative Space

When singer/songwriter Joni Mitchell needed to create music, she retired to a cabin in a remote part of Canada. Other creative types use similar approaches, taking themselves away from distractions and into environments that foster and feed their creative spirit. In the film *Love Actually*, a writer, played by Colin Firth, took himself off to Portugal and a rented cottage. Maybe this is a bit extreme, but the idea of a place or space where you can escape and think is a sound one. It might be why some men have sheds. You could try to develop a creative space too. The core of this idea is to create a sensory, stimulating environment.

Develop Your Sense of Humour

Having a creative bent means having a sense of fun and developing skills in, and an appreciation for, humour. Sometimes we need to see the funny side of things to allow the emergence of a new perspective about an issue we may have become too close to. De Bono (1985) describes humour as the most significant behaviour of the human mind, because it employs a different form of logic. Humour can therefore liberate our thinking and allow us to take different paths in our thinking journey, leading to greater creativity.

Define Your Problem

Know the problem you face. Often people struggle to find solutions because they have not taken time to define or name their problem. Once this is done, you might find that ideas come more freely. Brainstorming or mind mapping may be a useful tool to start this process.

Know Yourself Well

To a large degree, becoming more creative means being able to learn to listen to your inner voice or intuitive side. If you are not in tune with your inner monologue, then you may miss creative opportunities because your personality or beliefs might shield you from possible solutions or insights. The key here is to know yourself well.

Use Guided Reflection

This is reflection (see Chapter 15) with the use of a diary or notebook, or even the use of a mentor or guide, to support, direct or channel your thoughts and positive ideas.

Be Mindful

Mindfulness is about engaging in the 'now' and focusing on ways to open your mind to greater choices and possibilities (Goldstein 2014).

Focus

De Bono (2015, p. 149) suggests that 'simple focus' can be a powerful creative tool, as it allows you really to consider the issues you are hoping to be creative about. Goleman (2013) also describes focus as the hidden driver of excellence.

Do Not Be Afraid to Fail

Failure is likely in any endeavour, but even failure can lead to new positive insights and fresh possibilities. As mentioned earlier, there is no failure except in no longer trying. So even if the goal of becoming more creative takes time, attempting and failing is really only a way of finding other paths to your goal.

Develop Some Techniques for Creative Thinking

This might involve setting a measurable goal to a problem that requires a solution (e.g. streamlining the discharge process in the minor injury unit in which you work). The next step would involve establishing criteria related to reaching this goal, then gathering information that will help develop your creative response. You might want to read books, go to conferences, speak to other people, access networks, or search the internet or library resources. Once you have formulated some ideas, sound other people out about them and prepare yourself for the potential risk that you may be about to take. Celebrate your success and start thinking of yourself as a creative person.

Table 9.1 lists some of the other techniques that can be used to promote creative thinking, and there are many others. Like tools in the tool shed, these techniques can be used individually or collectively to bolster an individual or a group's collective creativity. The internet offers the greatest range of these ideas, and you can access a vast number by simply going to a search engine and entering 'Techniques for creative thinking'. I came across a

Table 9.1 Techniques for creative thinking.

Assumption smashing	Fuzzy thinking	Six thinking hats
Random input	Breakthrough thinking	Problem reversal
Attribute listing	LARC method	Ask questions
Storyboarding	Idea 'toons'	Imitation
Lotus blossom technique	Metaphorical thinking	Applied imagination
Roger Olsen's DO IT! method	Morphological analysis	Unconscious problem solving
Neuro-linguistic programming	Forced relationship	Visual thinking
Brainstorming	Discontinuity principle	Checklists

wide number in preparing this chapter; some I could recognise, many were a mystery, but most looked like they were worth considering or using in a number of situations.

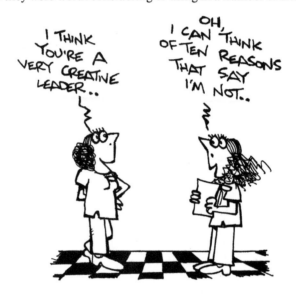

Barriers to Creativity

A number of barriers can hamper and hinder creativity. Evans (1993) suggests that we all carry with us culturally produced barriers to creativity. Many relate to our work or home environment or to the organisational structure; however, the main barriers are within the individual as a result of their cultural development.

Organisational Barriers

Competition

In the work environment, competition can hinder creativity if people focus more on their own advancement and share fewer ideas. There is a myth, particularly in finance and high-tech industries, that internal competition promotes innovation (Breen 2004). What was evident from Breen's (2004) research was that this belief can hinder productivity, research output or creative suggestions, as colleagues – who perceive themselves to be in competition for research funding or promotion – become less willing to share ideas, time or resources for fear of missing an opportunity or of helping a colleague to advance over them. Sharma (2010) adds that if the workplace is not risk free, creativity will be hindered. If people feel they have something to lose, their creativity will be stifled. Aligning with this, Weintraub and McKee (2019) suggested that a lack of group cohesiveness hindered orgaisational innovation and creativity.

Organisational Structure

Organisations that favour hierarchical structures over more democratic or meritocratic structures tend to support less- creative endeavour. In hierarchical organisations people feel that it is often up to those at the top to come up with the ideas, or they may have had ideas only to have had them taken by those above them as their own. Reward in these organisations is in the hierarchical climb and less in the joy of solving or addressing problems. Organisational restructuring is also counterproductive if creativity is to be fostered. When organisations downsize, creativity suffers (Breen 2004), and there can be residual effects on employee creativity for up to five months after the restructuring. Restructuring can be essential in times of economic hardship, but the impact on creativity can be negative, diminishing communication and collaboration (Breen 2004).

Being Too Busy to Address a Problem

Often, employees are kept so occupied that there is no time for them to have ideas or express these formally. Nurses working on a busy medical ward may recognise a solution to a problem but can be so caught up in their survival of the shift that the solution remains unvoiced and so unheard. Breen (2004) suggests that there is a myth that time pressure fuels creativity; however, the research demonstrated that when people work under great pressure their creativity went down – not only on that day, but remaining low for the next two days as well.

Too Hectic an Environment

Like being too busy, this implies that there is no time to stop and reflect, no place or time to have a 'quiet moment' and become introspective or to focus. It is often only on such occasions that solutions and ideas can germinate.

A Sterile Environment

I know operating theatres are meant to be like this, but this barrier allows no stimulation in the work environment to foster creativity and free thinking, such as whiteboards for mind maps or thinking exercises, places to relax, dream or contemplate, colour, variety, space, comfortable seats and places to talk. A sterile environment produces sterile thinking and stifles creativity. In the 1930s, Walt Disney commissioned and designed a new studio to house the increasing workforce at his company, but many of the older employees suggested that the new, specifically designed studio had lost the 'soul' of the original workplace and as a result creativity was diminished for a time. Sharma (2010, p. 236) suggests that setting up a 'contest committee' can help energise an organisation or department. This committee's role is to dream up all sorts of play and fun activities to help people laugh and smile and grow (and become more productive) while at work. This approach may motivate staff, improve communication and increase job satisfaction. The team, department or company that plays together stays together, and grows (Sharma 2010).

Poor or Harsh Feedback

People like to know that they are doing well. If they are not, telling them that in front of patients or other staff, or in a harsh way, will not foster their creative input. It may lead to very negative consequences for how they see or value themselves, or for the productivity and harmony of their work environment. Critique, if delivered poorly, can be a feeble motivator.

Rules

Rules are often essential for reasons of safety, to support economic constraints and to maintain order and production. Nevertheless, they can be a limiting factor if they are applied illogically, inhumanely or unfairly. Rules are great guides, but apart from some natural laws of nature, social rules that govern behaviour and other structures of the workplace may actually prevent staff from gathering information, meeting others or finding opportunities to develop. In the day-to-day running of an organisation this can lead to bureaucratic constraints and the proliferation of task forces, committees or think tanks with no power to act (Klein 1990). Rules or 'sacred cows' have had to be broken or slain for any sort of progress in almost every field of endeavour, and leaders have been pivotal to these occurrences (von Oech 1990).

Unrealistic Production Demands

As with being too busy personally or organisationally, if people are required to meet unrealistic targets and feel under pressure to perform at work, then stress and dissatisfaction can result, having a negative impact on creativity.

The Boss Is Always Right

If the 'boss', ward manager, team leader or head of department signals that they know they are always right and should not be challenged, this will hinder people's willingness to approach them with other and better ways of working or solutions to the problems of the area. Even the most creative people will not put their jobs at risk by challenging a boss who has an autocratic attitude (Klein 1990).

Poor Communication

When communication is open and information is shared effectively, teams and individuals are permitted to take risks and teamwork, creativity, innovation and empowerment result (Vogelsmeier and Scott-Cawiezell 2009).

Personal Barriers

Fear of Criticism/Fear of Failure

If we do not have an idea or take a risk, then no one will have a reason to be critical. When Breen (2004) studied the impact of fear on creativity, he initially set out to test the hypothesis that fear, sadness and depression fostered creativity, as some psychological literature had suggested. Breen found, though, that creativity was more positively associated with joy and love and negatively associated with anger, fear and anxiety.

Our Belief that We Are Not Creative

Many people see creativity residing in the domain of the creative arts, musicians and other people specifically assigned a creative role in society. They fail to recognise that creativity can be part of any occupation or job. In turn, this may lead to the belief that we are not, or do not need to be, creative.

Fear of Change

Being creative may imply that we are not happy with what we have or that we want things to change. Change can be a difficult thing to deal with, and being the instigator of change may compound the risks and threats. Initiating an idea brings with it responsibility and risk, and for many people this alone is enough to keep them from creativity's fire.

Ego

Having a powerful ego or identity can stop us from accepting new ideas or lead to us expressing our own ideas forcefully, to the point where people may even be threatened, less by the proposal and more by the style used to communicate it. Our ego, linked to our beliefs, may lead to an aggressive defence of our ideas, and this can hold us back from finding creative new ways to see where we might relate to the rest of the world.

Beliefs and Values

Beliefs and values can act in the same way as routines, if they become so entrenched that they cannot be challenged or reviewed. Our beliefs and values act like a filter for how we respond to information, gather data, perceive the world and process information. Like routines, holding fast to our beliefs can lead us to a personal reality tunnel that keeps us from seeing what else may be about us and from understanding 'reality' in new ways (de Bono 2016).

Lack of Confidence

Like fear of failure, some people may simply not feel confident enough about their place in an organisation to speak up, or they may lack sufficient faith in their talents to take the risk of putting them on display. Failure is the mother of invention, but in our workplace or society in general, failure is not valued. Richard Branson didn't get everything right on the first attempt – few people do. You may have tried before or may never have spoken up or taken the time to explore a new idea fully. People who lack confidence may find that their creativity is stifled because they are trapped by fear and lack the capacity to take a risk.

Stress

It is very difficult to be creative when we are stressed. Our mind is tied up with negative feelings or bound by the energy it takes simply to cope with the stress.

Previous Negative Experiences with Risk

If we have had negative experiences when we have attempted to be creative, it is not unreasonable to see that taking a further risk may require great courage. Overcoming negative emotions or simply gathering the courage to reapply your mind to the creative act can be a serious barrier.

Negative Self-Talk

Stress, previous negative experiences and a lack of confidence can all result in negative self-talk. Negative thoughts can lead us into false or hopeless traps, reinforcing our self-limiting belief that 'we are no good', 'our ideas are not right for the problem' or 'why would anyone listen to me?' Before the idea is expressed it is defeated by our mind's own limitation on ourselves – possibly the saddest of all barriers.

Routines

Having a set way of performing a task or job can lead to us becoming too entrenched in a way of life, a way of work or a way of thinking. This approach will limit the responses we can employ when faced with new problems and can result in a bureaucratic response to problems, in our personal and work life. Routines create the chains of habit that are too weak to be felt, until they are too strong to be broken. Being creative in these circumstances becomes very difficult.

Other Barriers

Daily Distractions

Being creative requires space for our brain to think, reflect, focus and mull over ideas without distractions and interruptions. Yet the modern world is overwhelmed with sounds, motion, activity and visual stimulation. Television, smartphones, radio, the press, magazines, movies and even advertising on billboards as we drive to work – or that pop up on our computer screen – never leave us with a minute's peace. The main issue that stifles creativity in the modern world is television and smartphones. Creativity and television rarely match. Routine activities also have a negative impact on creativity; childcare, school runs and housework can all sap our creative spirit, if we allow them to.

Not Having a Place to Go or Time to Get There

Many people lack a special thinking place or a hobby where we can think as we 'do'. Alternatively, we may not have a relaxing habit, like fishing, that allows us to reflect and think while we sit or stand in silent contemplation.

Drugs

Some 'creative' people see drugs (legal and illegal) as essential, but they rarely support significant creative developments. Medication of any kind is not helpful in this context.

> **Reflection Point**
>
> Look around your work or home environment. What do you recognise as barriers to your creativity? There may be none. If there are any, list them and, using the information in this chapter, see if you can make a list of potential barrier-busting interventions to help promote your creative output. Reflect for a moment on your relationship with creativity. Is it the environment or you? Do you feel the need to refrain from creativity in your home or work life? Are you the barrier?

Leadership and Creativity

There are two take-home messages from this chapter. As Weintraub and McKee (2019, p. 138) indicate, it is 'almost a cliché to say that health systems must constantly innovate'. Therefore, to be an effective leader it may be necessary to possess a highly developed creative streak. This is not always the case, and interestingly, in the clinical leadership research that underpins the theory of congruent leadership, creativity was not rated highly as a clinical leadership attribute (Stanley 2006, 2008; Stanley et al. 2012, 2014, 2015; Stanley and Stanley 2019). Indeed, clinical leaders were commonly not followed because of their creativity. This does not mean that they were not creative or did not offer creative solutions to the problems they faced, just that their creativity was not the reason or attribute that others used to identify them as a clinical leader. Nevertheless, this was not the case with Cook's (2001) research, in which clinical leaders were indeed identified as being 'shapers' who employed creativity in the fulfilment of their role.

The other message is that effective clinical leaders may be people who can recognise, stimulate, motivate or direct the creative energies of the people they lead, supporting them to contribute creative ideas and solutions that foster better client care, more effective processes or new and better ways of doing things (Price 2006). The key to this rests in clinical leaders' ability to use their communication and information-sharing skills to create a cohesive and empowered team (Reiter-Palmon and Illies 2004; Price 2006; Vogelsmeier and Scott-Cawiezell 2009). Clinical leaders may generate creative solutions of their own or support others to voice or develop creative contributions. However, if innovation and change are to develop, or if new and better healthcare is to evolve, it will only come from health professionals who are courageous or bold enough to speak out or propose their new ideas (Gentile 2010; Weintraub and McKee 2019) or if clinicians have the support and encouragement of clinical leaders to foster others' innovations.

There are a number of reasons why clinical leaders should foster creativity: it helps prevent obsolescence, it promotes productivity and innovation and it can help improve quality and reduce costs (Klemm 1990; Price 2006; de Bono 2015, 2016; Weintraub and McKee 2019). Organisations where creativity is rewarded and where new ideas are supported grow and develop, thrive and survive far more effectively than organisations that suppress creativity and reward people for maintaining the status quo (Klemm 1990; Reiter-Palmon and Illies 2004; Hall 2005; de Bono 2015; Weintraub and McKee 2019). We see creativity being rewarded in industries such as information technology or the arts, and in possibly the best-known internet search engine, Google, which is a great example of an organisation that thrives on the back of its creative and innovative drive.

Although healthcare or the healthcare industry is commonly not perceived in the same way, it is in fact no different. As Sharma (2010, p. 242) states, 'every human being is creative'. The role of the clinical leader is to foster a workplace or clinical environment that liberates and supports the expression of creativity. Price (2006, p. 54) is also clear that innovation is more likely to be successfully implemented in practice when the leader is 'clear about what they are doing and what they hope to achieve'. While the clinical leadership research results at the core of this book do not agree with Cook's (2001) findings, intuitively it makes sense for clinical leaders – who are at the forefront of client care – to be involved in the development of new and innovative ways to develop care practices or to support clinicians who have the ideas. Klemm (1990, p. 449) agrees, suggesting that leaders know 'in their gut' that creativity and innovation are the lifeblood of their organisation. It may be that this is not the reason clinical leaders are followed, but don't let that stop you. Brainstorm away!

Case Study 9.1   Jane Austen

Jane Austen was a female novelist. A number of health professionals have become successful writers or performers – Richard Hooker, who wrote the book *M.A.S.H.*, Joe Brand, a comedian and comedy writer who wrote the TV series *Getting On*, are just two examples. Jane Austen (although not a health professional) was a leader and writer with creativity – an elegant, witty and important female novelist. Her works of romantic, comedic fiction marked a shift in English literature away from the neo-classical style. Consider the description of her life and read the challenge that follows.

Jane was born in Steventon in Hampshire in 1775, the seventh of eight children. She was educated by her Reverend father who acted as a tutor to his children and other children of the district. However, in 1783 Jane and Cassandra, her older sister, were sent to Oxford to be taught by a Mrs. Ann Cawley. There, both girls caught typhus and Jane nearly died. The pair were inseparable almost throughout their lives, and they spent much of their childhood happily writing and performing plays and charades. Their father had a rich library, and Jane read widely and was encouraged to write from an early age. At the age of 14 she wrote her first novel, 'Love and Freindship' [sic]. This was followed by 'A History of England by a Partial, Prejudiced and Ignorant Historian' (with 13 illustrations by Cassandra), but Jane was in her 20s when she penned the first drafts of her novels *Sense and Sensibility*, *Pride and Prejudice* and *Northanger Abbey*. As a young woman, Jane enjoyed long country walks, attended church regularly, socialised frequently, supervised the family servants, made clothes and attended balls with local gentry. Between 1793 and 1795 she wrote *Lady Susan*, a short epistolary novel, described as her most ambitious and sophisticated early work.

She had many friends in Hampshire, and it was a shock when the family moved to Bath in 1801. The Reverend Austen moved there to retire, but he died in 1805, and Jane, her sister and their mother had to rely on their brother's support to survive. It was also during this time that Jane fell in love, but the young man died and she was heartbroken. Soon after she accepted a proposal of marriage from a wealthy landowner, Harris

(Continued)

Bigg-Wither, but she changed her mind the next day, leading to considerable upset for her family and friends. Jane, like her sister, Cassandra, was never to marry.

After 1805, Jane, her sister and their mother moved to Southampton, where Jane found herself unable to write. To some extent their fortunes changed for the better in 1809 when her brother Edward provided a small but suitable residence on his estate at Chawton in Hampshire. This cottage offered the stability Jane sought, and she revised *Sense and Sensibility* and *Pride and Prejudice* to the point where they were able to be published in 1811 and 1813, respectively. At Chawton cottage, Jane found time to focus on her writing, since her mother and Cassandra took a larger share of the domestic duties. The Austens socialised little apart from some teaching for local children or charity work among the poor of the estate, so their lives were commonly described by their relatives as 'quiet'.

In 1814, Jane wrote and published *Mansfield Park*, while *Emma* followed in 1816. She also worked on *Persuasion* and a redraft of *Northanger Abbey*, which were both published posthumously in 1818. She began work on *Sanditon*, but became ill before it could be completed. She died in 1817, with none of the books published in her lifetime bearing her name; instead, they were described as written 'By a lady'.

It is thought that Jane died from Addison's disease (although bovine tuberculosis is also suggested as the cause), and during her illness – as with the rest of her life – her sister Cassandra was never far from her side. In 1817, they moved together to Winchester to be near Jane's doctor, and it was in her sister's arms that Jane died in July, aged 41. She was buried in Winchester Cathedral.

Much of Jane's correspondence is missing and most of what is known about her comes from potentially biased family sources. Nevertheless, her literary works remain a vivid reminder of the contribution of women to the artistic world. Jane Austen was little regarded during her lifetime due to her decision to publish her works anonymously, and it took almost 50 years after her death for a popular appreciation of her work to take hold. However, she has since been recognised as a powerful author, achieving belated critical acclaim.

Challenge: Jane Austen's books are some of the most read and most beloved in English literature. They capture a piece of history, offering a critical commentary on the social practices of the period and with realism that brings the books to life. Her works focus on moral issues and women's dependence on marriage to secure social and financial security. Jane lived her entire life as part of a small, close-knit family unit, often facing financial insecurity, and it was not until she was in her mid-30s that she experienced success as a published author. Her books were out of print for a number of years after her death, but in 1832 her novels were republished as an illustrated set, and they have remained in print ever since. Jane kept her writing talent hidden by choosing to remain anonymous. It is possible that many health professionals do the same for different reasons. Is creativity, seeking new ways, finding new paths or being innovative valued in everyday clinical practice? Have you had a great idea about improving care or changing practice, but kept it to yourself or been dissuaded or discouraged from taking the idea forward? Why was this? How could you have managed the situation differently? As a leader, how can you draw good ideas from your colleagues in a way that supports and encourages them to

(Continued)

Case Study 9.1 (Continued)

feel safe and supported to contribute? Have you ever had a great idea? Have you thought of a new way to care for a particular client group or a new type of documentation that saved time or captured the right information in the right way? What was it? What did you do about it? Write a short reflection about your experiences of generating a new idea, positive or negative. What would you do differently if you had a similar idea in the future?

Summary

- Leadership and creativity are clearly linked.
- Developing creativity requires the application of the creative process, which includes being prepared, allowing ideas to incubate, illuminating the ideas and verification of ideas with their application.
- There are many ways to foster creativity. These include relaxing, keeping a notebook or journal, journaling, learning new skills, drawing, using mind maps, walking, looking at others' creative output, using a dictionary, studying creative thinking skills and attending courses, using associational thinking, facing your fears, grasping information, developing and releasing your imagination, recording your ideas, finding or making a creative space, developing a sense of humour, cartooning, defining the problem at hand, getting to know yourself well, not being afraid, using guided reflection and actively developing some creative thinking skills.
- There are many barriers that prevent the development or application of creativity. These include barriers at work such as competition, organisational structure, being too busy and a sterile environment. There are also personal barriers, which include fear of criticism, fear of change, lack of confidence and routines.
- There are often barriers to the development of creativity in our daily lives too. These include daily distractions like television, having no time or place to reflect or the inappropriate use of drugs.
- Clinical leaders are not often identified as such because of their creativity. Yet this does not mean that they are not creative or that creativity is not a highly valuable trait for clinical leaders to have.
- Clinical leaders can also be effective at facilitating or recognising creativity in others and helping them to develop their skills and talents to further promote change and innovation.

Mind Press-Ups

Exercise 9.1

Look at something as if you were a child: a policy, a relationship or a problem. Ask yourself 'What does this look like to me?' or 'What does this make me think of?' Try to consider the questions from a child's perspective.

Exercise 9.2

How do you find time to focus, to be mindful, to be present and deal creatively with the problems you face? Try looking now at one problem. Write it down. Give some time to considering it. Focus on it and really make finding a solution a priority. Imagine you are a detective. The problem is your 'case'. How might you solve it?

Exercise 9.3

Is failure an issue? What are the consequences of failure for you? For your clients? For your part in the health service? Clinical trials are often avoided by clients who may be afraid of becoming ill or being used as guinea pigs. Does fear of failure hold you back from embracing change or having a bold new idea? Start small, try a new dish in the kitchen. Will the benefits of a wonderful new meal be outweighed by the risk of making a mess or a meal that doesn't taste nice? Rate your risk / benefit score on a scale of 1–10. Where do you rate for each?

References

Barez-Brown, C. (2006). *How to Have Kick-Ass Ideas*. London: Harper Element.

de Bono, E. (1985). *Six Thinking Hats*. London: Penguin.

de Bono, E. (2015). *Serious Creativity*. London: Penguin.

de Bono, E. (2016). *Thinking to Create Value*. Malta: Kite Group.

Breen, B. (2004). The 6 myths of creativity. *Fast Company*. p. 75.

Cook, M. (2001). The attributes of effective clinical nurse leaders. *Nursing Standard* 15 (35): 33–36.

Doyle, R. (1993). *Develop Your Creative Skills*. London: Dorling Kindersley.

Evans, J.R. (1993). Creativity in MS/OR: overcoming barriers to creativity. *Interfaces* 23 (6): 101–106.

Gentile, M.C. (2010). *Giving Voice to Values: How to Speak Your Mind When You Know What's Right*. New Haven, CT: Yale University Press.

Goldstein, E. (ed.) (2014). *Mindfulness Made Simple*. Berkeley, CA: Calistoga Press.

Goleman, D. (2013). *Focus: The Hidden Driver of Excellence*. London: Bloomsbury.

Hall, M.L. (2005). Shaping organizational culture: a practitioner's perspective. *Peak Development Consulting* 2 (1): 1–16.

Klein, A.R. (1990). Organisational barriers to creativity, and how to knock them down. *Journal of Consumer Marketing* 7 (1): 65–66.

Klemm, W.R. (1990). Leadership: creativity and innovation. In: *Concepts for Air Force Leadership*, 2e (ed. A.F.B. Maxwell), 426–439. AL: Alabama Air Force University.

Mukerjea, D. (1997). *Braindancing*. Oxford: Oxford University Press.

von Oech, R. (1990). *A Whack on the Side of the Head: How You Can Be More Creative*. New York: Warner Books.

Price, B. (2006). Strategies to explore innovation in nursing practice. *Nursing Standard* 21 (9): 48–55.

Reiter-Palmon, R. and Illies, J. (2004). Leadership and creativity: understanding leadership from a creative problem-solving perspective. *The Leadership Quarterly* 15 (1): 55–77.

Rickards, T., Runco, M.A., and Moger, S. (ed.) (2008). *The Routledge Companion to Creativity*. London: Routledge.

Sharma, R. (2010). *Leadership Wisdom from the Monk Who Sold His Ferrari: The 8 Rituals of Best Leaders*. London: HarperCollins.

Stanley, D. (2006). In command of care: clinical nurse leadership explored. *Journal of Research in Nursing* 2 (1): 20–39.

Stanley, D. (2008). Congruent leadership: values in action. *Journal of Nursing Management* 16: 519–524.

Stanley, D. and Stanley, K. (2019). Clinical leadership and rural and remote practice: a qualitative study. *Journal of Nursing Management* 27 (6): 1314–1324.

Stanley, D., Cuthbertson, J., and Latimer, K. (2012). Perceptions of clinical leadership in the St John Ambulance Service in WA. *Response* 39 (1): 31–37.

Stanley, D., Latimer, K., and Atkinson, J. (2014). Perceptions of clinical leadership in an aged care residential facility in Perth, Western Australia. *Health Care: Current Reviews* 2 (2): 121–129.

Stanley, D., Hutton, M. and McDonald, A. (2015). *Western Australian Allied Health Professionals' Perceptions of Clinical Leadership: A Research Report*. http://www.ochpo. health.wa.gov.au/docs/WA_Allied_Health_Prof_Perceptions_of_Clinical_Leadership_ Research_Report.pdf (accessed 1 July 2016).

Tulloch, S. (1997). *The Oxford Dictionary and Thesaurus*. Oxford: Oxford University Press.

Vogelsmeier, A. and Scott-Cawiezell, J. (2009). The role of nursing leaders in successful technology implementation. *Journal of Nursing Administration* 39 (7/8): 313.

Weintraub, P. and McKee, M. (2019). Leadership for innovation in healthcare: an exploration. *International Journal of Health Policy and Management* 8 (3): 138–144.

Wolff, J. (2009). *Creativity Now: Get Inspired, Create Ideas and Make Them Happen*. Sydney, NSW: Pearson.

Zuber, C. and Moody, L. (2018). 'Creativity and innovation in healthcare: tapping into organizational enablers through human centered design. *Nursing Administration Quarterly* 42 (5): 62–75.

10

Leading Teams

Alison H. James and Clare L. Bennett

'I do not think there is any doubt that we all owe our lives to his leadership and his power of making a loyal and coherent party out of rather diverse elements'
Reginald W. James, Physicist, The Endurance.
(Morrell and Capparell, *Shackleton's Way*, 2017, p. 13)

Introduction: Identifying Dynamics and Self-Role within Teams

Whatever your role in healthcare, you will be a component of a team, as healthcare is constructed and depends upon teamwork in the majority of contexts (Jones and Bennett 2018). While we acknowledge that some healthcare professionals work remotely and in isolation, the overall construct of healthcare involves a network of relationships composed of the organsiation, professionals, patients, patients' families and significant others. Because of this, the role of clinical leader can vary, from taking responsibility for a team to being part of the team decision making. Identifying what is required of your role, being self-aware of what is needed of you from a team, can be challenging. However, being aware of the emotional labour of this relationship dynamic can support the challenging aspects of clinical leadership and teamwork. Remaining emotionally aware of self, of the relationships of the team and of the context or culture of the environment, can provide insight and allow adaptation to the shifting requirements of being an effective leader. This requires humility and maintaining professional values central to the team aims. A reflective perspective can create a culture of *'psychological safety'*, which enables inclusive, supportive and safe teamworking (West 2021), and realigns clinical leadership from a status and authoritarian approach much further towards an appreciative role.

To some extent, considering clinical leadership implies attention to the power of one: to the self, to your values and beliefs. Aspects of clinical leadership such as motivation, conflict resolution, clinical decision making, innovation and managing change imply a need for the leader to gain personal insight and a grasp of their own values and beliefs, strengths

Clinical Leadership in Nursing and Healthcare, Third Edition.
Edited by David Stanley, Clare L. Bennett and Alison H. James.

and weaknesses. However, teamwork relates to the power of many: to the leader's capacity to recognise the strengths and limitations of those about them. In modern healthcare environments, an ideal organisation is made up of cohesive teams in which people pool their skills, talents and knowledge to address complex problems and come up with creative solutions. Effective teams are able to develop a unified purpose and cohesive ethos, so that the barriers they face are few or easily overcome, resulting in consistently high quality work. Effective teams promote a sense of shared responsibility, mutual respect, safety and identity. It is also known that clinical leadership can be central to establishing the cultures of teamworking by promoting shared values, which influences team behaviours (Akhtar et al. 2016; Manley et al. 2019).

Developing effective teams can be challenging, and if the leadership is poor, it may be that the only team output is in a shared sense of dissatisfaction as disgruntled workers pull together against ineffective management or weak leadership (Cantwell 2015). This can also result in unsafe cultures and serious safety outcomes for patients (Francis 2013; Kirkup 2015). In many cases, teams may have the public face of cohesion, but if you scratch the surface, explore them further or put them under a little pressure, they stretch to a breaking point. You may even find that people within them are unsupportive, uncooperative, in competition, have personal grudges or are in open conflict. As a result, talented, skilled people, frustrated by the limitations of a poorly performing team, fail to deliver their best work. So, teamwork in healthcare is central to its effectiveness in delivering safe and high-quality patient care. Leaders must consider their roles and responsibilities within teams, rather than sitting outside and remote to the relationships on which patients place their trust.

This chapter looks at teams within the current context of healthcare and the importance of psychological safety. It also considers the role of the leader in a team, how to build and manage effective teams, and considers the value of support and challenge in helping teams work well.

Do We Really Need Teams?

There are many tasks that can be done either through good allocation of work to individuals or by a group working more or less cooperatively (Lessard et al. 2008). Before the decision is taken to establish a team, consider the degree of complexity of the work and the extent to which a group is required to work cooperatively.

Teams are not really needed if the task relates to a simple exchange of information, or if it involves simply sharing out work, updating each other and/or making simple operational decisions. These interactions relate mainly to reference and consultation groups with low levels of interaction, requiring only clear lines of communication (Lessard et al. 2008).

Teams are needed if the work is uncertain, difficult and complex, or where a high degree of collaboration and interdependence is required (Casey 1993). The effectiveness of teamwork is crucial within healthcare, and it is the connection of core values and aims which bind healthcare teams and can make them highly capable. We know that a supportive, encouraging work environment can have positive effects and allows individuals to thrive and cope within challenging environments (Bliese et al. 2017). In contrast, incivility and bullying have the opposite effect, so enabling cultures and environments which are safe and supportive is essential to achieve safe and effective patient outcomes (Razzi and Bianchi 2019). For clinical leaders to enable effective teams, it is important to consider both the requirements and challenges, some of which are complex and unexpected.

Are We a Team or a Group?

A **group** is defined as a number of individuals assembled together or having some unifying relationship (e.g. members of a church, or all the people in a cohort of students). These are groups because all the various members are related in some way because of their involvement and interest in a certain endeavour or subject.

A **team** is described as a number of people associated together in specific work or a particular activity. Ellis (2021) define a team as the organised unit, which aims to effectively and efficiently achieve a task. Parker (1990) indicates that a group is not a team, and that a team is based on a highly interdependent set of people that:

- have defined goals and objectives (Markiewicz and West 2011)
- have an ongoing relationship
- are focused on accomplishing a task

Added to this is the idea that teams work best if they recognise the value of:

- effective communication (Vogelsmeier and Scott-Cawiezell 2009)
- a singleness of mission
- a willingness to cooperate
- a commitment to each other

The attributes of effective teams include the following:

- clarity of purpose/shared objectives or goals (Markiewicz and West 2011)
- informality
- participation
- listening
- meeting regularly
- interdependent working
- civilised disagreement
- consensus decisions
- clear roles and work assignments
- shared leadership
- diversity of styles/life experiences/thought
- small to moderate size
- self-assessment and self-regulation

By referring to 'real' teams, we mean they have:

- shared values and aims
- regular performance review
- strategies for improvement

- psychological safety
- climates and cultures of trust and mutual respect
- are inclusive
- both inward and outward looking
- demonstrate shared leadership approaches

'Pseudo' teams do not possess these characteristics and are often considered as failing teams and relate more to a group of people with separate agendas. While the concern of 'pseudo' teams within health and social care has been a concern, during the pandemic, bonds have formed and some teams have demonstrated greater effectiveness, creativity and innovation, a sense of shared purpose and improved communication through determination in the face of adversity (West 2021). In many areas, hierarchies have had to be relinquished and professions integrated, and values have been forced to the fore by the challenges faced. This has only resulted in enlightened teams and a realisation of their power to advocate and provide the best care for patients, and leadership characteristics have been clear in these achievements.

Reflection Point

Do you work in a team? Look at the attributes of 'real' teams described in this chapter. Does your team meet these attributes? If not, what are the consequences for your workplace, the clients or patients and your own work satisfaction?

Established Teams

Established teams usually fall into three basic sets. These are:

- high-performance teams
- OK teams or functional teams
- struggling teams

High-Performance Teams

These teams need recognition and resourcing. They have their own (good) working habits and address their own learning and development needs. These teams tend to offer what is called 'synergy' (where $2 + 2 = 5$), or what Leanne (2010) calls an 'all-hands' culture, with the rules for creating synergy related to:

- an established and clear purpose
- active listening
- compassion and collaboration
- truth telling
- being flexible
- commitment to a resolution (agreeing to disagree, but moving on)

- high levels of passion and commitment
- a sense that team members' perspectives and efforts are valued
- a strong sense of 'ownership' of the team/organisational goals/values (Guttman 2008, p. 35)

High-performance or effective teams demonstrate good team cohesion, where team members stick together and remain focused on the pursuit of their common goal. Effective teams are also described as self-directing, where members are seen to work together, sharing leadership and decision making (West et al. 2014). Self-directing teams excel at using their team members' differences and sharing the team resources and assets to their overall advantage (Guise and Segel 2008; Andersen et al. 2010; Capella, et al. 2010; Siassakos et al. 2011; Steinemann et al. 2011). West (2021) suggests a Compassionate Leadership approach supports an inclusive, trustful and psychologically safe team environment by representing shared professional values such as humanity, empathy and compassion. The Compassionate Leader provides clear direction and co-production, invoking trust rather than fear, and supporting high-performance and achievement of positive patient outcomes (West and Markiewicz 2016).

While strong teams are desirable, they can have negative aspects too. The main areas of concern are that they can become exclusive, complacent, competitive and big-headed. Another issue with strong, high-performing teams is that they may lose sight of the big picture and focus on their own goals. They may build power through loyalty to the team

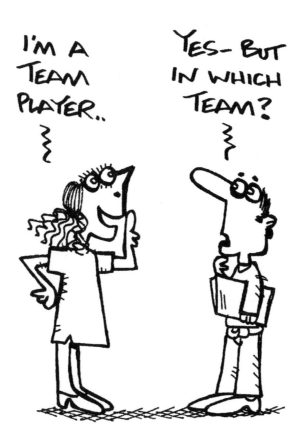

and create barriers and competition with other teams to the detriment of the organisation as a whole. They may hold on to their own staff, stifle adaptability or innovation and reject newcomers. Thus, the balance between the potentially positive and the potentially negative issues needs to be monitored carefully for success to be sustained, with professional values clearly visible in the philosophy.

OK or Functional Teams

A large number of teams can be described as OK or functional. They may need no intervention at all, and some OK teams do not want or need to adjust their dynamics. They may work well and they have a competent balance. These teams may have tried-and-tested ways of addressing problems but lack the confidence to be innovative. Functional teams are based on a traditional hierarchical composition with a supervisor and subordinates, usually with formal communication and authority lines. These teams can be recognised right across the health service in wards, departments and a raft of clinical environments and are often evident as they are commonly uni-professional in membership.

These sorts of teams can be good at puzzles and are made up of people with the skills to know the way to find answers. However, these same teams may struggle with complex problems. A lack of confidence might mean that they are unable to create new partnerships, motivate each other and fail to act collectively or collaboratively. These teams carry the risk of slipping towards becoming struggling teams, as a lack of innovation and confidence, with a stagnated approach to change, can result in compromised standards and reluctance to act on negative attitudes and unprofessional behaviours.

Struggling Teams

Struggling teams pose the biggest challenge and may offer the closest reflection of a pseudo-team. These teams often display:

- attempts to establish hierarchy and prevent individual contribution and ideas
- in-fighting or turf wars
- individuals avoiding any work activity that will make them look bad
- avoiding addressing negative attitudes and behaviour
- lack of collaborative decision making
- poor-quality and non-visible leadership
- poor personal relationships
- unresolved conflicts
- poor communication and hidden agendas
- protecting information to establish small wins

The main issue is often a lack of trust or commitment or fear of personal ability. Teams that are not committed to working together will not learn together and will often fail to develop. In these cases, the collective output may be less than if the individuals had acted alone. Thompson and Kusy (2021) in considering team effectiveness during the pandemic consider lack of clarity and mistrust, miscommunication and uncertainty, remoteness by the leader and lack of vision as contributing to team break down. Also, due to the pressures of the pandemic, the overwhelming pressure on the leaders and team members and guilt in addressing failure at such challenging times, Thompson and Kusy (2021) state that acting to deal with incivility and negative behaviours became even more challenging.

If a team is not working well, it may be that the team as a whole is failing to function, or it may be that there are some pernicious individuals within it that are – through bullying or controlling behaviour – bringing down the contribution of the whole team. It may also be a reflection of leadership style or effectiveness. Assessing the core problems with struggling teams is vital before taking action, because if the issue is destructive individuals, reforming the team without addressing that will only transfer the problem to the newly created team, making its formation a more difficult process. While this may be challenging, the following may save deteriorating relationships and ineffectiveness:

- Be visible and present as much as possible
- Communicate messages clearly and to all team members
- Acknowledge the challenges through compassion
- Deal with unprofessional, negative or uncivil behaviour

Reflection Point

There are three basic types of teams described in this chapter: high-performance teams, OK or functional teams and struggling teams. Which type of team do you think you work in? Why is this? How can you change the team's effectiveness if necessary?

'Teaming' for Healthcare

Healthcare is a high-stakes environment. Therefore, the demands on healthcare teams are constant, complex and dynamic, and we have witnessed this at a much higher level during the pandemic. These characteristics of teamwork have been discussed, theorised and studied for many years now; however, the effects on our professions and how we are able to deliver care during this time has meant teamwork taking on even more challenging dilemmas, mobilising and reshaping on demand and responding with speed. Professor Amy Edmondson presents the uniqueness of teams having to suddenly form, made of diverse and groups of individuals from varying professions and with no prior planning as 'Teaming' (Edmondson 2018). This approach has been used to explore how the sudden formation of a number of people can operate effectively as a team, rather than just a group, and achieve positive outcomes. The scenario used by Edmondson (2018) is detailed in the Reflection Point below, and it is useful to understand the elements of this approach as well as other characteristics which can be enabled for more planned and established teams. It is also useful to reflect on how leaders respond in this situation. Where it is perhaps not fully clear who is taking a leading role, should this be shared, and who establishes this?

'Teaming' supports individuals to work and achieve outcomes effectively, while faced with fast-changing landscapes and challenges. This approach also supports individual well-being when effective and strong leadership supports it (West 2021). Recognising that working in large teams with multi-professions and differing communication methods and processes, as is seen, for example, in health and social care in the UK, is complex and challenging. So here the concepts of 'teaming' can be highly supportive, ensuring 'real' teamwork is established, rather than 'pseudo' teamwork. This means having clearly defined objectives and aims, shared values and regular communication, and checking in to review performance by the leader (West 2021; Lyubovnikova et al. 2015).

Reflection Point

Professor Amy Edmondson studied organisational responses to challenges to gain an understanding of the psychological mindset and behaviours that enable varied professions and groups to collaborate, share and work effectively without prior planning. She calls this **Teaming** and presents the situation of the San Jose mining disaster in Chile in 2010. Thirty-three miners were trapped 2000 ft underground with two days' supply of food. Chances of survival were estimated at less than 10%. Seventy days later, all the miners were rescued alive, attributed to effective teamwork and leadership. Consider a situation where you have had to form as a team with others quickly, and then watch/ listen to the YouTube video at https://www.youtube.com/watch?v=3boKz0Exros. Consider these characteristics and how they may support you as a leader in a similar situation.

'Teaming' identifies the following important characteristics for effective teams in this situation.

- Define and provide clarity on aims and common goals
- Curiosity – when we think we know everything, we should be curious to learn from others
- Be appreciative of others' talents and connect through shared aims
- Share knowledge and experience so that others may learn
- Be open and transparent, have no hidden agendas
- Be humble in the situation and know its ok to not know all the answers

Source: Amy Edmondson, How to turn a group of strangers into a team | Amy Edmondson - YouTube

---

Creating Powerful and Positive Teams

Creating a new team, while difficult and time consuming, can often be very rewarding because it avoids the sort of historical baggage that can interfere with working practices and allows communication channels and subcultures to develop as the new team does. Creating a team requires a number of essential elements, some of which are presented here:

- Clarify the team's purpose (objectives and goals) and task (Hart 2010; MacDonald 2010)
- Agree on shared professional values
- Establish and understand the team vision (Whitehead 2019)
- Create working processes and ground rules
- Set the expectation for regular meetings and reviews
- Establish shared decision making
- Establish effective communication (Whitehead 2019)
- Share learning and openly discuss errors, complaints and near misses (West 2021)

- Practice problem-solving approaches such as action learning (James and Stacey-Emile 2019)
- Establish a quality improvement agenda

Tuckman (1965) proposes that teams go through forming, storming, norming and performing stages, which illustrates that it takes time to achieve a status quo; however, teams are often in continuous flux. Not allowing time for a team to develop creates problems, as the team members are thrown together and expected to be at their peak performance at once. The forming stage is vital and is too often a neglected element of team building, and here the development of psychological safety can be an advantage to the process.

Clinical Leader Stories: 10 Communication Skills

During a clinical placement at an emergency department, my preceptor nurse displayed positive attributes of a clinical leader. During the shift, we had a patient that was deteriorating at a steady rate. Unfortunately, the doctor did not agree when I raised this concern with them. Although, as my preceptor nurse was concerned about the patient, they spoke to the doctor highlighting strong interpersonal skills and strong communication skills, and as the doctor knew them to be clinically proficient, they agreed to undertake further assessments on the patient. After this discussion, my preceptor made appropriate decisions regarding further assessment. Due to these additional assessments, a new provisional diagnosis was given to the patient. As a result, their decline was slowed with new treatments and the patient was well enough to talk to family members. After this my nurse gave me a debrief of the event and highlighted important questions of deterioration along with tips on how to communicate my concerns to other team members. This was a positive experience that left me feeling prepared for similar situations and excited to learn more from my preceptor. Through analysing this scenario, it is clear that my preceptor showed clinical leadership through multiple traits, all of which indicates that she was a congruent leader, as my preceptor was able to demonstrate and action out their values. The first attributes they showed were that they were approachable, a role model and a motivator. This was seen after the scenario when they took the time to discuss the events in detail so that I could learn from my experience. They demonstrated that they were an effective communicator and focused on quality patient outcomes; through their communication with the doctor they showed their concern for the patient. Finally, they demonstrated that they were decisive in their decisions and clinically proficient. This was done through the additional assessments they initiated to confirm their suspicion of an alternative health concern.

After reflection on the clinical leadership attributes that my preceptor possessed, there are several implications for my practice. Firstly, it has allowed me to develop better clinical judgement concerning a patient's condition; secondly, my preceptor's example has motivated me to develop better interpersonal communication skills, especially when talking to other members of the multidisciplinary team. Thirdly, they have supported me to develop more ways of expressing my concerns about patient conditions, which will be important for better patient outcomes. Finally, my preceptor supported me to see the attributes that will allow me to become a better clinical leader.

Ryan: Student Nurse

Psychological Safety

Psychological safety in teams can be defined as a shared, inclusive, interpersonal and trusting culture where trust and mutual respect are intrinsic (West 2021). Developing a philosophy and culture which supports this can enable teams to establish a social capital in which they can invest, cooperate and participate (Whitehead 2019). A non-threatening and safe culture enables individuals to form the bonds that distinguish a team from a group. As a result, everyone feels included, valued, trusted and respected. West (2021) suggests compassionate leadership supports this ethos, and the establishment of shared values is core to this approach, along with building a reflexive approach to learning and innovating.

Leaders who are change-focused, are role models for innovation, transparency, trust and taking interpersonal risks are effective in enabling psychological safety in their teams (O'Donovan and McAuliffe 2020). Enabling individuals to have a shared experience of psychological safety by feeling valued, listened to and respected through effective leadership can support the process of team cohesion and positivity, even in adverse and challenging circumstances.

Team Building

Often, when there are problems within a team, the proposed solution is to engage in 'team building' in one form or another; indeed, in healthcare environments strategies to improve teamwork commonly include team-building or teamwork training (Dietz et al. 2014). Dyer (1987) and Dietz et al. (2014) suggest that team-building and teamwork training can be enhanced by:

- Setting the goals or priorities for the team
- Employing a team-building/training framework
- Defining the parameters within which the team works
- Allocating or describing the way in which work is performed
- Considering the manner in which the team works: its processes, norms, decision making and communication
- Focusing on the relationships among the people doing the work

However, these approaches often generate no more than minor, short-lived improvements in morale and performance (Holland 2008) and are only of use after some sort of assessment has been undertaken to identify the team's problem. There is also a view that team building can be a 'bit of a laugh', avoiding the real 'at work' issues. This perspective has grown from a number of 'play-like' approaches to team building, with paintball and similar adventure activities used to build team spirit and cohesion. Another issue may be that the team seems to function well while away from the work environment during the team-building activity, but old habits prevail when back in the thick of a negative work culture that has not been addressed.

For team-building and teamwork training (or indeed team work) to be successful, clear and present leadership is required (Holland 2008). When groups are struggling, effective leadership is even more important, as is understanding what matters to team members

(Andersen et al. 2010). Leaders need to know, at least in part, what the problems are so that they can avoid becoming defensive and simply window-dressing the problem. The advantage a clinical leader has is that they are often very much a part of the team and can support and facilitate better communication and more attention to problems and solutions. Whitehead (2019) suggests creating emotionally intelligent teams by exploring and being open about the realities of emotion in work, which could certainly be explored further in the context of healthcare. While we often manage and empathise with patients' emotions, we are perhaps not always as good with managing and empathising with our own. Encouraging the sharing of emotional upheavals can allow individuals to relate and connect rather than take home the emotions of the day and be left feeling isolated with those feelings.

Team Roles

One key to effective teamworking is to support and promote diversity. To achieve this, teams need to be made up of a variety of different people with a variety of skills and talents (Handy 1999; Frandsen 2014). Imagine a soccer team made up of 11 goalkeepers. Their potential for match success would be limited by their over-specialisation. Belbin (1981) undertook research into team roles that suggested the idea that a team made up of the brightest and best did not always produce the best results; this was called the Apollo syndrome. He also proposed, after considerable research, that successful teams are composed of people who fulfil a number of different roles, identifying eight (or nine) key team roles.

The result of the research was a questionnaire used to support team members to identify their 'preferred' team role and to help teams gain an insight into their composition and development needs. Belbin's (1981) approach to team role assessment offers a robust and highly effective insight into how teams work and represents an accurate approach to assessing individual behaviour and its impact on team functioning. In Belbin's words, 'Nobody is perfect . . . but a team can be'. Therefore, gaining an understanding of teams and how they are made up and of individual team roles can be of great benefit to team success (Belbin 1981; Frandsen 2014). The eight key team roles described by Belbin (nine including the role of the 'specialist') are:

- **Plant:** Introverted, but intellectually dominant. The source of original ideas and described as creative, imaginative and unorthodox.
- **Coordinator:** Presides over the team and coordinates its efforts. Described as mature, confident and clarifies goals.
- **Monitor/evaluator:** Intelligent and directed towards analytical rather than creative energies. Described as sober, strategic and an accurate judge.
- **Implementer:** Turns ideas into manageable tasks. Schedules, charts and plans are their thing. Described as disciplined, reliable and a doer.
- **Completer/finisher:** Checks details and makes sure that schedules are met, drives others on to complete their tasks. Described as painstaking, conscientious and delivers on time.

- **Resource investigator:** Usually a popular member of a team. Described as sociable, relaxed, extrovert and enthusiastic. Their role is to make or bring in new contacts, acting as a salesperson or liaison for the team.
- **Shaper:** Described as highly strung, outgoing and dominant; can also be challenging, dynamic and courageous.
- **Team worker:** Holds the team together, supporting others, listening, encouraging and acting as a link person for others. Described as diplomatic, mild and cooperative.
- **Specialist:** Often called into a team for special knowledge or skills, and frequently does not stay in the team beyond its immediate requirements. May be seen as single-minded.

Significantly, no one role is affiliated with leadership in the team, and the advantage of understanding team roles from Belbin's perspective is that the team needs will often dictate the most appropriate leader at the most relevant time. Thus, different roles may be required to different degrees at different times. For example, when the team is struggling it may be that a coordinator is needed to focus the team's efforts on its goals and objectives. Or if a team is being formed, it may require a strong shaper or plant to motivate team members or generate ideas. Times of competition may demand the intervention of a plant with good ideas or an evaluator to avoid high-risk activities.

It is not essential that teams have eight people, each undertaking one of the eight main Belbin roles, but teams do need people to be aware of these various roles and find ways to fulfil them. In small teams people can assume more than one role, while in larger teams it would be reasonable to expect that different people undertake the same team role. Establishing team roles is also beneficial when it comes to team decision making. At times, teams struggle to make effective decisions, so having set ground rules and clear team roles can facilitate confidence and allow teams to reach alignment in decision making (Frisch 2008).

The point of Belbin's (1981) team roles is that teams are made up of a variety of different people with different skills and that the most effective teams recognise this and act to include these various roles. To function well, teams need all types, team workers, coordinators and finishers. This perspective was supported by Leggat (2007), who suggested, after a significant research project among Australian health service personnel, that team-working competencies were perceived to be different for management and clinical teams, further reinforcing the value of having different people with different skills populating teams. However, it should be remembered that in spite of having well-defined team roles, the interaction of people in teams and the impact of their personalities can – and often does – have an effect on team friction or relationships within the team. The key in these circumstances is to manage conflict constructively.

Reflection Point

Consider Belbin's team roles. Can you identify with one or more? Think of other members of your team and how they display these characteristics. How well does your team function and balance in view of this?

Leadership and Teams

We have discussed styles of leadership such as compassionate leadership, which supports the creation of safe and inclusive cultures. So, considering the recent challenges of the pandemic, what lessons have been learnt in leading teams? It is useful to consider how leading teams may now be approached differently, given the sudden and magnified challenges many healthcare teams have experienced.

Thompson and Kusy (2021) explored leadership and the effects during the pandemic and identified two common issues which contributed to 'dysfunction' in teams: *losing trust* and *ignoring disruptive behavior*. As the impact was sudden, leaders were often unprepared for the impact and disruption, leaving little time to think and plan for their approach to leadership in this new context. Making promises and sharing misinformation were also identified as inducing a lack of trust, while some felt they had lost authenticity and integrity because they were asked to share decisions that they did not agree with. Because of the challenges and stress of the staff, some leaders did not address negative behaviours, and this also had negative effects (Thompson and Kusy 2021). The lessons from this study are clear; however, as we continue to experience dips and peaks in the pandemic globally, there are some long-term lessons here for clinical leaders, perhaps:

- Read widely, as much research is now emerging on the effects of the pandemic on leadership, teams and individuals
- Consider how a pandemic disrupts your 'usual' leadership style and have a back-up plan
- Always remain values-focused in your approach as these are the shared principles which bond us in healthcare

Leaders are often people who care about people, and this care translates into a willingness to focus time and energy on members of the team. From this perspective, caring is risking being with the team and sharing both suffering and joy. Behaviours that demonstrate caring include giving of oneself in terms of warmth, passion and, particularly, time. The second aspect of caring is truly listening to team members, really hearing and understanding them. The third aspect is being 100% present for them. The fourth is to honour team members and see their wholeness, their possibilities and their hope.

Leading a team is one of the most difficult things to do. Being a team member is also difficult, because the reality is that being part of a team is the same as being part of a relationship and, as with any other relationship in our lives, involves risk and requires commitment, trust and character, both personal and professional. Acknowledge and recognise these aspects of teams.

Case Study 10.1   Emmeline Pankhurst

Emmeline Pankhurst, as the leaders of the Women's Social and Political Union (WSPU) led a campaign to gain equal votes for women in the UK and has since inspired women and men in the struggle for equality. She also brought together women from across class and race, age and education, urban and rural environments to campaign, often with severe personal consequences. While her approach was considered militant and legally

---

(Continued)

Case Study 10.1 **(Continued)**

---

disobedient, she demonstrated a transformational and authentic style of leadership bringing this once disparate group of women together, all committed to campaigning and suffering for the cause. The Suffragette movement finally achieved its aims in 1928 with woman gaining equal suffrage. While the methods of this movement are still considered as extreme, the benefits to women's rights have been significant for future generations.

Considering Emmeline Pankhurst's approach to building the movement, it is possible to identify her key leadership approaches which made this such an effective team of its time:

- Influence and role modelling – she was present and had a clear purpose for the movement. She highlighted the importance of all working together to achieve the aims, and was visible and active with her fellow women in protests.
- Enthusiasm and optimism – she communicated the strategy and actions clearly and effectively.
- Challenging and stimulating – she challenged assumptions and questioned bigotry and tradition, encouraging others to seek information and learn.
- Nurturing – she nurtured others into leadership roles and had a vision for the future through her followers.
- Core values – She maintained her values core to the cause, suffering with her followers to achieve the aims.

Challenge: Emmeline Pankhurst demonstrated a style of leadership which ignited a movement and brought women together to form an efficient and effective team. She empowered women to aim for equality and to be leaders within their own communities by demonstrating vision and optimism, focused on actions. How do you think she has enabled women and men to aim for change? She also came across criticism for her approach and methods to mobilise her 'team'. What can be learnt from her key leadership approaches and for keeping her authenticity and visibility core to her approach?

Summary of Suffrage: The right of women to vote has been achieved at various times in countries throughout the world.

In many nations, women's suffrage was granted before universal suffrage, so women and men from certain classes or races were still unable to vote. Some countries granted suffrage to both sexes at the same time.

Some women in the Isle of Man (geographically part of the British Isles but not part of the UK) gained the right to vote in 1881.

New Zealand was the first self-governing country in the world in which all women had the right to vote in parliamentary election, from 1893. Women could not stand for election until 1919.

The colony of South Australia allowed women to both vote and stand for election in 1894.

In Sweden, conditional women's suffrage was granted between 1718 and 1772, but it was not until the year 1919 that equality was achieved, where women's votes were valued the same as men's.

(Continued)

Case Study 10.1   (Continued)

The Australian Commonwealth Franchise Act 1902 enabled women to vote at federal elections in Australia and also permitted women to stand for election to the Australian Parliament, making the newly federated country of Australia the first in the modern world to do so (although some states excluded Indigenous Australians – both men and women).

In 1906, in what was to become Finland was the first country in the world to give all women and all men both the right to vote and the right to run for office.

In Saudi Arabia, women were first allowed to vote in December 2015.

Summary

- Teams are essential in healthcare and can be effective when values are clearly defined.
- Teams and groups are different.
- Effective teams have a clear purpose; are informal; meet regularly; feature interdependent working, civilised disagreement, consensus decisions, shared leadership, a diversity of styles; are usually small to moderate in size; and employ self-assessment and self-regulation.
- Teams can sometimes stifle dissent and creativity.
- Teams fall into three basic sets: high-performance teams, OK or functional teams and struggling teams.
- Creating a new team can be liberating or even inspiring. It can also be difficult and require considerable time. Creating a new team requires clarity of purpose, the establishment of team roles, clear working processes and ground rules, clear decisions, effective communication and the establishment of support and trust.
- Enabling psychological safety in teams can support cohesion and trust.
- There are a number of different roles that team members can take to make the team function effectively: plant, coordinator, monitor/evaluator, implementer, completer/finisher, resource investigator, shaper, team worker and, in some circumstances, specialist.
- The key to effective teams is to create a balance between support and challenge.
- Teams involving a variety of people undertaking different roles offer strength and diversity.
- Team leaders care about team members by listening to them, giving of their own time and being present. This is expressed as trust in the team.

Mind Press-Ups

Exercise 10.1

Look for the Belbin Team Role questionnaire online (or go to Belbin's original text, Belbin 1981) and complete the questionnaire. Assess what your team role is.

Exercise 10.2

Watch the You Tube video on 'Teaming' here:

How to turn a group of strangers into a team I Amy Edmondson – YouTube
How do you think these strategies may be helpful for you as a leader?

Exercise 10.3

Do teams from different professional disciplines work differently or are their team-working principles the same? Does it matter?

Exercise 10.4

Are you a leader within your team? If so, how do you use support and challenge to strengthen or achieve team cohesion?

References

Akhtar, M., Casha, J., Ronder, J. et al. (2016). Leading the health service into the future: transforming the NHS through transforming ourselves. *International Practice Development Journal* 6 (2): 5. https://doi.org/10.19043/ipdj.62.005.

Andersen, P.O., Jensen, M.K., Lippert, A., and Ostergaard, D. (2010). Identifying non-technical skills and barriers for improvement of teamwork in cardiac arrest teams. *Resuscitation* 81: 695–702.

Belbin, R.M. (1981). *Management Teams: Why They Succeed or Fail*. Oxford: Butterworth-Heinemann.

Bliese, P.D., Edwards, J.R., and Sonnentag, S. (2017). Stress and wellbeing at work: a century of empirical trends reflecting theoretical and societal influences. *The Journal of Applied Psychology* 10 (3): 389–402.

Cantwell, J. (2015). *Leadership in Action*. Melbourne, VIC: Melbourne University Press.

Capella, J., Smith, S., Philip, A. et al. (2010). Teamwork training improves the clinical care of trauma patients. *Journal of Surgical Education* 67 (6): 430–443.

Casey, D. (1993). *Managing Learning Organisations*. Buckingham: Open University Press.

Dietz, A., Pronovost, P.J., Menddez-Tellez, P.A. et al. (2014). A systematic review of teamwork in the intensive care unit: what do we know about teamwork, team tasks, and improvement strategies? *Journal of Critical Care* 29: 908–914.

Dyer, W.G. (1987). *Team Building Issues and Alternatives*. Reading, MA: Addison Wesley.

Edmondson, A. (2018). How to Turn a group of Strangers into a Team. You Tube, Amy Edmondson: How to turn a group of strangers into a team I TED Talk: https://www.youtube.com/watch?v=3boKz0Exros.

Ellis, P. (2021). *Leadership, Management and Team Working in Nursing, Transforming Nursing Practice Series*. London: Sage.

Francis, R. (2013). *The Report of the Mid Staffordshire NHS Foundation Trust Public Inquiry: Executive Summary*. London.: The Stationery Office.

Frandsen, B. (2014). *Nursing Leadership: Management and Leadership Styles*. Denver, CO: American Association of Nurse Coordination (AANAC) https://www.aanac.org/docs/white-papers/2013-nursing-leadership---management-leadership-styles.pdf?sfvrsn=4 (accessed 1 July 2016).

Frisch, B. (2008). When teams can't decide. *Harvard Business Review* 86 (11): 121.

Guise, J.-M. and Segel, S. (2008). Teamwork in obstetric care. *Best Practice and Research in Clinical Obstetrics and Gynaecology* 22 (5): 937–951.

Guttman, H.M. (2008). Leading high performance teams. *Chief Executive* 231: 33–35.

Handy, C. (1999). *Understanding Organizations*, 4e. London: Penguin.

Hart, J. (2010). Team purpose. *Leadership Excellence* 27 (3): 15.

Holland, K. (2008). How to build teamwork after an awful session. *New York Times* (28 December), p. 9.

James, A.H. and Stacey-Emile, G. (2019). Action learning: staff development, implementing change, interdisciplinary working, and leadership. *Nursing Management* 26 (3): 36–41.

Jones, L. and Bennett, C.L. (2018). *Leadership in Health and Social Care: An Introduction for Emerging Leaders*, 2e. Banbury: Lantern.

Kirkup, B. (2015). The report of the morecambe bay investigation. http://publishing.service.gov.uk.

Leanne, S. (2010). *Leadership the Barack Obama Way: Lessons on Teambuilding and Creating a Winning Culture in Challenging Times*. New York: McGraw-Hill.

Leggat, S. (2007). Effective healthcare teams require effective team members: defining teamwork competencies. *BMC Health Services Research* 7 (17): 1–10.

Lessard, L., Morin, D., and Sylvain, H. (2008). Understanding teams and teamm work. *Canadian Nurse* 104 (3): 12–13.

Lyubovnikova, J., West, M.A., Dawson, J.F., and Carter, M.R. (2015). 24-karat or Fool's gold? Consequences of real team and co-acting group membership in healthcare organsiations. *European Journal of Work and Organisational Psychology* 24 (6): 929–950.

MacDonald, N. (2010). How to set up a new team. *Estates Gazette* 1 (4): 75.

Manley, K., Jackson, C., and Makenzie, C. (2019). Microsystems culture change: a refined theory for developing person-centred, safe and effective workplaces based on strategies that embed a safety culture. *International Practice Development Journal* 9 (2): 1–21. http://fons.org/library/journal-ipdj-home.

Markiewicz, L. and West, M. (2011). Leading groups and teams. In: *ABC of Clinical Leadership* (ed. T. Swanwick and J. McKimm). Oxford: Wiley-Blackwell.

Morrell, M. and Capparell, S. (2017). *Shackleton's Way: Leadership Lessons from the Great Explorer*. London: Nicholas Brealey Publishing.

O'Donovan, R. and McAuliffe, E. (2020). A systematic review of factors that enable psychological safety in healthcare teams. *International Journal for Quality in Health Care* 32 (4): 240–250. http://doi.org/10.1093/intqhc/mzaa025.

Parker, G.M. (1990). *Team Players and Teamwork: New Strategies for Developing Successful Collaboration*, 2e. San Francisco, CA: Jossey-Bass.

Razzi, C.C. and Bianchi, A.L. (2019). Incivility in nursing: implementing a quality improvement program utilizing cognitive rehearsal training. *Nursing Forum* 54: 526–536. http://doi.org/10.1111/nuf.1236.

Siassakos, D., Fox, R., Crofts, J.F. et al. (2011). The management of a simulated emergency: better teamwork, better performance. *Resuscitation* 82: 203–206.

Steinemann, S., Berg, B., Skinner, A. et al. (2011). In situ multidisciplinary, simulation-based teamwork training improves early trauma care. *Journal of Surgical Education* 68 (6): 472–477.

Thompson, R. and Kusy, M. (2021). Has the COVID pandemic strengthened or weakened health care teams? A field guide to healthy workforce best practice. *Nursing Administration Quarterly* 45 (2): 135–141. http://doi.org/10.1097/NAQ.0000000000000461.

Tuckman, B. (1965). Development sequence in small groups. *Psychology Bulletin* 63 (6): 384–399.

Vogelsmeier, A. and Scott-Cawiezell, J. (2009). The role of nursing leadership in successful technology implementation. *Journal of Nursing Administration* 39 (7/8): 313.

West, M.A. (2021). *Compassionate Leadership: Sustaining Wisdom, Humanity and Presence in Health and Social Care*. London: The Swirling Leaf Press.

West, M.A. and Markiewicz, L. (2016). Effective teamwork in healthcare. In: *The Oxford Handbook of Healthcare Management* (ed. E. Ferlie, K. Montgomery and R. Pederson), 231–252. Oxford: Oxford University Press.

West, M.A., Lyubovnikova, J.R., Ekert, R., and Denis, J.L. (2014). Collective leadership for high-quality healthcare. *Journal of Organizational Effectiveness: People and Performance* 1 (3): 240–260.

Whitehead, C. (2019). *Compassionate Leadership: Creating Places of Belonging*. West Yorkshire: Solopreneur Publishing.

11

Networking and Delegation

Tracey Coventry

> *You can delegate authority, but you can never delegate responsibility by delegating a task to someone else. If you picked the right man, fine, but if you picked the wrong man, the responsibility is yours – not his.*
>
> Richard E. Krafve, General Manager Edsel Division,
> Vice-President Ford Motor Co., in Eigen and Siegel (1991), p. 222

Introduction: Strength in Numbers

This chapter looks at the topics of networking and delegation. Networking is explored and its importance in terms of clinical leadership for health professionals. It also considers what delegation is and the skills essential for effective delegation. For health professional leaders, networking is a useful way to extend professional connections and opens up lines of communication with others (Weberg et al. 2019). Networking is about placing people in touch with friends, friends of friends, their friends, parents, partners, co-workers and so on. In addition, networking supports the success of an organisation (or the people in it), because it brings knowledge, information and influence to both the organisation and the people who belong to it. With information technology (IT) and the widespread use of social media, the ability to network is continually enhanced. Delegation supports networking, because when it is done well and with the right motives it can be a powerful boost to team-building and leadership in healthcare.

Networking

Networking can be defined in a number of ways, such as 'the exchange of information or services among individuals, groups, or institutions, specifically the cultivation of productive relationships for employment or business' (Merriam-Webster 2021). Increasingly, the term networking is associated with information technology (IT) and the development of social

Clinical Leadership in Nursing and Healthcare, Third Edition.
Edited by David Stanley, Clare L. Bennett and Alison H. James.

networks or in reference to the interconnection of computers. However, in its broadest sense, a network can be defined as an interconnected system of things or people. Networks can be informal interconnections (Marquis and Huston 2021) or associations between individuals or groups of people where the association can be personal relationships with family, friends, members of a sporting club or social group, or indeed anyone. Networks can be formed with people with whom we have a business relationship, a professional relationship or the clients and customers encountered in the course of our professional activities.

Opportunities for networking happen whenever people meet, and, in many respects, networking is about how things get done (Drake 2017). This applies to our personal life, the business world, in industry, in sports and entertainment, and in our professional life. Networking is a formal term for the informal connections and interconnectedness that come about as we move through our lives as social beings.

We are networking when we:

- talk with a product representative who visits our place of work
- meet a former colleague at a conference
- engage with friends and friends of friends on social networks
- talk to the person behind us in the line at the checkout
- strike up a conversation with someone while waiting in the doctor's waiting room
- talk over the fence with our neighbour
- attend a meeting at work
- stand on the sidelines at our child's soccer match at the weekend
- take up an evening class
- interact socially in any way

Bresnen (2017, p. 140) suggests the primary purpose of networking is to acquire or share knowledge, followed by networking for support, such as 'emotional reassurance, personal validation, consolation or the expression of feelings outside of the immediate work context'. The role of networking for career advancement is also through connecting with new opportunities and is useful to secure influence over decision making and desired behaviours or actions. Marquis and Huston (2021) suggest that networking increases power and influence by forming alliances with peers, senior and junior co-workers, and colleagues outside the organisation. Therefore, establishing effective networks is an essential aspect of a clinical leader's role, particularly if formal power is not an option. Networking gives a clinical leader access to contacts, information, resources and support so that they can accomplish a range of tasks, employ creativity and offer innovative solutions to clinical and other problems. In the same way that evidence-based information can facilitate power and influence or clarify decision making, the collective wisdom and influence of a successful network can support clinical leaders by adding to their capacity to get things done. Indeed, the creation of informal networks provides vital sources of knowledge, energy and information on current happenings, within an organisation and in wider health professional associations.

The Skills of Networking

Becoming a good networker can be achieved with a minimal amount of effort, but if you want to foster a specific network for a specific purpose, it may take a degree of attention and focus and require some thought to set up. Although networking may not come naturally to some people, being a good networker by simply interacting and exchanging ideas can be an easy thing to achieve (Kaweckyj 2019). One of the reasons to network is to establish a level of influence or personal power that may help you to achieve your personal and professional goals.

Here are some ideas for establishing an effective network or developing professional networking skills.

Get Yourself Known

Successful networking requires you to find people with whom you want to be known and using this time effectively to your advantage (Kaweckyj 2019). This can involve a number of approaches, such as finding common interests and using technology to communicate more widely. You may want to develop local hospital, local community, clinical specialism, national or, indeed, international networks.

Volunteer

Make yourself available for volunteer tasks, for example, as a minute taker on a committee, giving your time on open days or offering support for educational forums. This can be an effective strategy if you want to be noticed in your hospital community or by the influential people in your clinical specialism or organisation. The advantage of this is that you can then influence or gain experience in decision making and debate or meeting approaches.

Join a Professional Organisation

Membership of professional organisations, such as the Royal College of Nursing (UK), Australian Nursing Federation, Australian College of Nursing or other peak professional bodies, can bring credibility, keep current with best practices, and give you access to a voice for effecting changes in subjects that interest you. Also, you will be recognised as enthusiastic and keen, as well as building a more diverse curriculum vitae and broadening your contacts and interests. Professional organisations have within them local interest groups for active engagement and offer educational support as well as conferences, which also encourage greater networking opportunities (Kaweckyj 2019; Houston 2020).

Look Beyond Your Own Organisation

While you may work in one place or department, your networks are richer if they stretch beyond these boundaries and even beyond one organisation. There is a need to be aware of and understand external trends, to be informed of critical developments and anticipate implications to your current role and career progression and even post-retirement plans. In the area of interprofessional education and multi-professional working environments, looking to gain networks in other organisations or with other professional groups can be an effective way of developing interesting and rewarding contacts.

Be Professionally Committed and Have Clear Messages

Clinical leadership requires clear communication, not cliché heavy declarations, but explicit explanations of intentions and directions. Similarly, know what it is you stand for and be prepared to express your views clearly if called on. This is about knowing what you can offer and what you are looking for from a networking relationship.

Join Professional Discussion Groups

These are especially relevant if they are associated with your clinical specialism. Thus, if you are a health professional involved predominantly with cardiovascular care, joining a relevant discussion group or special interest group will give you access to others in this specialism, allow you to gather information and contacts to support your professional development and have a positive impact on the care and service you could offer your clients and patients (Houston 2020). Professional organisations often function similar to social networking sites and include forums and chat rooms to engender interactions and ideas and encourage collaborative practice.

Use Social Networks

Social media as a communication tool offers active engagement through sharing ideas, knowledge, and support in informal and formal links with professionals from across the globe. Social networks present both opportunities and risks for communication and networking with the ever-increasing growth of worldwide connectivity in interprofessional and intraprofessional groups and associations. Web-based platforms provide the opportunity to augment professional practice and education and link to research, with risks of misuse managed to increase the benefits. However, maintaining confidentiality of client and patient details and ensuring ethical practice is an important component of professionalism (Marquis and Huston 2021). Many health professional associations have established principles for social networking to guide professionals on the boundaries on their participation in relation to posts, privacy settings, patient rights, and institutional policies on online conduct (Weberg et al. 2019). Social networking platforms use a profile that allows your education, work experience, publication, and conference presentation history to be visible. This information can be used by health professionals seeking topic experts for collaboration, speakers for conferences, and recruiters looking to fill positions. A detailed profile can be beneficial and may support your ongoing career goals.

Engage with Professional Development

Completing a course and acquiring more information is an excellent way to learn more and meet new people who have similar interests. Professional development covers many options, from formal courses, which add to your skill base and include application to practice activities that may broaden your organisational networks, to informal professional development such as workplace mentoring or coaching by a more experienced colleague who can help to broaden your connections to others with similar interests or ideas. Digital platforms for professional development can also increase the opportunities for building capacity as a health professional and encourage exploration and engagement in easily accessible ways. The benefits of the online space include immediate, relevant, updated content and resources, and access to social connections, which encourage multi-directional interactions and sharing (such as videos, blogs) which can be accessed on digital devices in any location.

Go to Conferences

Conferences play a critical role in the professional development of health professionals and provide many opportunities to network and build relationships (Lindsay 2018). Generally, at a conference you will meet people within your professional group and often beyond it, and from a wide range of locations, frequently international. Attendance allows opportunities to talk formally and informally and incorporate a social aspect to the occasion, facilitating greater discussion and more possibilities to make links and foster professional relationships. Attending conferences – even those that at first glance seem only peripheral to your professional sphere – can offer up wonderful new perspectives on old problems and exciting new ideas or contacts (Drake 2017).

Mentor Others or Be Mentored

Acting as a mentor or seeking out and engaging with a mentor for yourself can enhance your leadership and learning skills and show your commitment and support for others (Houston 2020). Gaining a mentor means that you will have access to experienced and reliable clinical experts who can help shape and direct your career and offer advice or support when times are difficult or when you may need to make career-changing decisions. Supporting people in this way builds your profile as a person willing to help others and promotes the growth of neophyte professionals.

Travel (for Professional Reasons)

A radical way to widen your networks is actually to go and work in other countries and locations. Nursing and other health professions are global and, apart from some language issues, the practice of nursing and healthcare is generally universal. Techniques change and skills may vary, but interacting with nursing or healthcare colleagues internationally enriches both you and them and has positive impacts on the whole profession. You can do this as a volunteer or as a paid employee.

Develop a Clinical Supervision Process

Clinical supervision has a focus on progressing the professionals' reflective skills on clinical practice and competence with the support and guidance of a more experienced professional to enhance accountability and patient safety in complex situations (King et al. 2020). This leads to increased confidence, less isolation and personal development. Clinical supervision also supports the workforce during challenging times, when moving to different roles or workplaces in response to demand, and can have a positive impact on health professional well-being (Martin and Snowdon 2020). Clinical supervision supports networking because you are mixing with professionals who have considerable experience and insights into the clinical and professional issues that may arise in your career (Houston 2020).

Expand Your Informal 'Coffee' Network

Health professionals often meet over coffee or tea, and making an effort to have informal social meetings with professionals from other areas or departments will significantly expand your professional network and give you access to information from other parts of the organisation. Ensure you are prepared to make the most of this type of valuable networking exercise; update your social media profiles and invite them to connect, research any of their recent work, have some points ready for discussion, keep to a short time frame to respect their time, take notes and follow up on any suggestions (Drake 2017). Similar to physical meeting, a chat over coffee can still occur through digital means and be no less useful for expanding your networks.

Publish

When something is published it enters the global network of professional work, enriching others' knowledge and allowing them to recognise your professional contribution. When an article or book is published, it leaves a trail that can lead back to you. Opportunities for further collaboration on your topic of interest with other like-minded health professionals may develop and provide a greater platform for change of practice or thinking and lead to further publications.

Other Ideas

Drake (2017) states successful organisational, personal and strategic networking is about relationship building in order to achieve goals. Suggestions to improve your networking success include the following. Being genuine and authentic so that you can build trust in your relationships, being clear about your goals when you network so that you can focus on the right networks, connecting with groups and interests that spark your interest and attention, listen and ask open-ended questions in networking conversations, become known as a powerful or useful resource for others, regularly follow up on the contacts you have made, and be clear about how you can be of help to others, rather than just focusing on what the network can do for you.

Reflection Point

This chapter offers a considerable list of activities that can enhance your capacity to network. What are you doing now, and what might you think to include for an enhanced or improved networking capacity?

Networking Through Social Media

Working on developing personal and professional networks can also help with your personal and professional development. Indeed, Pizzuti et al. (2020) in their study of healthcare workers (nurses, pharmacist, administrators and doctors) believe that social media is an effective tool for healthcare education. It allows an opportunity to meet new people, contribute to new ideas and influence professional developments. The continuing advancement of technology, especially connectivity through smartphones, has allowed people a greater opportunity to network globally and to share ideas and information that will help any profession improve and develop. Social media uses web-based technologies that allow connection and interaction in real time to share and exchange information to enhance and support practice. Extending your network encourages professional discussion, critique and debate. Social media use is not without its associated risks, however, and in particular health leaders need to be mindful not to breach confidentiality or professional boundaries. A general rule of thumb is that if you would not want someone to read a particular statement, never, ever post it.

As a professional social network, LinkedIn is gaining ground. Established in 2003, it now has over 400 million users worldwide (Higgs et al. 2019). LinkedIn members create their own personal profile and link with others based on shared interests, education, career development and professional affiliations, which enables broader connections across multiple groups. Other social media platforms include, but are not limited to, Facebook, Twitter, YouTube, Instagram, WhatsApp, Snapchat, Reddit, and Pinterest. Through the use of social media, reaching out to people far beyond your everyday contacts is beneficial, although, remember that social media networks are a tool and are incredibly valuable, but only when used appropriately and wisely.

To become skilled at networking, it is important to know where you may or may not have any influence, so that you can apply your personal resources prudently. Like most nurses and other health professionals, you will have other demands on your time, and reaching a suitable work/life balance means focusing your networking attention appropriately. Choose where best to make your contributions and focus on professional activities that will challenge, enrich and offer the greatest impact from your energies. Networking can increase your circle of influence or allow you to take charge of situations, or indeed influence others.

Clinical Leaders Story 11:   A Time to Shine

I had not been a nurse educator long, but I was encouraged by the Head of School to attend a conference in another country. I had been working on my doctoral thesis and had published some papers related to my methodology and findings. I had not travelled outside of my home country before (other than a short holiday in Bali), and I was unsure how I could present my findings in such a short time and to an international audience.

First, I spoke with colleagues who had travelled to international conferences in the past and gathered what information I could about what to expect and how they might work. They also gave me tips about long haul international travel and making the most of my experience overseas. My more experienced colleagues proved both helpful and informed.

I also spoke with my research supervisors about what specifically to present and how to condense my findings into a meaningful presentation. Feeling as prepared as I could, I set off for the United States. There, I met a host of other like-minded professionals, from the United States and from other countries. All were encouraging and supportive and many expressed their interest in my research topic or in my methods. I made some excellent international links, and I'd go so far as saying that I learnt that the study challenges I was facing were similar to those faced by colleagues in other countries, and that we were facing similar challenges with research funding and growing student expectations. Knowing this and with the encouragement and support of the wider nursing community, I gained greater confidence and the boost I was looking for to progress towards the completion of my doctoral studies and even led to an international post-doctoral collaborative research opportunity

– Terry, Nurse Academic.

Networking Tips

A number of approaches can be employed to support and enhance effective networking, but they all involve a commitment to building relationships with the people with whom you connect and remembering that our first impressions count, whether face to face or online. Look for opportunities when you meet people online through professional discussion groups or at conferences or meetings. Experienced health professionals will use networking to extend their influence by meeting new colleagues. Think about extending your network to include health professionals from a range of disciplines and at various stages of their professional careers. New starters can bring fresh perspectives; experienced colleagues can provide a wealth of information (Prado et al. 2020). If you are not an experienced networker, try the following icebreakers to open conversations with someone you wish to know or meet:

- Where are you from?
- What is your area of clinical specialism?
- How do they do things at your facility or organisation?
- What do you think about the outcomes of the meeting?
- Is there anything on the conference programme that particularly interests you?
- What professional interest groups would you recommend?

Once you have got beyond the initial opener and the conversation is coming to an end, do not forget to ask for either a phone number or an email address, and to offer a business card with your contact details. With the use of smartphones, there are many ways of keeping in contact, thus making networking even easier.

After this initial engagement, remember to follow up. Here are some suggestions:

- Send a quick text
- Send a short email
- Make a phone call to discuss something of mutual interest
- Check out the other person's LinkedIn account and send an invitation to connect

There are so many people you are yet to meet – those who are willing to network and continue working with you will let you know.

Delegation

Delegation is an important management/leadership tool that requires decision-making skills to decide who should receive an assignment, to explain what is required and to ensure the delegate completes the work with the desired outcome (Cole 2018). Weberg et al. (2019, p. 463) suggests delegation has increased importance in healthcare related to 'increased complexity, new technologies and innovations in this field', with the ability to delegate a critical competency for all healthcare leaders. Delegation saves time and maximises the skills and expertise of team members. Giving staff respect, trust and real responsibility, together with a degree of independence, can be powerful in team building and to enhance leadership. This was stated succinctly by Woodrow Wilson, the 28th U.S. President: 'I not only use all the brains that I have, but all that I can borrow'.

According to Marquis and Huston (2021), delegation can be described as achieving goals through the work of others, although the person who delegated the work remains accountable for the outcome. Delegation allows for a shift in decision making, and, done well, is not abdication or dodging responsibility. Effective delegation uses trust with only the minimum controls; however, there must be a balance between trust and control depending on the situation. The opposite of successful delegation is micro-management, a practice that confines and restricts the 'creativity and problem-solving potential' and leads to the frustrating of competent delegates (Weberg et al. 2019, p. 472). Building trust is therefore essential for effective delegation. Trust comes from:

- having confidence in your staff or team members
- being willing to take a risk
- having confidence in yourself

Control is about appropriate levels of freedom according to experience and it relates to accountability. Delegation is not simply handing over a task that you do not want to do, and it means that you need to know the skills and abilities of the person to whom you are delegating. Clinical leaders need to be able to describe the task, know what is required, display interpersonal skills, offer training, and monitor the team member's capacity to undertake the task. Delegation should ideally be positive for both the clinical leader and the person to whom the task has been delegated.

Reflection Point
Reflect on a time when a task was delegated to you. How was this undertaken? How did you feel? Did you feel empowered or suppressed? Liberated or used?

Effective Delegation

Effective and successful delegation allows clinical leaders to foster communication that develops the skills and confidence of the staff involved. Weberg et al. (2019) suggests delegation includes elements of accountability (individual and organisational), assignment, and authority, which require preparation and practice. Successful delegation follows these steps:

- Define the task: Be sure it is suitable for delegation.
- Select the correct individual or team: Are they the most appropriate person/people?
- Assess ability and training capability.
- Explanation: Why is the job being delegated? What is its relevance to the unit/ward/ department objectives?
- Results wanted: What must be achieved?
- Resources: Agree what is needed to achieve the task (people/equipment/money).
- Deadlines: Agree when the job needs to be completed.
- Support: Offer support when necessary and make sure everyone knows that a task is delegated and that you are there to support them.
- Feedback: It is essential to give feedback and review the situation if the task is not on track.

When delegating, the following tips may also be useful:

- Give the person the whole task. Handing over part of a task or continually returning to meddle will not be helpful and will lead to frustration.

- Make sure that the delegate understands exactly what you want them to do.
- Share your picture of what a successful outcome will look like.
- Identify how success will be measured.
- If possible, determine in advance what reward the person will get or how you will thank them.
- Identify key points in the project when you want feedback about progress.

The 'five rights' to employ for successful and effective delegation (Barrow and Sharma 2021) are:

1) *Right task:* Does the delegated task conform to established policies, procedures and standards?
2) *Right circumstances:* Does the staff member have the right education, resources, equipment and supervision to complete the task safely?
3) *Right person:* Is the staff member qualified and competent to perform the task delegated?
4) *Right direction and communication:* Are the directions given with the task clear and does the staff member understand these directions?
5) *Right supervision and evaluation:* Are appropriate monitoring, intervention and evaluation provided?

In nursing and other health professions, delegation is commonly related to the matter of sharing tasks and duties in terms of clinical work. In this regard it is linked to how teams work (see Chapter 10) and is also regulated by law (enforced by Acts of Parliament) in relation to the appropriateness of certain tasks that can, or cannot, be delegated to various types of healthcare professionals. Therefore, all health professionals need a clear understanding of delegation and the legislation that supports its use.

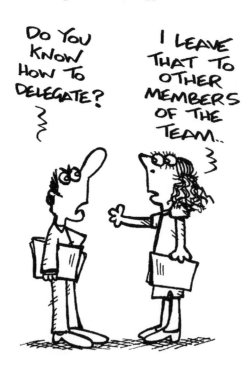

Common Mistakes in Delegation

Delegation is a skill that can be learnt. Errors that are commonly seen are under-delegation, over- delegation, inappropriate delegation and failing to provide sufficient supervision. The following discussion draws on Marquis and Huston (2021) description of these common mistakes.

Under-Delegation

Sometimes leaders will be reluctant to delegate tasks as they perceive that if they do so, this may show an inability to perform their job. It often reflects a lack of trust or a desire to hold on to power and authority (Weberg et al. 2019). Delegation is about letting go, and this can sometimes be very difficult for clinical leaders who are passionately invested in their role or responsibilities. Confident leaders despise micro-management; instead, they set achievable goals and give people the freedom to act independently.

Over-Delegation

Leaders who are poor time managers, disorganised or feel insecure about performing tasks themselves will tend to over-delegate. Often, this means making decisions on the task themselves despite the delegation and frequently checking-in to monitor the task and the delegate. This often leads to conflict and mistrust of the leader, which in turn results in reduced team productivity.

Inappropriate Delegation

In appropriate delegation is assigning tasks to the wrong person at the wrong time for the wrong reason. Allocating tasks to someone who is not qualified or does not have the training needed to undertake the requested task can have significant consequences in relation to safety of both patients and staff.

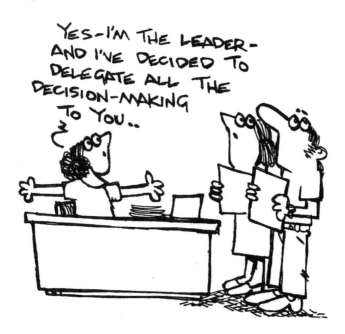

Failing to Provide Sufficient Supervision

If the task has been delegated and insufficient supervision provided, particularly when the person delegating does not support or build trust, the person may feel abandoned and unsupported. This generates feelings of mistrust and is likely to result in conflict between the leader and the person to whom the task has been delegated.

When delegating, you should avoid the following:

- Offloading – delegating a task just because you do not want to do it
- Mixed messages – delegating then retaining too much control (micro-management)
- Offering a poisoned chalice – a task that you know is fraught with nasty surprises or is very difficult to achieve
- Too much too soon – involving inexperienced staff ahead of time
- Imprecise definition of the task

Resistance to Delegation

Not all team members will see the opportunities that delegation offers as a benefit; indeed, resistance to delegation is not uncommon (Marquis and Huston 2021). Some team members will feel over-burdened due to existing work pressure, being unprepared to take on new tasks, lacking in self-confidence, being reluctant to cooperate with 'new' initiatives and a perception that the task, although delegated, will be overseen too closely or micro-managed.

When faced with resistance, the clinical leader may be tempted simply to reallocate the task or undertake it themselves to avoid conflict or to get the job done. Nevertheless, it would be a mistake to miss the opportunity to investigate the reason behind the resistance. There may be legitimate reasons for team members feeling the need to resist delegation, and these should be explored and addressed appropriately. These types of opportunities may be the key to facilitating greater trust within the team and building greater team cohesion.

Reflection Point

Speak with colleagues in the area where you work. Have any of your colleagues had any formal education or training in how to delegate effectively? Have you? Reflect for a moment: what impact might the results of your informal survey have on the quality of delegation where you work?

Delegation and Clinical Leadership

Effective clinical leadership is directly related to the skills of delegation (Marquis and Huston 2021). Clinical leaders need to be aware of the relevant legislation affecting what is and what is not permissible in terms of intra- and interprofessional delegation. Clinical leaders should also act as role models for effective delegation, supporting team members and colleagues and acting as a resource person if needed. Effective clinical leaders see delegation as a time management and team-building tool and are able to identify tasks and situations that are appropriate for delegation (Marquis and Huston 2021). Clinical leaders also use effective communication skills, including assertiveness and support, to build trust so that patient safety remains a primary focus of the delegated task. Clinical leaders need also to be conscious of the potential impact of cultural issues on delegation across cultures, should this be needed.

Leaders who demonstrate congruent leadership delegate as an act of congruence, leading through delegation by demonstrating their values and beliefs in their trust and support (faith) in team members and colleagues. In this way, clinical leaders use their colleagues and team members' potential, not their job title, to decide whether delegated tasks are relevant or appropriate (Walker et al. 2021). Delegation then becomes an act of elevation, lifting others' performance and confidence as they feel supported and guided to higher levels of participation.

The skills required for delegation improve with practice, and clinical leaders will become more effective at delegation as their confidence and competence grow. There are real benefits from delegation for clinical teams, since team members gain new skills, develop more self-confidence, develop greater responsibility and broaden their scope of practice.

Case Study 11.1   Edith Dircksey Cowan

Edith Cowan was a networking pioneer. She lived in an age when men dominated politics and yet she was able to use her connections and networks to help her to do more for her community, and specifically for children. Read about Edith Cowan and consider how she struggled to make a difference for single mothers and young children and the impact that having effective networks had on her success.

Born Edith Brown in 1861, Edith is worthy of note as the first female member of the Australian Parliament and a true Western Australian pioneer. She was born at Glengary, near Geraldton in Western Australia, the second daughter of a pastoralist, Kenneth Brown, and a teacher, Mary. Her childhood was unhappy, with her mother dying in childbirth when Edith was seven and her stepmother being murdered by her father eight years later. He was hanged for the offence.

Edith attended boarding school in Perth where she met James Cowan, whom she married in 1879. James was the registrar and master of the Supreme Court. His appointment in 1890 as police magistrate gave them economic security as well as a place in Perth society where they were able to network with the great and the good. Edith also gained an insight into society's wider problems. Between 1880 and 1891, the couple had four daughters and a son.

In the 1890s, Edith became involved in a number of voluntary organisations, including the North Fremantle Board of Education, the Karrakatta Women's Club, the House of Mercy for Unmarried Mothers and the Ministering Children's League. In addition, in 1906 she was one of the founding members of the Children's Protection Society and pioneered a day nursery for working mothers in 1909. The Children's Protection Society was instrumental in supporting the State Children's Act in 1907, which led directly to the Children's Court. In 1915, Edith was among the first women appointed to the bench, and she became a Justice of the Peace in 1920.

In 1909, she helped initiate the Women's Service Guild, which undertook fundraising activities and government lobbying, a function of which was the opening of the King Edward Memorial Hospital for Women in 1916. Edith became secretary of the advisory

(Continued)

Case Study 11.1   (Continued)

---

board to the hospital. In 1911, she was instrumental in the creation of the National Council of Women of Western Australia, serving as president from 1913 to 1921 and then vice president until her death in 1932. She was also a foundation member of Co-Freemasonry in Western Australia in 1916, the first female member of the Anglican Social Questions Committee from 1916, and a co-opted member of the synod from 1923.

Edith supported amendments to the Health Act that proposed the compulsory notification of venereal disease. She travelled to Britain and Europe between 1903 and 1912, and in 1925 she went to the United States. During World War I she took part in a wide range of social activities, including the Red Cross, which saw her recognised with the award of OBE in 1920. The political scenery after the war also led to changes in legislation that barred women from parliament. As such, in 1921 Edith stood as an endorsed Nationalist for the Legislative Assembly seat of West Perth. She campaigned on her community service record, the need for law and order, and for the place of women in parliament to 'nag a little' on social issues. She won, narrowly, and became the first woman member of the Australian Parliament.

During her first term in office, Edith proposed improvements in migrant welfare, the development of infant health centres and the promotion of women's rights. She was also an advocate for sexual education in state schools. Sadly, she lost the 1924 election, and she was defeated again in 1927, so ending her political career.

In 1926, Edith was a founder of the (Royal) Western Historical Society, and in 1929 she was active in planning the state's 1929 centenary celebrations. She continued her social and committee involvement until ill health became too much of a burden. She died in 1932 aged 71. Edith Cowan is an example of an articulate and driven woman who spent the majority of her life fighting for women and children's rights, and finding ways to develop social and community support systems from within contemporary political and social structures. Edith was a genuine pioneer, forging a path and networks not previously trodden by women in both politics and social reform in Australia.

Challenge: Could Edith have done all this alone or without connections? In a political landscape dominated by men, could she have managed to make the progress she did without their support or engagement? There are parallels here to interprofessional working and interprofessional education. Can the health service grow and prosper, or will better patient or client outcomes be possible without different professional disciplines finding effective ways to work together? How can we better network with different professional disciplines?

Summary

- Networking is about the interconnectedness of things and people.
- Networking is about 'how things get done'.
- Becoming an effective networker is important for success in the health arena.
- There are a number of strategies that can be employed to enhance your networking skills. These include getting yourself known, volunteering, joining a professional

organisation, looking for contacts beyond where you work, being clear about your professional views, joining a professional discussion group, use of social media, engagement with professional development, going to conferences, mentoring others, travel, engagement with clinical supervision, expansion of your 'coffee' network, publishing and developing trusting professional relationships.

- Networking is not always easy or natural, and it takes energy and focus to do it well.
- Delegation is an important leadership tool.
- Delegation is the assignment of authority and responsibility to another person to carry out a specific activity.
- Effective delegation relies on a relationship of trust.
- Successful delegation requires that the task be clearly defined, that the right people or person be selected, that training be offered if needed, that the task be explained clearly, that rewards and resources be agreed in advance, that deadlines be set and that support and feedback be offered.
- Effective delegation can be summarised as the 'five rights': right task, right circumstances, right person, right direction and communication, and right supervision and evaluation.
- Effective clinical leaders require the skills of delegation.
- Done correctly, delegation becomes an act of elevation, lifting others' performance and confidence as they are supported and guided to higher levels of participation.
- Common errors of delegation include under- and over-delegation, inappropriate delegation, delegating too late, not delegating enough and failing to support or supervise the delegate or to build trust.

Mind Press-Ups

Exercise 11.1

Are there tasks that you could delegate to others? How do you go about it? Are people generally receptive to your requests, or do they respond with resentment? Why do you think people respond the way they do?

Exercise 11.2

When delegating to people from other cultures, it is important to consider how you communicate, interpersonal space, issues related to social organisation, time, environmental issues and biological variations. How might these factors be important in your delegation to transcultural team members?

Exercise 11.3

How easy or difficult do you find the act of delegation? Reflect on why you might feel this way. Is it about your clinical competence, confidence, authority or experiences with previous delegation episodes? What has influenced your approach to delegation?

References

Barrow, J. M. and Sharma, S. (2021). Five rights of nursing delegation. https://www.ncbi.nlm. nih.gov/books/NBK519519 (accessed 15 October 2021).

Bresnen, M. (2017). *Managing Modern Healthcare: Knowledge, Networks and Practice*. Londong: Routledge http://doi.org/10.4324/9781315658506.

Cole, K. (2018). *Leadership and Management: Theory and Practice*, 7e. Cengage Learning Australia Pty Ltd.

Drake, K. (2017). 'The power of networking. *Nursing Management* 48 (9): 55–56. http://doi. org/10.1097/01.NUMA.0000522184.39403.65.

Eigen, L.D. and Siegel, J.P. (1991). *The Manager's Book of Quotations*. New York: Amacom.

Higgs, J., Cork, S., and Horsfall, D. (2019). *Challenging Future Practice Possibilities*. Leiden: Brill.

Houston, C.J. (2020). *Professional Issues in Nursing: Challenges and Opportunities*, 5e. Philadelphia: Wolters Kluwer.

Kaweckyj, K. (2019). 'It's all about networking. *The Dental Assistant* 88 (3): 12–14. f9f9e14f19c44083b9dc87aeffda08d4.pdf.

King, C., Edlington, T., and Williams, B. (2020). The 'ideal' clinical supervision environment in nursing and allied health. *Journal of Multidisciplinary Healthcare* 13: 187–196. https://www.ncbi.nlm.nih.gov/pmc/articles/PMC7034973.

Lindsay, E. (2018). 'Importance of attending conferences: being aware of what is happening around you. *British Journal of Community Nursing* 23 (Sup6): S40–S41. https://doi. org/10.12968/bjcn.2018.23.Sup6.S40.

Marquis, B.L. and Huston, C.J. (2021). *Leadership Roles and Management Functions in Nursing: Theory and Application*, 10e. Philadelphia: Wolters Kluwer Health.

Martin, P. and Snowdon, M. (2020). Can clinical supervision bolster clinical skills and well-being through challenging times? *Journal of Advanced Nursing* 76: 2781–2782. http://doi.org/10.1111/jan.14483.

Merriam-Webster. (2021). Networking. Merriam-Webster.com Dictionary. https://www. merriam-webster.com/dictionary/networking. (accessed 6 October 2021).

Pizzuti, A.G., Patel, K.H., McCreary, E.K. et al. (2020). 'Healthcare practitioners' views of social media as an educational resource. *PLoS One* 15 (2): e0228372. http://doi.org/10.1371/ journal.pone.0228372.

Prado, A.M., Pearson, A.A., Bertelsen, N.S., and Pagán, J.A. (2020). 'Connecting healthcare professionals in Central America through management and leadership development: a social network analysis. *Globalization and Health* 16 (1): 34–34. http://doi.org/10.1186/ s12992-020-00557-4.

Walker, F.A., Ball, M., Cleary, S., and Pisani, H. (2021). 'Transparent teamwork: the practice of supervision and delegation within the multi-tiered nursing team. *Nursing Inquiry, vol. 4* e12413. http://doi.org/10.1111/nin.12413.

Weberg, D.R., Mangold, K., Porter-O'Grady, T., and Malloch, K. (2019). *Leadership in Nursing Practice: Changing the Landscape of Health Care*, 3e. Burlington, MA: Jones & Bartlett Learning.

12

Dealing with Conflict

Kylie Russell

> *For good ideas and true innovation, you need human interaction, conflict,*
> *argument, debate.*
>> Margaret Heffernan, US entrepreneur and documentary producer, b. 1955

Introduction: Collaboration or Clash

Conflict is part of life. It is a natural and normal aspect of both home life and the workplace (Scannell 2010). We can be in conflict with ourselves or with others. Conflict is derived from the Latin word *conflictus*, meaning 'the act of striking together', and all interactions offer the potential for discord and strife, with differences over values and beliefs or behavioural issues having an influence on relationships and outcomes. In the health arena, conflict can lead to poor working relationships, a degeneration of communication, negative impacts on client or patient care and poor patient outcomes. Bad relationships and inappropriate use of conflict resolution skills can increase stress and limit innovation (Johansen and Cadmus 2015). Conflict can also result in competition or 'turf wars' that strangle communication and teamwork. All these can diminish the effectiveness of clinical leaders and reduce their capacity to inspire, innovate and successfully initiate or lead change.

In more positive terms, Labrague et al. (2018), in an integrative review, found that organisations that managed conflict benefited from effective workplace relationships through innovation, staff commitment, and positive attitudes towards change. Johansen and Cadmus (2015) noted similar results, with a reduction in the stress of emergency department nurses resulting from a more positive approach to conflict resolution, following opportunities and interventions to build conflict resolution skills. A key to building successful relationships is the application of emotional intelligence (see Chapter 15). This chapter suggests that it is clinical leaders who are in an ideal position to recognise and deal with conflict in the clinical environment (Angelo 2019) and that collaboration, effective conflict resolution skills and the use of emotional intelligence may be the ideal approach

Clinical Leadership in Nursing and Healthcare, Third Edition.
Edited by David Stanley, Clare L. Bennett and Alison H. James.
© 2023 John Wiley & Sons Ltd. Published 2023 by John Wiley & Sons Ltd.

for working through, managing or dealing with conflict. However, it also requires the application of a range of other skills.

For clinical leaders to have a positive impact on conflict or manage their own styles of dealing with conflict and relationships, they need to determine what conflict means, understand conflict and know how it can be recognised and managed (Almost et al. 2016). This chapter explores approaches to dealing with conflict and why recognising and building skills in emotional intelligence can be vital for managing and minimising conflict. Specifically, it considers approaches for dealing with conflict such as 'self-talk' and 'I-messages'. It also discusses the value of active listening in reducing conflict and the tools for recognising and building emotional intelligence.

Reflection Point

Reflect for a moment about conflicts you may have had at work or at home. Think about what the conflicts have been about and how they were dealt with or resolved. How do you feel thinking about them now? Do you usually feel that conflict is resolved positively, or are your dominant feelings about conflict negative? Are your responses to conflict at work different from those to conflict at home or in your personal life?

Past Conflict

We tend to learn our dominant style of dealing with conflict early in life, and to a large extent these responses stem from watching or being involved in conflicts within the family or in our formative social experiences. Everybody uses different strategies for managing or dealing with conflict, and once they have been learnt we tend to employ them automatically, almost naturally. Usually, we are not aware at the time how we act in conflict situations, but we commonly employ our 'preferred' strategy (Marquis and Houston 2017).

A number of styles can be identified for dealing with conflict. These conflict styles relate to our preferred response or natural inclination when faced with conflict. It may be that we respond in different ways to different types of conflict situations. However, we do have a general tendency to respond to conflict in particular 'preferred' ways. As our 'preferred' response grows from learnt behaviours, understanding our strategies for dealing with conflict can allow us an opportunity to recognise positive or combative approaches and modify our strategies as needed. Learnt behaviours can always be unlearnt if they are non-productive.

Influencing Factors

One of the strongest influencers on our style of conflict management is gender. Men are often categorised as competitive rather than collaborative; in contrast, women place relationships at the forefront of importance (Marquis and Houston 2017). Evidence further suggests that conflict management is multifactorial, influenced by the personal character-istics of age, nationality, principles, experience, resilience, emotional intelligence, and personality in combination with the workplace context, including staffing levels, workload, stress, patient acuity, culture, executive leadership, teamwork, position level, education, and support (Almost et al. 2016; Labrague et al. 2018).

Conflict Styles

The Thomas–Kilmann Conflict Mode Instrument (Thomas and Kilmann 1974; Thomas 1992) helps people assess their own preferences for dealing with conflict. Thomas and Kilmann (1974) propose that by assessing our own or others' conflict styles, an appropriate intervention can be initiated to engage, manage or diffuse conflict. The basic proposition of the model is that conflict resolution is orientated to either assertiveness or cooperation. The Thomas–Kilmann Conflict Mode Instrument is also known as the 'Conflict Behaviours Style Questionnaire', and it offers an insight into our tendencies for dealing with conflict. According to Thomas and Kilmann (1974), there are five potential strategies for dealing with conflict:

1) **Withdrawing (the turtle – avoiding):** Turtles withdraw from conflict and tend to give up their goals and relationships. They stay away from people with whom they are in conflict as they believe that it is hopeless to try to resolve the conflict. The withdrawal can be physical or emotional, and this strategy is seen as easier than dealing with conflict face to face (Thomas et al. 2008; Losa Iglesias and Becerro de Bengoa Vallejo 2012).

2) **Forcing (the shark – competing):** Sharks compete and try to force their solution on others. Their goals are highly important, relationships less so. As such, they seek to achieve their goals at all costs and are not overly concerned with others' feelings or needs, or whether others like them. Sharks see conflict as having only two outcomes – winning and losing – and sharks want to win. Their approach to conflict is to attack, intimidate, overwhelm or overpower (Thomas et al. 2008). In the long term this approach impacts team dynamics, increasing stress for the wider team and ultimately is detrimental to patient care (Labrague et al. 2018).

3) **Smoothing (the teddy bear – accommodating):** Teddy bears are the opposite to sharks. For them the goal is less important than the relationship. They seek harmony from conflict and try to help people discuss conflict without harming their relationships. They worry that if conflict persists, people may get hurt and relationships may be damaged. They like to smooth things over and tend to give up their goals to preserve the relationship. Although it may initially smooth potential conflict, long term, gratifying others' needs first can be determinantal to one's self-esteem, elevating stress levels and impacting on an individual's ability to problem solve (Thomas et al. 2008; Labrague et al. 2018).

4) **Compromising (the fox – compromising):** Foxes are concerned both with their goals and their relationships with others. They are prepared to give up part of their goals if

others in the conflict will give up part of theirs. They seek the middle ground where both parties gain something. They compromise and are willing to relinquish a little to maintain the relationship and find common ground (Thomas et al. 2008).

5) **Confronting (the owl – collaborating):** Owls value their goals and relationships highly. They view conflicts as problems to be solved and seek a solution that will support their own and others' goals. Owls see conflict as an opportunity to improve relationships by reducing tension and by focusing on a discussion that identifies the conflict as a problem to be solved. They seek solutions that satisfy everyone and at the same time maintain their relationships. They work hard to find a solution that addresses the conflict and that supports positive feelings and healthy relationships (Thomas et al. 2008; Labrague et al. 2018).

The relationship between each of these strategies can be expressed as tension between assertion (concern for self) and cooperation (concern for others). Figure 12.1 demonstrates this. The Thomas–Kilmann Conflict Mode Instrument is offered in a modified form in Box 12.1. However, before you consider it, reflect on the following five statements. Which do you agree with most? Once you have attempted the Thomas–Kilmann Conflict Mode Instrument, revisit these statements and determine whether your instinctive response corresponded with your results.

- The best way of handling conflict is to avoid it (turtle).
- Put your foot down where you mean to stand (shark).
- Soft words win hard hearts (teddy bear).
- When both give halfway a fair settlement is achieved (fox).
- Every person has a piece to contribute (owl).

The Thomas–Kilmann Conflict Mode Instrument is useful in that it often clarifies or explains our preferred conflict strategy. Knowing your preferred strategy may help you communicate more effectively, work more cooperatively or be less judging of others' behavioural or conflict styles. It is worth considering whether you employ different styles in different situations. Or should we all be aspiring to be collaborators (owls) in all situations?

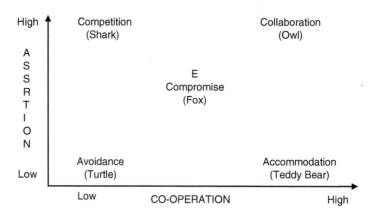

Figure 12.1 Conflict styles. *Source:* Thomas (1992). Copyright 1992 by LM Hough. Adapted by permission.

Box 12.1   Thomas–Kilmann Conflict Mode Instrument

Read the following proverbs and use this scale to score how typical each of your actions is when in conflict: 1 = never do this, 2 = seldom do this, 3 = sometimes do this, 4 = frequently do this, 5 = usually do this.

No.	Statement	Score
1	It is easier to refrain than to retreat from a quarrel	
2	If you cannot make a person think as you do, make them do as you think	
3	Soft words win hard hearts	
4	You scratch my back, I'll scratch yours	
5	Come now and let us reason together	
6	When two quarrel, the person who keeps silent first is the most praiseworthy	
7	Might overcomes right	
8	Smooth words make smooth ways	
9	Better half a loaf than no bread at all	
10	Truth lies in knowledge, not in majority opinion	
11	He who fights and runs away lives to fight another day	
12	He hath conquered well that hath made his enemies flee	
13	Kill your enemies with kindness	
14	A fair exchange brings no quarrel	
15	No person has the final answer, but every person has a piece to contribute	
16	Stay away from people who disagree with you	
17	Fields are won by those who believe in winning	
18	Kind words are worth much and cost little	
19	Tit for tat is fair play	
20	Only the person who is willing to give up their monopoly on truth can profit from the truths that others hold	
21	Avoid quarrelsome people as they will only make your life miserable	
22	A person who will not flee will make others flee	
23	Soft words ensure harmony	
24	One gift for another makes good friends	
25	Bring your conflicts into the open and face them directly: only then will the best solution be discovered	
26	The best way of handling conflicts is to avoid them	
27	Put your foot down where you mean to stand	
28	Gentleness will triumph over anger	
29	Getting part of what you want is better than not getting anything at all	

(Continued)

Box 12.1   (Continued)

No.	Statement	Score
30	Frankness, honesty and trust will move mountains	
31	There is nothing so important you have to fight for it	
32	There are two kinds of people in the world, the winners and the losers	
33	When someone hits you with a stone, hit them with a piece of cotton	
34	When both give halfway, a fair settlement is achieved	
35	By digging and digging, the truth is discovered	
	Total	

Scoring

Copy your scores from the proverbs to the appropriate place on the scoring grid. Then total each column. The total for each column relates to a preference for that conflict strategy. The higher the number, the stronger the preference.

Withdrawing	Forcing	Smoothing	Compromising	Confronting
Turtle	Shark	Teddy bear	Fox	Owl
1	2	3	4	5
6	7	8	9	10
11	12	13	14	15
16	17	18	19	20
21	22	23	24	25
26	27	28	29	30
31	32	33	34	35
Total	Total	Total	Total	Total

Conflict at Work

Coan (2010) suggests that at work people commonly experience conflict around who should do what and how things should get done. Conflicts over style and personality and conflict that is unresolved can have a negative impact on teamwork or group dynamics (Labrague et al. 2018). Group working and teamworking are also frequent areas in which conflict arises (Kelly and Tazbir 2021). The signs that conflicts exist are not always as blatant as might be assumed. It may be that colleagues are in open dispute, with loud verbal exchanges, but the other signs could relate to there being a drop in motivation or productivity, an increase in absenteeism or changes in behaviour. Bauer and Erdogan (2015) identify six main causes of conflict within the workplace:

- **Organisational structure** – where unclear reporting lines confuse staff as to who they should report to
- **Limited resources** – money, time and equipment may be scarce
- **Task interdependence** – where you rely on others to complete their tasks in order to achieve your goals
- **Incompatible goals** – your priority may not be the same as someone else's
- **Personality differences** – these are common within workplaces; people coming from different cultures have different values and beliefs, and the key is to understand how they see the world
- **Communication problems** – the way a message may either be delivered or interpreted is often a cause of misunderstanding, leading to conflict; the written word (emails) can be readily misinterpreted

These causes are reflected in Almost et al.'s (2016) integrative review of managing and mitigating conflict, where a lack of emotional intelligence, poor working environments, role ambiguity, certain personality traits, a lack of support and poor communication are seen as influencing poor conflict management. We can choose or defer to our preferred style of conflict resolution when faced with any or all of these types of conflict.

Conflict Resolution

An organisation where staff are encouraged to adopt a conflict resolution style based on collaboration supports a more positive organisational culture and facilitates better staff relationships (Labrague et al. 2018; Peng et al. 2021). This is enhanced if employees are resilient and have strong personal characteristics, an ability to organise their work and personal life and strong support networks (McDonald et al. 2016). Dreachslin and Kiddy (2006) add that there are several steps that leaders can take to manage or minimise conflict and build resilience:

- **Recognise hot and cold conflict:** Identify the continuity of events. Cold conflict is formed by suppressed or passive anger, harbouring a grudge or underlying resentment. To deal with this, warm it up by bringing it to the surface so that the issue can be addressed and resolved. Hot conflict is the expression of anger or the voicing of concerns without thinking them through. Here the conflict should be cooled down and then dealt with.
- **Develop emotional intelligence** (see Chapter 15): This is about knowing how to recognise and manage your feelings to build stronger relationships, enhance self-awareness and achieve a greater work/life balance (Goleman 2011, 2014). The four building blocks of emotional intelligence are self-awareness (our own feelings), self-management (managing our emotions), social awareness (recognising others' feelings) and social skills (managing emotions in others).

- **Determine who you are managing (leading):** This involves being sensitive to the different people you are leading, acknowledging cultural differences, gender differences and historical issues in the workplace.
- **Reduce community conflict:** Recognise and appreciate that you may not be dealing just with one individual and that they are usually part of a wider community; conflicts or solutions may have an impact on that community too.
- **Build strong personal networks**: You need a range of support from both a personal and work life perspective (McDonald et al. 2016).
- **Pre-empt and resolve conflict:** In relation to the principles of congruent leadership, how you are seen to deal with conflict will reflect on how your values are perceived. Doing something about conflict will usually produce a more positive outcome than doing nothing or trying to suppress it. Dreachslin and Kiddy (2006) suggest that leaders should find time to talk (and listen), plan for dealing with the conflict, talk the issues out, keep all parties engaged and make a deal to ensure that the problem will not be repeated.

The keys to managing conflict are to be prepared to deal with it when it occurs and to employ clear, open and honest communication (Kelly and Tazbir 2021). Engage in positive self-talk and rehearse conflict encounters. Understand the value of emotional intelligence and your own conflict style. Dreachslin and Kiddy (2006) conclude that one of the main things people can do to resolve conflict is to listen to each other more effectively.

Kohlrieser (2007) supports Dreachslin and Kiddy's (2006) view by suggesting that there are six essential skills for managing conflict:

- Create and maintain a bond, even with your 'adversary'
- Establish a dialogue and negotiate
- Put the fish on the table (raise the issue without aggression or hostility)
- Understand what causes conflict
- Use the law of reciprocity
- Build a positive relationship

Kohlrieser (2007) feels that conflict can be productive if managed properly and that leaders who use these six essential skills efficiently can reduce conflict or manage it well.

Responding to Conflict

While we may have a preferred method or response to conflict, there are a number of ways in which we respond. Kohlrieser (2007) and Coan (2010) summarise these as follows:

- **Flight** – running away (turtle style) or avoidance of the conflict.
- **Diversion** – delay, deflection or simply changing the subject.
- **Fight** – imposing one's will on another (the shark approach). This can take the form of control, verbal abuse and even violence. It is never an appropriate way to resolve conflict. People get hurt. Conflict does not get sorted, it just goes underground and festers.
- **Deny the conflict** – wait until it goes away.

- **React emotionally** – this may involve becoming aggressive, abusive, hysterical or frightened. It may also involve finding others to blame or creating excuses. These are rarely appropriate responses and lack the potential for a successful resolution.
- **Constructive conflict resolution** – resolving conflicts in a way that is mutually satisfying allows problems to be dealt with positively and involves a commitment to dealing with the issue. This only works if both parties are genuinely willing to resolve the conflict.

Clearly, the last approach is recommended as it allows leaders to determine the real source of the conflict, decide whether this is the correct source, set time aside to deal with the conflict and search for agreement together by negotiation, mediation or compromise. The other methods are non-productive and can even be counterproductive or destructive, implying that the correct approach to conflict is vital to diminish negative consequences and build the best chance of an effective resolution.

To reach a collaborative solution to problem solving, the following steps are suggested:

- **Define the problem:** Everyone involved needs to reach a clear agreement on what the problem is before it can be addressed.
- **Establish what everyone wants to get from the conflict (what are the goals):** For example, the goals could be 'a voice at the table', 'respect from a senior colleague' or 'influence in clinical decision making'.
- **Separate emotion and feelings from the solution/problem:** When feelings and emotions are tied up in the solution, a decision is much more difficult to reach. This does not mean that you may not have strong feelings, but you should not let those feelings get in the way of a potential solution. Using I-messages (see later in this chapter) during the discussion will help keep emotions and feelings in check.
- **Self–awareness:** Identify any of your behaviour that contributes to the conflict.
- **Brainstorm options for mutual benefit:** There may be a raft of solutions, many of which could work, but often the first solution suggested is settled on as a technique to resolve the conflict. Keep ideas coming and suggestions on the table so that creative and innovative ideas flow and are well discussed.
- **Find objective criteria to evaluate the solutions proposed:** Look at the pros and cons, and establish a criteria set or standards on which all parties can agree. This may take time and care and requires considerate negotiation. It will mean being open to good ideas and closed to threats, yielding to sound arguments rather than pressure or intimidation.
- **Reach a mutually acceptable solution:** Once this is decided on, ensure that each party takes responsibility for the decision, and clarify that a collaborative solution has in fact been reached.

These steps require participants to listen to each other and check what they have heard. I-messages and self-talk can be used so that topics stay on track and remain future orientated. These steps should be followed with action, the sharing of responsibility and the wisdom to seek help if needed.

The key is to intervene early and recognise that the process may lead to understanding rather than agreement (Archee et al. 2013). A good relationship is not one without conflict, but one in which the participants can resolve conflicts so that no one is hurt or oppressed.

Kelly and Tazbir (2021) maintain that to be an effective leader, it is essential to be able to handle (manage) conflict. This implies that leaders are able to offer constructive responses to problems and conflict, recognising their styles and overcoming or using them as necessary. These skills are implied by Dotson (2007) when she suggests that 'self-management', 'networking', 'flexibility', 'synergy with others', 'being coachable' and 'using a mentor' are all keys to conflict success. They all rely on avoiding or controlling conflict and, as such, make conflict management a central issue in developing clinical leadership skills.

Conflict Management and Clinical Leaders

Successful conflict management requires clinical leaders (champions) who demonstrate key conflict resolution principles and the ability to influence rather than wield power and authority. Clinical leaders need to bring conflict into the open (Marquis and Houston 2017) so that it can be effectively addressed in a collaborative style. This will result in greater organisational or departmental creativity and innovation and lead to satisfaction for all parties involved. Clinical leaders need to value their goals and professional relationships highly and view conflicts as problems to be solved. Solutions should be sought that satisfy all involved, allowing everyone to meet their goals and at the same time maintain collaborative relationships.

Conard and Franklin (2010) suggest that this approach requires clinical leaders to show:

- a willingness to acknowledge conflict
- open communication and support throughout
- an attitude and environment of mutual respect when dealing with conflict
- understanding, tolerance and acceptance of different perspectives
- a commitment to fairness
- support for educating or sharing conflict management strategies with others
- commitment to the policies and procedures established to support conflict management
- encouraging accountability for all involved to employ these principles when dealing with conflict

When individuals know how to employ a collaborative approach to conflict, the conflict can actually be turned into a constructive force (Conard and Franklin 2010). Collaboration fosters team working and facilitates understanding that leads to a genuine appreciation of differences, resulting in a system of shared values, shared decision making and effective communication (Bauer and Erdogan 2015), all of which facilitate the application of congruent leadership.

Boateng and Adams (2016) state that conflict is common in all workplaces and that in nursing it is a frequent source of work-related stress and disharmony. Added to this are growing tensions in the make-up of the healthcare workforce, with greater interprofessional education and workplace dependence (creating power clashes) that mix and heighten tensions around gender, race, ethnicity, age and generational values. These factors in themselves do not necessarily contribute to conflict, but they can add tension to an already stressed and highly charged clinical environment. Effective communication techniques may not resolve conflicts; therefore, it is important that managers or leaders understand when conflict resolution requires escalation to the next level through negotiation and mediation. We examine this more closely in the next section.

Building Bridges: Negotiation and Mediation

According to Pruitt (2011), negotiation is where two or more parties come together to reach an agreement to resolve a conflict. Leading and participating in the negotiation process is part of the role of clinical leaders and managers (Marquis and Houston 2017). Becoming a skilled negotiator takes practice, and leaders should look to undertaking additional education programmes to gain these skills (Marquis and Houston 2017). There are three phases to the negotiation process: pre-negotiation, negotiation and post-negotiation. All phases are equally important if successful conflict resolution is to occur.

Pre-Negotiation Phase

- Build bridges between the two parties so that they can communicate – decide whether the meeting is to be on neutral ground, ensure that it is a suitable venue that meets all party's requirements, talk to both parties to gauge an understanding of the issues that have created the conflict (Pruitt 2011).
- Agree on preconditions before entering the negotiation, such as acceptable behaviours; aggressive (both verbal and physical) behaviour will not be tolerated in any form.
- Identify the problem clearly and gain an understanding of each side's goals or needs.
- Set an agenda for what issues will be discussed and in what order.
- Choose a spokesman for either side (when two or more people exist on either side).
- Decide on who the facilitator of the negotiation should be – this person could either be neutral or be someone whom both parties respect.
- Set a mutually agreed date and time for the meeting to occur, allowing both parties to be equally prepared to 'come to the table'.
- Make sure that all relevant information is available at the time of the meeting (Pruitt 2011).

Negotiation Phase

For the leader involved in the negotiation, it is important to think about the following (Marquis and Houston 2017):

- Maintain your composure.
- Facilitate pauses in the conversation.
- Be a good role model for communication, be assertive and flexible and emulate good speaking and listening skills.
- Avoid using destructive negotiation techniques and be prepared to counter these in others if required. Such techniques include ridicule, ambiguous or inappropriate questioning, flattery, feigned helplessness or aggressive behaviour.

General rules described by Marquis and Houston (2017) to follow during the process of the negotiation are:

- Be factual and do not give hearsay any credibility.
- Listen carefully and observe non-verbal communication.
- Keep an open mind and do not take sides.
- Seek to understand both parties' viewpoints.
- Discuss the issue, do not personalise the topic of conflict.
- Do not fix blame on either party.
- Be honest and open (deception will destroy any trust).
- Be firm and clear about expectations.
- Know the bottom line, the non-negotiable aspects, particularly if they breach safety or industrial agreements.

Post-Negotiation Phase

- Notice body movements or indications that the person is forming a response and wait for them.
- Summarise accurately the meaning of what you have heard.
- Paraphrase key points and, if your paraphrasing statement was not well received, try again or ask for clarification.
- Give feedback on feelings as well as content.
- Put the focus of your attention totally on the speaker.
- Record key aspects of the meeting for future reference or for reflection.

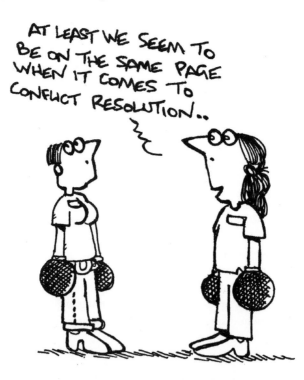

The success of any agreement relies on having the needs of both parties met in some way (Pruitt 2011). It is important that all parties understand the outcomes of the agreement and that they commit to upholding their part of it. After a pre-determined period of time, follow-up should occur with both parties to ensure that the agreed outcomes are being maintained.

If either party does not hold up their end of the agreement or if negotiation is unsuccessful, mediation should be considered. Mediation is an extension of the negotiating process whereby an external party arbitrates with both conflicting parties in order for an agreement to be reached (Pruitt 2011). In my experience, mediation is the last resort in managing conflict. Where decisions about the outcome are taken away from the conflicting parties, neither party may be satisfied with the outcome, as generally both parties lose something that they felt was important. This may potentially lead to disgruntled and dissatisfied employees.

Non-Productive Behaviour

Not all conflict is managed well, and often this is the result of non-productive behaviour. Clinical environments are not free from non-productive behaviours, and they can occur in meetings, at handovers, in educational situations and indeed in any forum where health professionals interact (Layne et al. 2019). Some non-productive behaviours are described in the following.

Negativity

Do not put other people's ideas down, such as saying 'It will never work'. Instead, ask the question 'How do the rest of you see this?' Or the person with a new idea could be asked to offer further explanation or even a replacement idea for the one that got zapped. Nothing kills creativity more than negativity.

Being Talkative

Some people love the sound of their own voice and use it all the time. This can be addressed by referring these people to team rules, by stating a time frame for talking before starting a meeting or by politely saying 'Sorry if I interrupt you ...', then making your point.

Attention Seeking

People may clown around and disrupt the team effort. Counter such behaviour by restating the purpose of the work or discussion, or by asking them to contribute in a serious way or to offer more serious dialogue. Then reward their serious side by complimenting the desired behaviour.

Arrogance

People can be highly assertive and prefer to get things done in the way they know best. This behaviour can be very controlling and self-assured, but it can alienate others in the team. It can be dealt with by using questions to get them to expand on their ideas, or by paraphrasing to repeat their ideas, so that they can see you know what they are suggesting.

Arguing

When questioning goes beyond clarification or thoughtful debate, or when people are obviously looking for an opportunity to disagree or pick at an idea, it becomes annoying and disruptive. Change the focus of the discussion by acknowledging the person's ideas, or feelings, and limiting the speaking time so that there is an equal opportunity for all to speak. This behaviour can also be handled by paraphrasing the various positions expressed or by dealing with people individually at a later date.

Withdrawing

Some people may act indifferently or passively, or simply not get involved in discussions. They may also occupy themselves by doodling or whispering to others or getting off the subject or being distracted by a mobile phone or tablet. These behaviours can be addressed by getting the person to share their ideas in the meeting, or by asking them to contribute their ideas in advance so that you can call on them during the meeting. If they are simply not confident, they could tell someone else their ideas or views, then contribute to the team themselves once their ideas have been 'tried'. Their participation can also be encouraged by simply asking open-ended questions.

Aggression

This can be expressed in going after others' ideas in a critical or vicious manner, blaming others or showing hostility and anger, or putting other people's ideas or status down. Keep cool and say something like 'I see you have strong opinions, but let's hear what others think'. It may also be appropriate to respond to the whole team and not just to this person or to remain neutral. However, when you respond, make it clear that this behaviour is unwelcome.

Complaining

Some people will find fault, blame others or whine that things are unfair, and will express dissatisfaction with the way things are being done. A response could be to remain patient and compassionate, ask the person to focus on solutions, listen for their main points or concerns, and shift the focus of the discussion to solutions.

There may be other non-productive behaviours, and the solutions offered here are not exhaustive, but in general the key is to listen to the person and try to understand what might have prompted the behaviour in the first place. This requires the application of active listening, considered next.

Active Listening

One of the main reasons that conflict occurs is that we either do not hear what is communicated, or what we are trying to say is not understood or heard clearly. In order to promote more effective communication, active listening will facilitate greater attention to what is being communicated. The benefit of active listening is that it enables the demonstration of understanding by one person to another and clarifies feelings about the communication (Kristinsson et al. 2019). Active listening can be used as a successful approach to avoiding conflict by ensuring that communication is effective and focused.

Active listening involves:

- concentration (energy)
- focus on the speaker
- listening to the whole message
- suspended judgement
- taking note
- making eye contact
- checking and reflection
- using paraphrasing
- separating fact from feeling
- elimination of distractions (telephones, computers, loud noises etc.)

Employing active listening may be difficult if some of the following barriers are encountered:

- being unable to hear all the time
- not understanding the topic
- being confused
- a noisy or distracting environment
- having other things on your mind or IT equipment in your hand (e.g. iPhone or laptop)
- not liking what is being said
- finding the content boring
- the talker's tone of voice, or speed and manner of speech
- poor paraphrasing skills

Active listening may not come naturally, and some practice may be needed. This may seem an odd statement, given that health professionals are commonly heavily involved in communication. Yet are we always listening actively? Here are some hints to help with your development of active listening (similar to the suggestions for the post-negotiation stage discussed earlier):

- Allow silences in the conversation.
- Notice body movements or indications that the person is forming a response and wait for them.
- Summarise accurately the meaning of what you have heard.
- If your paraphrasing statement was not well received, try again or ask for clarification.
- Give feedback feelings as well as content.

- Put the focus of your attention totally on the speaker.
- Position yourself so that you can see and hear the speaker clearly.

Consider these helpful hints, and in your next conversation (at work or at home) make an attempt to employ active listening skills. It can feel a little strange at first (unless you do this already), but try to follow the advice here and really focus on what the other person is saying.

Self-Talk

Managing conflict means, in many cases, managing ourselves. Grant (2003) suggests that we can choose not to be victims of our emotional reactions to events, and that we have a conscious reaction or process and a subconscious reaction or process. What we have been taught is that a particular event leads to feelings, and this has an impact on our communication. In this model we are potentially victims, controlled by what happens. Thus:

Event = Feelings = Communication

However, what really happens is that after an event we have the thought, belief, and interpretation of the event in our mind. This leads to an emotion and then we have a reaction seen as behaviour, and it is this that affects our communication. Thus:

Event + (Interpretation / Thought / Belief)
+ Emotion = Reaction / Behaviour = Communication

If we can modify our reaction (our thinking) and behaviour, we can promote more effective communication by catching faulty thinking. Examples of faulty thinking are exaggeration, over-generalisation, should/must thoughts, having to be right, catastrophising, self-blaming, mind-reading and the misperception of being treated unfairly. These fuel negative thinking and result in miscommunication, which can lead to conflict. I can recall getting an email from a senior colleague indicating that they were taking over a project I had been running successfully. I felt upset, as I had invested heavily in the project and I felt as if they were just taking over at the project's conclusion to get the credit for it. This resulted in my feeling unfairly treated, and I sent a sharp and inappropriate email in response. My feelings had led to an assumption about the reason I was being taken off the project. I had acted without clarifying the reason, and this led to conflict (not about the issue, but about my feelings), as my colleague could not understand my response.

Here is another example of this process in play:

- **The event is activated** – in this case, giving a presentation in front of colleagues.
- **Belief** (in this case negative) – I must perform exceptionally well or my colleagues will think I am incompetent.
- **Consequences of this belief** – anxiety, poor concentration, defensiveness.
- **Disputing the self-limiting belief(s)** – just because I want to perform exceptionally well does not logically mean that I must. If I do not perform exceptionally well, will my colleagues really think that I am stupid?

- **Effective new beliefs** – there is no evidence that my colleagues think that I am stupid if I do not perform exceptionally well. I have given great presentations before. I have received positive feedback from peers in the past.
- **New feeling** – more confident, able to approach the presentation as a challenge rather than an ordeal.

The process outlined is really the process of self-talk or mindfulness. It is a concept that can be understood and developed and relates to an individual's capacity to become more competent by identifying negative thoughts and replacing them with positive self-talk, which in turn has a positive impact on communication. Eunson (2015) describes the concept of self-talk, recognising that leaders need to learn to analyse and manage three things: internal dialogue (self-talk), mental images (visualisation), and beliefs and assumptions. Eunson (2015) identifies that distinguishing between unhelpful or negative self-talk as opposed to helpful or positive self-talk can enable an individual to move away from patterns of self-talk that are limiting or damaging in some way. Once you engage in positive self-talk opportunities, you can focus on constructive ways of managing and dealing with change and challenging situations, including conflict. Once you have rethought and want to communicate effectively, another approach to developing clear communication is to use I-messages.

I-Messages

I-messages mean speaking for yourself and not for others. At first this will sound odd, and if your first reaction to this is like mine, you will be thinking 'But I already speak for myself, who else do I speak for?' You may be surprised when you really consider it, but often our conversations are aimed at speaking for others, frequently to avoid conflict. Do you ever start a conversation with 'sorry'? I did so the other day in a restaurant when a waiter dropped a fork and I said 'Sorry, I'll get that', as if it had been my fault.

I-messages use words like 'I, me, my, I think, I believe, I want to know that, I want to, I don't want you to'. The key is that they all start with 'I'. The communication is about what *you* want, feel or think. It is constructed so that you own what is being said and the listener is directed to how you feel, the behaviour of concern and its effect. As such, I-messages are structured as follows: 'I feel ... (describe your feelings) when you ... (describe a behaviour) because ... (describe the effect).' For example, 'I feel upset when you don't fill up the car with petrol because it means I was late for work as I had to stop and do it.' Or 'I feel fed up when you say you are coming to bed and instead you stay up and watch television for another hour, because you wake me up coming to bed later.'

Relating to each other in this way all the time may make conversations sound a little fake or stilted, but in terms of addressing or stalling conflict it is a very effective way of demonstrating the impact of a set of actions and owning the feelings related to them. Practice some I-messages at home or at work and consider the results.

Conflict often sets people up on different sides of a discussion and leads to further division. Wheeler (2006) suggests that it is better to find common ground, and in many respects the proposed approach to dealing with conflict already set out is designed to help clinical leaders recognise their own conflict styles and search for common ground when they encounter conflict.

Reflection Point

Think about a conflict you have had recently at work. Was it resolved positively or could the outcome have been improved? If it could have been improved, how might I-messages, self-talk or active listening have affected the outcome?

Clinical Leader Stories 12: Roadside Warrior

The local ambulance service has just initiated a new role called 'clinical leader'; however, the managers within the service positioned the role in offices to develop policies and processes and not on the road, where the clinical and client-focused activity takes place. While the policies and processes will be used to influence and guide practice and will make a significant contribution to clinical care, I think it's a shame that the potential clinical leader skills will not be used where I see them being more effective. I expressed my views at a team meeting and was told it had already been decided. My view is that the clinical leaders would be better employed as roadside experts, where they could support, guide and role model excellent paramedic practice, and where junior paramedics and volunteer ambulance officers could see and be helped directly by their clinically focused and highly skilled paramedic colleagues with great decision-making abilities and real-world paramedic insights.

I also feel that the office-based role would soon erode the senior paramedic's skills and make them less relevant to roadside practice. I also considered that their many years of experience and well-honed clinical skills could be better employed and be seen to be employed by other paramedics (visible), and they will act as better leaders because they will be seen doing what paramedics aspired and are trained to do. Work with clients on the roadside.

I had thought of applying for one of these new roles. But I value working in a road crew too much, and I value what I can do on the roadside more than what might occur in an 'office job'. It is not just that I would rather be on the road and not in an office, and even though the 'the pay will be better in the office job'. I believed that I have more to offer my colleagues and the public by being seen performing what I believed are the key and clinically appropriate actions of a senior paramedic in practice. I think I can do more by being visible, approachable and by role modelling excellent paramedic practice. I thought about taking my concerns further but knew that I would face opposition from the senior managers, so I simply did what I could and stayed in a roadside crew. I feel I can better be a congruent leader if I stay mobile and with the clinical team at the roadside.

Tony - Paramedic

Communication Styles

There are several communication strategies and tools to support difficult conversations, to reduce conflict, and improve patient care, including graded assertiveness and mindful communication. Mindful communication supports open dialogue to reduce conflict, and graded assertiveness challenges unsafe practice. Both techniques support communication dialogue, in particular for junior staff, in a safe way that focuses on clinical observation and fact rather than a perceived criticism of an individual's practice (Hanson et al. 2020).

Mindful Communication

Mindful communication uses the principle of mindfulness. Mindful communication takes time, it is a habit and practice that we use during our communication with others to be in the moment, to listen, and demonstrate the attributes of honesty, curiosity and tolerance. We engage in these conversations with our colleagues, our patients and their families (Dobkin 2015). During mindful communication, we are self-aware of our internal thoughts and emotions, and how these relate to external stimuli, being purposeful to form non-judgmental conclusions. Whilst we must make a decision based on our judgement of the situation, we take the time to consider the experience, to step outside of our own experiences, to observe, and not simply react. Arendt et al. (2019) summarised these attributes as three *mindfulness in communication* behaviours: (p. 4)

a) being present and paying attention in conversations,
b) an open, non-judging attitude, and
c) a calm, non-impulsive manner.

Assertive Communication

Assertive communication refers to an individual's capacity to communicate in a direct way, being respectful of others' opinions, and taking ownership of ones ideas and thoughts. Within health, patient safety is dependent on good communication; however, given the hierarchical nature of the professions, junior staff can find it difficult to speak up and be heard. Assertive communication is one strategy to support junior staff and members across disciplines. Graded assertive communication provides a staged approach of assertive communication, supporting junior staff to escalate concerns through guiding questions, which display a curiosity of learning, while being respectful and collaborative (Dobkin 2015).

Communication Tools

Questioning members of the healthcare team is an essential skill to prevent patient harm. There are a number of communication tools to support clinical handover and escalation of care. The CUS and PACE models provide a graded assertive approach to support junior practitioners communicating with senior staff. While these models promote a safety net of care, their endorsement must not shift the focus of communication to junior staff; instead, these models work in unison with senior staff communication strategies to break down perceived or actual communication barriers (Weller and Long 2019). A study of first year nursing students (n = 535) identified that teaching assertiveness, using the CUSS and PACE models, provided a toolkit for junior nurses that supported their overall confidence in speaking up to protect patient safety (Hanson et al. 2020).

CUS/S

The communication tool CUS/S is a graded assertive verbal alarm to communicate patient care. Using the CUS/S words indicates to the team the severity of your concern. Effective implementation of CUS/S requires a shared understanding of the words and their intent. The tool is one part of an evidence-based toolkit for healthcare professionals to support communication developed by the Agency for Healthcare Research and Quality. There are slight variations of the tool, but all have the same intent (Agency for Healthcare Research and Quality 2017).

CUS

- I am **C**oncerned: At this stage you may have a concern related to patient's status or an intervention and want to voice this. You may communicate this concern beginning with the statement 'I am concerned...' Followed by your reasons, that is, why you feel concerned.
- I am **U**ncomfortable: If your concern remains unresolved, you can re-emphasis this concern with 'I am uncomfortable. ...' Again, clearly articulate why you feel uncomfortable.
- This is a **S**afety issue: If you remain concerned and uncomfortable by a patient situation, or an intervention, you restate your concern with greater conviction in your choice of words. You communicate these concerns starting with the words 'This is unsafe. ...'

The following CUSS version includes STOP:

- **S**top: By now, if your concern remains unheard you need to take the final action and state 'Stop'.

PACE

The PACE communication tool provides another example of using specific words to effectively communicate with members of the healthcare team to question care or seek an intervention. The PACE model has been endorsed by the Australian and New Zealand College of Anaesthetists (Weller and Long 2019):

- **P**robe: gain attention or raise a concern.
- **A**lert: repeat this concern. Increase your volume.
- **C**hallenge: formally state concerns and challenge the individual's decision.
- **E**mergency: get eye contact and potentially take over the task.

Benefits of Conflict Management

There are a number of benefits for healthcare professionals and clients or patients if conflict is dealt with more effectively. Cullati et al. (2019) found in the clinical area 4 out of 10 conflict situations potentially affected patient care, in particular timeliness of care, patient-centred care and efficiency of care. This supports previous findings by Bearden (2009) that conflict management led to more culturally appropriate care, improved communication, greater staff satisfaction and increased nurse retention. For clinical leaders who can deal with their emotions and react in a collaborative style when faced with a conflict situation, the result can be communication that is more effective and better opportunities to proceed with practice improvements, innovation and change.

Case Study 12.1   Cathy Freeman

Cathy Freeman is an Australian woman who overcame many of the barriers faced by indigenous people to represent her culture and country as a sporting icon. Her cultural heritage dominates her life and how others see her achievements. Consider Cathy's story and the challenge that follows.

Catherine (Cathy) Astrid Salome Freeman was born on 16 February 1973, in Mackay, Queensland, Australia. Her father was Norman Freeman, an ex-rugby player from Woorabinda. He was a loving father, but was prone to excessive drinking and violent outbursts. When Cathy was five years old he moved to the Aboriginal Mission three hours west of Mackay, where he lived away from his wife and children for the rest of his life. He was soon diagnosed with diabetes and became further depressed, drinking more frequently. Cathy's mother Cecelia was known to be very strict with her children, always for their own benefit, of course. However, early on Cathy found her mother overbearing and even domineering. This lead to frequent arguments and Cathy sometimes ran off at night to hang out with her cousins. Her mother was nevertheless a constant in her life, and Cecelia proved to be a great source of support when Cathy was troubled or upset. She also encouraged the young girl with her running and from an early age Cathy was prompted to write out, 'I am the world's greatest athlete' as a positive affirmation on which to build her athletics dreams.

Cecelia married Bruce Barber, a white railway worker, and initially this new relationship upset the children. Eventually, though, Bruce was to become one of Cathy's greatest supporters, and even though the family had to move frequently because of his job, it was Bruce who recognised Cathy's potential and became her first coach. He took an interest in positive psychology and counselled or supported Cathy during some niggling injuries and a bout of glandular fever that threatened to stall her early career. It was also Bruce who raised money to allow Cathy and her younger brother, Norman, to attend various national athletics championships.

Bruce also knew his limitations, and once he was sure Cathy would excel in her sporting career with more guidance, he put his energies in 1987 into securing her a place at Fairholme College in Toowoomba where, with the aid of a scholarship and better coaching and facilities, she did indeed improve.

It is for her sporting prowess that Cathy is best known. She won her first gold medal at her school championships when she was eight, although she faced frequent discrimination for being an Aboriginal. Once she had to watch the first-place trophy being given to another girl, even though Cathy had won the race, because it was

---

(Continued)

Case Study 12.1   (Continued)

inconceivable that a black child could win. Her first international race was at the Commonwealth Games in Auckland in 1990. She ran as part of the Australian 4 × 100 m relay team. In doing so, she became the first female Aboriginal Australian to win a gold medal in any international athletics event.

In 1991, Cathy was named Young Australian of the Year. After more intensive training, she took part in the 1992 Olympic Games in Barcelona, Spain, becoming the first Aboriginal to represent Australia at the Olympics. She did not win a medal, but the competition offered vital insights into how to prepare for later competitions.

In 1994, Cathy again excelled at the Commonwealth Games, this time in Victoria, Canada, where she won the 200 m and 400 m Gold medals. In terms of heightened international recognition, she came under more intense scrutiny at the 1996 Olympics in Atlanta, Georgia, USA. Here she ran her personal best of 48.63 seconds to win a Silver medal in the 400 m event. This was followed by a Gold medal in the 400 m at the World Athletics Championships in 1997.

Off the track, Cathy was also making waves as a successful Indigenous ambassador, supporting and promoting Aboriginal culture. Much of this off-field work contributed to her being named 1998 Australian of the Year.

Next, she competed in the 1999 World Athletics Championships in Seville, Spain, and was successful with a Gold medal in the 400 m event. However, her real target was the Gold medal at the Olympics, and as the year 2000 rolled around, the world watched with fascination and anticipation as she stormed to victory in the 400 m final. Cathy had also carried the Olympic flame at the opening ceremony, but her highlight in these games was her fantastic victory. She stood out too in a specially designed green and gold running suit, in complete contrast to the ill-fitting and poor running equipment that she had been offered or was able to secure as a young athlete.

Her dream of winning Olympic Gold had come true, and she had done it in front of her friends and family in Australia. Her only regret was that her father, Norman, had died before her greatest win. Cathy retired from competitive running in 2003 and began to concentrate more on her domestic responsibilities and on the Cathy Freeman Foundation, which focuses on making life better for Indigenous Australians.

Challenge: Cathy Freeman is a great athlete in spite of her cultural heritage not because of it, although her upbringing, her cultural background and the circumstances of her youth clearly affected her athletic development. Culture can be a point of conflict and is one that health professionals need to be aware of as they navigate the challenges of working in the health service. How can you be your best self? How do you manage conflict to be and do the best for your patients or clients?

Summary

- Conflict is part of life.
- Clinical leaders are in an ideal position to recognise and deal with conflict in the clinical environment.

- It is vital that clinical leaders understand what conflict means and how it can be recognised and managed.
- There are a number of ways in which people tend to respond when faced with conflict: they can withdraw, compete, become accommodating, compromise or collaborate.
- Clinical leaders who use a collaborative approach to conflict resolution deal more effectively with conflict.
- Conflict at work is often the result of unclear expectations, poor communication, unclear boundaries, conflicting interpersonal styles, conflicts of interest or change within an organisation.
- To reach a collaborative solution, clinical leaders are encouraged to define the problem, establish the goals, separate emotion from the problem or solution, brainstorm options for mutual benefit, find objective criteria to evaluate the solutions proposed and reach a mutually acceptable solution.
- Clinical leaders seeking a collaborative approach to conflict resolution should also employ integrity, honesty and superior listening skills.
- These approaches should reduce non-productive behaviours such as negativity, talkativeness, attention seeking, arrogance, arguing, withdrawal, aggression and complaining.
- Communication can be enhanced with active listening, self-talk, I-messages and being mindful
- Employ effective communication strategies such as mindful or assertive communication / PACE or CUS/S.

Mind Press-Ups

Exercise 12.1

How was conflict resolved in your family when you were growing up? What lessons have you learnt about conflict resolution from your experiences with family, friends and co-workers?

Exercise 12.2

When you have a conflict with someone, how do you prefer to handle it? What approaches to dealing with conflict are you less comfortable with or would rather not use?

Exercise 12.3

Think of someone with whom you often find yourself in conflict. What is the behavioural style or conflict strategy that you often notice them using? How can understanding this help with the conflict in future?

References

Agency for Healthcare Research and Quality. (2017). CUS Tool – Improving communication and teamwork in the surgical environment. https://www.ahrq.gov/hai/tools/ambulatory-surgery/sections/implementation/training-tools/cus-tool.html (accessed 14 October 2021).

Almost, J., Wolfe, A.C., Stewart-Pyne, A. et al. (2016). Managing and mitigating conflict in healthcare teams: an integrative review. *Journal of Advanced Nursing* 72 (7): 1490–1505. http://doi.org/10.1111/jan.12903.

Angelo, E. (2019). 'Managing interpersonal conflict: steps for success. *Nursing Management* 50 (6): 22–28. http://doi.org/10.1097/01.NUMA.0000558479.54449.ed.

Archee, R., Gurney, M., and Mohan, T. (2013). *Communicating as Professionals*, 3e. South Melbourne, VIC: Cengage Learning Australia.

Arendt, J., Verdorfer, A., and Kugler, K. (2019). 'Mindfulness and leadership: communication as a behavioral correlate of leader mindfulness and its effect on follower satisfaction. *Frontiers in Psychology* 33 (2): 187–193. http://doi.org/10.1097/NCQ.0000000000000282.

Bauer, T. and Erdogan, B. (2015). *Organizational Behaviour*. Washington, DC: Flat World Education.

Bearden, M.T. (2009). Conflict resolution for nurses. MA dissertation, Royal Roads University, British Columbia, Canada, http://search.proquest.com/docview/305160349 (accessed 6 Oct 2021).

Boateng, G. and Adams, T. (2016). '"Drop dead. ... I need your job": an exploratory study of intra-professional conflict amongst nurses in two Ontario cities. *Social Science & Medicine* 155, 35–42. http://doi.org/10.1016/j.socscimed.2016.02.045.

Coan, G. (2010). *Managing Workplace Conflicts*. Casselman, Ontario: Bacal Associates, http://conflict911.com/guestconflict/manworkplaceconflict.htm (accessed 1 July 2016).

Conard, J.R. and Franklin, J.F. (2010). Addressing the art of conflict management in health care systems. *Dispute Resolution Magazine* 16 (3): 14–17.

Cullati, S., Bochatay, N., Maître, F. et al. (2019). When team conflicts threaten quality of care: a study of health care professionals' experiences and perceptions. *Mayo Clinical Proceedings: Innovations, Quality & Outcomes* 3 (1): 43–51. http://doi.org/10.1016/j.mayocpiqo.2018.11.003.

Dobkin P. (2015). *Mindful Medical Practice: Clinical narratives and therapeutic insights*, Springer. https://doi:10.1007/978-3-319-15777-1 (accessed 27 October 2021).

Dotson, T. (2007). Top 10 secrets to career success. *Black Collegian* 37 (3): 28–30.

Dreachslin, J.L. and Kiddy, D. (2006). From conflict to consensus: managing competing interests in your organisation. *Healthcare Executive* 21 (6): 9–14.

Eunson, B. (2015). *Communicating in the 21st Century*, 4e. Milton, QLD: Wiley.

Goleman, D. (2011). *The Brain and Emotional Intelligence: New Insights*. Northampton, MA: More Than Sound.

Goleman, D. (2014). What it takes to achieve managerial success: four facets of emotional intelligence epitomize the necessary competencies. *T+D* 68 (11): 48.

Grant, A.M. (2003). The impact of life coaching on goal attainment, metacognition and mental health. *Social Behavior and Personality* 31 (3): 253–263.

Hanson, H., Wllsh, S., Mason, M. et al. (2020). "Speaking up for safety": a graded assertiveness intervention for first year nuring students in preparation for clinical placement: thematic analysis. *Nurse Education Today* 84: 104252–104251, 7, 104252. http://doi.org/10.1016/j. nedt.2019.10425.

Johansen, M.L. and Cadmus, E. (2015). Conflict management style, supportive work environments and the experience of work stress in emergency nurses. *Journal of Nursing Management* 24 (2): 211–218.

Kelly, P. and Tazbir, J. (ed.) (2021). *Nursing Leadership and Management*, 4e. New York: Wiley.

Kohlrieser, G. (2007). Six essential skills for managing conflict. *Perspectives for Managers* 149: 1–4.

Kristinsson, K., Jonsdottir, J., and Snorrason, S. (2019). Employees' perceptions of supervisors listening skills and their work-related quality of life. *Communication Reports* 32 (3): 137–147. http://doi.org/10.1080/08934215.2019.1634748.

Labrague, L., Hamdan, Z., and McEnrie-Petitte, D. (2018). 'An integrative review on conflict management styles among nursing professionals: implications for nursing management. *Journal of Nursing Management* 26 (8): 902–917. http://doi.org/10.1111/jonm.12626.

Layne, D., Nemeth, L., Mueller, M., and Martin, M. (2019). 'Negative behaviors among healthcare professionals: relationship with patient safety culture. *Healthcare* 7 (23): 1–11. http://doi.org/10.3390/healthcare7010023.

Losa Iglesias, M.E. and Becerro de Bengoa Vallejo, R. (2012). Conflict resolution styles in the nursing profession. *Contemporary Nurse* 43 (1): 73–80. http://doi.org/10.5172/conu.2012.43.1.73.

Marquis, B.L. and Houston, C.J. (2017). *Leadership Roles and Management Functions in Nursing*, 9e. China, PA: Wolters Kluwer Health.

McDonald, G., Jackson, D., Vickers, M., and Wilkes, L. (2016). Surviving workplace adversity: a qualitative study of nurses and midwives and their strategies to increase personal resilience. *Journal of Nursing Management* 24: 123–131.

Peng, J., Lou, H., Ma, Q. et al. (2021). Association between workplace bullying and nurses' professional quality of life: the mediating role of resilience. *Journal of Nursing Management* http://doi.org/10.1111/jonm.13471.

Pruitt, D.G. (2011). Negotiation and mediation in intergroup conflict. In: *Intergroup Conflicts and Their Resolution* (ed. D. Bar-Tal), 267–289. New York: Taylor & Francis.

Scannell, M. (2010). *The Big Book of Conflict Resolution Games*. New York: McGraw-Hill.

Thomas, K.W. (1992). Conflict and negotiation process in organizations. In: *Handbook of Industrial and Organizational Psychology*, 2e, vol. 3 (ed. M.D. Dunette and L.M. Hough), 652–717. Boston, MA: Nicholas Brealey Publishing.

Thomas, K.W. and Kilmann, R.H. (1974). *Thomas–Kilmann Conflict Mode Instrument*. Mountain View, CA: Xicom.

Thomas, K.W., Fann Thomas, G., and Schaubhut, N. (2008). Conflict styles of men and women at six organization levels. *International Journal of Conflict Management* 19 (2): 148–166. http://doi.org/10.1108/10444060810856085.

Weller, J. and Long, J. (2019). 'Creating a climate for speaking up. *British Journal of Anaesthesia* 122: 710–713.

Wheeler, P. (2006). Whose side are you on? *Leadership Excellence* 23 (11): 8.

13

Motivation and Inspiration

David Stanley

> *If your actions inspire others to dream more, learn more, do more and become more, you are a leader.*
>
> John Quincy Adams, 6th US President, 1767–1848

Introduction: Inspiring Others

To be effective, clinical leaders need to be able to motivate and even inspire others. As many clinical leaders are not in positions of 'power' over others (indeed, controlling others is strongly seen as a trait of non-clinical leaders), they need to consider other more appropriate and effective motivational approaches. In the research that underpins this book, most participants described clinical leaders as guides and teachers, indicating that they should be open, approachable and help people to feel part of a team (Stanley 2006a, b, 2008, 2010, 2011, 2012; Stanley et al. 2012, 2014, 2015; Stanley and Stanley 2019). Many suggested that leaders should provide support and motivation and be individuals they could look up to or admire, even be inspired by. One participant in Stanley's (2006a) study said 'you need to be motivated I think to be a leader'. The researcher then asked 'And do you need to motivate others?' to which the research participant responded, 'Definitely'.

In light of this vital aspect of clinical leadership, approaches to motivating and inspiring others are considered in this chapter. The key to motivating others, from a clinical leader's standpoint, is to allow them to see and be inspired by the leader's values and beliefs about care and patient health management. In this way, followers who identify with the clinical leader's values and beliefs will be prompted to align themselves with those values and be motivated to support and follow the clinical leader. West and Bailey (2019) add that if we impose a 'dominant command and control style' with 'the effect of silencing. . . voices, suppressing. . . ideas for new and better ways of delivering patient care and suffocating. . . intrinsic motivation and fundamental altruism' then 'motivation and creativity will. . . fail' as it ignores the reality of day-to-day care.

Clinical Leadership in Nursing and Healthcare, Third Edition.
Edited by David Stanley, Clare L. Bennett and Alison H. James.
© 2023 John Wiley & Sons Ltd. Published 2023 by John Wiley & Sons Ltd.

This chapter will also consider something more significant than motivation for the clinical leader. It will briefly explore the issue of inspiration and how clinical leaders might inspire others to follow and engage with steps to improve patient care and the health service.

What Is Motivation?

Motivation is that extra, often intangible element that gets us up in the morning, the fire in the belly, the joy of getting 'stuck into something'. Daft and Pirola-Merlo (2009, p. 230) refer to motivation as 'the forces, either internal or external to a person, that arouse enthusiasm and persistence to pursue a certain course of action'. Heller (1998) supports this and describes motivation simply as the will to act. Health Direct (2021) an Australian government website, suggest that motivation is the drive to achieve your goals or needs. Clinical leaders are responsible for enabling a culture where motivation can flourish. Goleman et al. (2002, p. 41) link motivation with emotional intelligence and self-awareness (see Chapter 15) and explain that motivation is guided by values that are represented in emotionally toned thoughts, which can either appeal to us or repel us. The appealing elements can translate into motivators that drive us to do and achieve what we want.

Motivation is closely aligned to values. Kpanake et al. (2019), when exploring what motivated volunteers to respond to an Ebola epidemic, found that after a feeling of patriotic duty, seeing the act of volunteering as a moral responsibility emerged as the second most powerful motivator. If you work in an environment where your own values resonate with that of the health agency, then there is an increased likelihood that you will display the behaviours of motivation. So, what are these behaviours and what do they look like? Examining some models and theories of motivation may help explain this.

Models and Theories of Motivation

Motivation theory has been around since the 1940s, although it is only in recent times that its relationship to the work environment, and specifically leadership, has been recognised. Therefore, it will be useful to gain an overview of several theories of motivation. The earliest theories were Maslow's hierarchy of needs, theory X and theory Y and the two-factor theory, and more contemporary models include expectancy theory, the job characteristics model (JCM), McClelland's theory of need, cognitive evaluation theory, goal-setting theory and equity theory. Only three of these will be discussed here, so for more detailed information, see the explanations of various motivation models on the site for ChangingMinds (http://changingminds.org/explanations/theories/a_motivation.htm).

Maslow's Hierarchy of Needs

One of the best-known and earliest theories of motivation is Abraham Maslow's hierarchy of needs. Maslow believed that there are five main needs that drive our motivation: psychological security, safety, belonging, self-esteem and self-realisation (Rouse 2004, p. 27; see

Table 13.1). Within these stages are intrinsic (internal) and extrinsic (external) aspects of motivation. Amabile (1993, p. 185) examines intrinsic and extrinsic motivation in the workplace and suggests that 'unmotivated employees are likely to expend little effort in their jobs [and] avoid the workplace as much as possible'. The upside is that motivated employees are creative, persistent and productive.

Motivation and creativity are closely attuned. Giugni (2004, p. 69) comments that 'creative individuals also demonstrate some degree of self-satisfaction' and that 'they are enthusiastic, attracted by the challenge and feel that they are working on something important'. Intrinsic motivational factors tend also to be more linked with creativity as extrinsic factors are with task achievement. Both are important; however, intrinsic factors are driven from within and are therefore aligned with the individual's personal values. MacKenzie (2004, p. 143) describes Maslow's hierarchy of needs as well suited to the workplace environment, highlighting, for example, that primary needs are met in the form of remuneration (the safety stage) and more complex needs in areas such as knowledge, morality and creativity (the self-actualisation stage). For leaders, it is noteworthy to appreciate what sits beneath motivation, how powerful it can be and why it can influence how someone behaves and performs in the workplace.

Table 13.1 Maslow's model adapted for motivating workers.

Maslow's model	Motivating through
Basic needs	Remuneration – they will go where the pay is good Safe workplace and appealing environment Incentive schemes for employees
	Treated as individuals
Relatedness needs	Show respect
	Give responsibility and autonomy
	Recognise good work – for example, publicly acknowledge and express this at staff meeting; privately send a 'well done on a good job' note or email
	Communicate – when things are going well and not so well
	Decision making – involve others
	Encourage ideas – open engagement, healthy debate
	Praise people
	Get to know the team – address people by name; genuine 'small talk' is just as important as talking 'work'
	Team-building events – not just something only managers do
	Celebrate – announce publicly, reward and acknowledge
Growth needs	Support to complete new tasks
	Present challenges, invite debate
	Encourage people to think for themselves
	Avoid predictable routines
	Ask people what motivates them
	Provide opportunities for self-development
	Reward good work

Source: Adapted from PRLog (2008).

Expectancy Theory

Expectancy theory is one of the most widely accepted contemporary models of motivation. Developed by Vroom in the 1960s (Holdford and Lovelace-Elmore 2001), it is focused on outcomes rather than need and consists of three factors: the strength to act in a certain way depends on the expectation of the reward or the attractiveness of the motivator. Robbins et al. (2004, p. 184) support this with an example: 'An employee will be motivated to exert a high level of effort when he or she believes that effort will lead to a good performance appraisal'.

Job Characteristics Model

The JCM is a framework developed by Hackman and Oldman (1976) for defining job characteristics that are important to employee motivation (see the description in Daft and Pirola-Merlo 2009, p. 176). The framework is divided into five core dimensions: skill variety, task identity, task significance, autonomy and feedback. Examples of the JCM from a fictitious ward setting are offered in Table 13.2. All the dimensions have a low value and a high value, and motivation results from a high level of satisfaction.

The first three dimensions merge to become purposeful work, when the work is more meaningful to the worker. As the person's autonomy is increased, so too is their level of personal responsibility and satisfaction. This was supported in a study of motivational factors in the health and human services professions by Shannon (2019), who found that the most significant factors for motivation were effective communication and a sense of being included, respected and valued in the workplace. Job characteristics act more widely to influence the individual's critical psychological state (meaningfulness, responsibility and knowledge of outcomes) and outcome (high motivation).

Reflection Point

Who motivates you? Take a moment to consider people whom you find motivational or inspirational. This can be someone you know personally or someone you know about. Consider at length what attributes or behaviours they display that you find appealing. What can you learn from this?

What motivates you? Take a moment to consider what it is that gets you out of bed each day. Is it the joy of being with someone you love? Doing a job you love? Being in a place you love? Working towards a dream? Building a relationship? Making a better life... for you or your family? It's cold, the frost is on the ground, you are warm in bed... Why get up? Reasons can change, but right now... What is it that is inspiring you to get up and get going?

How to Motivate Others

Toode et al. (2010) conducted a literature review on nurses and motivation and found that motivated nurses have reported stronger empowerment in behaviour, words and outcomes than unmotivated nurses. They also go on to say that this attitude is positively reflected in

Table 13.2 JCM: Examples of high- and low-level job characteristics.

Job characteristics	Level	Examples
Skill variety	High	Community mental health nurse, providing services to a range of clients, designing client interventions, collaborating with health professionals and families providing a mobile, flexible service.
	Low	Taking temperature and blood pressure only.
Task identity	High	Identifying an improvement activity and implementing a change in a health setting, for example, identifying a need for an orientation package for graduate nurses working in the emergency department. Forming a project team, running a pilot project and leading the project to its conclusion, including evaluation of the effectiveness.
	Low	Completing an audit by ticking boxes on a form without knowledge of the subsequent improvement activity.
Task significance	High	Coordinating an intensive care unit or managing a residential aged-care facility.
	Low	Collecting meal trays.
Autonomy	High	Community nurse who manages own workload based on client need. Ability to be flexible without asking permission. Outcomes-based approach.
	Low	A nurse who cannot be flexible with client needs unless permission is given.
Feedback	High	Wound care specialist nurse adjusting wound care interventions and evaluating effectiveness through evidence via observation, data and patient feedback.
	Low	A nurse applying a dressing, while a wound care specialist evaluates its effectiveness and discusses with the patient.

Source: Johns and Saks (2008).

patient health outcomes, which is a good argument for harnessing motivational attributes in the workplace.

The research that supports this book also reinforces the importance of motivation in leadership and identifies motivation and inspiration as key features of congruent leadership. A number of other studies have searched for the motivational factors that drive nurses and other health professionals (Bengtsson and Ohlsson 2010; Lambrou et al. 2010; Sung 2010; Kudo et al. 2011; Rose 2011; Moghimian and Karimi 2012; Millar et al. 2017; Sewdas et al. 2017; Abbiati et al. 2019; Nguyen et al. 2020; Macdiarmid et al. 2021; Smith and Williams 2021). As a clinical leader, it is important to recognise that different things motivate different people, with nurses mainly motivated by autonomy, positive relationships and access to resources (Germain and Cummings 2010; Smith and Williams 2021), while for other health professionals it is about money (Kudo et al. 2011; Millar et al. 2017). For others, it is the satisfaction of connecting with others or accomplishing something complex (Macdiarmid et al. 2021). Motivation is not a 'one size fits all' approach. Blanchard et al. (2003), Toode et al. (2010), and Smith and Williams (2021) support this view, indicating that one should never assume what motivates someone else. They add that establishing motivation relies on building trust, focusing on the positive and redirecting energy when mistakes occur.

In the past, organisations have been dependent on a command-and-control approach to motivation, with reward or punishment used as the dominant motivational tool. However, partly in response to generational workforce issues (Stanley 2010), organisations have moved more towards advise-and-consent cultures or approaches. These are based on the premise that rewarding 'good' work is more effective than threatening punitive measures for 'poor' work (Handy 1999). Toode et al. (2010) also identified five themes that affect work motivation: workplace characteristics, working conditions, personal characteristics, individual priorities and internal psychological states. These are useful strategies to consider when motivating others and are summarised in Box 13.1.

Another motivation dynamic has been promulgated by author and analyst Daniel Pink (2009), who examined the traditional approach of businesses and compared it to the science of motivation. Pink (2009) found that the business world traditionally used extrinsic rewards as motivators to increase performance, such as bonuses, increased leave and share percentage. His research discovered that intrinsic rewards are far more motivating, suggesting that basically people do things they like if they align with their values and if they have meaning for that individual. Pink (2009) suggests that there are three core elements of motivation: autonomy, mastery and purpose:

- **Autonomy** – the ability to decide and control what you do, when you do it and how you do it
- **Mastery** – the thrill at becoming better at something and increasing one's knowledge through engagement
- **Purpose** – the yearning to do something bigger than ourselves

Building these elements into clinical roles may enable motivation to occur. A motivated individual and team are far more effective and efficient and can provide better patient outcomes than a demotivated team (Pink 2009).

Another approach to motivating people is offered by Lundin et al. (2000), who describe the four principles of the FISH! philosophy. The motivational approach of FISH! originated in the Pike Place fish market in Seattle and has grown into an international motivational movement. The FISH! philosophy is about producing a constant flow of positive energy that motivates and empowers people at work. The four principles are:

- **Play** – a way to have fun, creating energy and engaging people's playful and creative sides.
- **Be present** – engaging with clients, patients, customers and colleagues in a way that focuses on their needs in each moment.
- **Make their day** – again focusing on the needs of clients, patients, customers and colleagues in a way that energises them and creates feelings of involvement, belonging and support.
- **Choose your attitude** – a reminder that whatever you are doing it is important to be conscious of your attitude and that this is at the control of your will. We can choose to be sad, or upset or miserable, or happy. The circumstances in which we find ourselves at work may be sad, or disappointing or happy, but we all have a choice about how we respond. We can choose to be 'world famous' or to be down. It is up to us.

Box 13.1   Five Themes of Work Motivation

1) In terms of **workplace characteristics**, nurses and other health professionals are motivated by:

- good collaboration between members of the healthcare team
- social support inside the team
- positive team spirit on the ward or in the clinical area
- each health professional having equal status as a valued health professional in a team
- high level of autonomy, especially in regard to decision making
- variety of skills and combination of different talents
- performing 'whole care' rather than 'part care'
- opportunities to learn

2) **In terms of working conditions**, nurses and other health professionals are motivated by:

- the coordinator's ability to manage changing demands on a ward or clinical area
- suitable working hours and the possibility of combining work and private matters
- appropriate remuneration and job security

3) **Personal characteristics** that are attributed to motivated nurses and other health professionals include:

- a variety of correlations with age and work environment
- high levels of motivation and awareness of professional knowledge and ability among tertiary qualified professionals, who are internally motivated

4) **Individual priorities** for motivation of health professionals include:

- whether their work meets certain individual needs and values that are important to them
- the ability to meet their own needs and have control over their use of time
- the opportunity to help others
- positive opinions on ethical factors in the work environment

5) **Internal psychological states** influencing motivation include:

- knowledge of actual results of work and experiencing outcomes of work
- perception of work as being meaningful

Signs that People Are Demotivated

As a clinical leader, it is important to recognise potential signs of reduced motivation among ourselves and others. For example, the workplace culture may not be an ideal one where motivation and inspiration are valued or flourish. The clinical leader will need to be not only an expert clinician but also an astute detective of motivation. The signs, reasons for and costs of demotivation are summarised in Box 13.2.

Clinical Leader Stories: 13 – Love

I am going to talk about one of my favourite clinical placements so far. It was during my second year of nursing. I met a person who exhibited many clinical leadership skills and attributes. She was my clinical facilitator at that time. She really inspired and changed my view about being a leader. She was not trying to be a leader, but her words and actions made her a great leader. She always greeted us with a warm smile and asked about our day. On the very first day of placement, she gave us a very structured plan and asked us to work through it at our own pace. She was always approachable and inspiring. She motivated all the students throughout the placement period. She always made an extra effort to bring out the best in us. Halfway through the placement, one of the students had face a sad event. Her brother, who lived overseas, died. The student was devastated but couldn't travel to be at the funeral. As such, she experienced a lot of grief. During those days, I witnessed how a true leader should behave. Our facilitator took her to one side and listened while the student talked about her feelings and expressed her grief. She stood beside her and advocated for her when needed. The student was able to successfully complete her placement. We all loved and followed our facilitator not just because of her leadership qualities, but because of her values and actions. Congruent leadership is when a leader's activities, actions and deeds are consistent with and motivated by the leader's values and beliefs about care and nursing. Congruent leaders may have a vision and a plan for where they want to go, but that isn't why people follow them. Congruent leadership is founded on the values, principles, and beliefs of the leader. Congruent leaders are inspiring, motivational, organised, relation builders and effective communicators. Those leaders can be found at many levels of an organisation, and they aren't always in management roles. Compassion, passion, and qualities of the heart seem to guide congruent leaders. They cultivate long-term connections with others, uphold their values, and are more concerned with empowering others than with preserving their own authority or status. My experience has positively impacted me both as a student and as healthcare professional. I discovered that leadership is not just about leading, but it can also change the lives of people. Looking forward to my clinical career, I would like to practice more of these qualities and be a great asset to healthcare.

Kiran: Student Nurse

The Motivational Power of Failure

Failure is not something that people aim for, but when it occurs it need not always be seen as negative. There is a Chinese proverb, 'Failure is the mother of success', and Cantwell (2015 p. 19) states simply that teams 'learn from their mistakes', adding that in 'rapidly changing situations, they will respond more effectively to, and recover better from, setbacks'. Moreover, Japanese engineer Soichiro Honda is known to have said that 'success is 99 percent failure'. Failure, then, can be regarded as a motivational force, if it is viewed as an experience that can be learned from. Martin Seligman (2006) suggests that setbacks can

---

Box 13.2   Demotivation Uncovered

Signs of demotivation:

- increased sick leave
- increased absenteeism
- lateness
- decreased work quality
- decreased communication
- sloppy attire or poor attention to presentation
- change in attitude from positive to negative

Why staff become demotivated:

- lack of recognition
- lack of job stimulation and involvement
- inadequate education and training at work
- work overload
- being micro-managed
- lack of autonomy
- lack of decision-making ability
- high workload with limited support

Costs of demotivation in the workplace can be:

- staff replacement, such as retraining, readvertising
- emotional contagion of working where motivation is low – negativity spreads quickly
- interruption to job routines, for example, through frequent orientation of new staff to a ward, unit or department
- the word gets out, 'please don't send me to ward 93G' and so on
- a knowledge drain, as the repository of intellectual information leaves

---

be viewed optimistically, depending on our capacity to recognise them as remote from ourselves. If people feel that setbacks are due to their own inadequacies and cannot be overcome, then those setbacks become a genuine barrier to progress. However, if failures are seen as being related to individual or specific circumstances, or as temporary in nature and able eventually to be overcome by greater effort and more application, then the response may be to effect a solution or do better next time (Tan 2013).

Taking an optimistic view of failure can be learnt, with the result being that even failure can be seen as a motivational force. Some of the greatest medical advances have come about because of apparent failure (e.g. the discovery of Viagra as a potent treatment for erectile dysfunction when the drug was being tested for its impact on heart problems, such as angina). Furthermore, humans have a greater tendency to pay more attention to negative than positive occurrences (Tan 2013), since such failures can be used to help us learn not just what did not work well but what might be best avoided in future. In the health service, mistakes and errors are (sadly) not uncommon, but the lesson to take from them

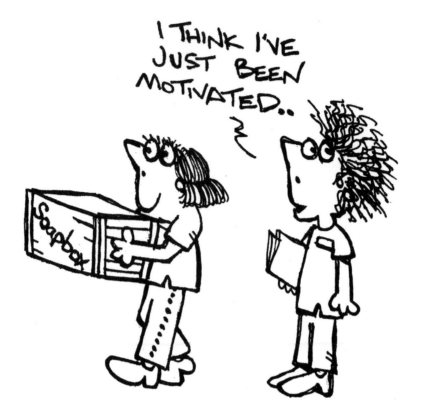

is to recognise them, acknowledge them and use them to learn. Clinical leaders are not perfect, but the mark of a great clinical leader is likely to be their capacity to see setbacks optimistically and to use them to try harder and not give up. Recognise that sometimes to find new and innovative paths you need to get lost first, if not most of the time.

Inspiration

Inspiration is described as the arousal of the mind to a special or unusual activity or creativity, or the arousal of a particular emotion or action. In my opinion, it holds a key place in the role of a clinical leader. Goleman (2013) is of the view that leaders who inspire can articulate a shared set of values that resonate with and motivate the group. Inspiration and motivation are closely related, but there is something about inspiration that takes people to a higher plane. In terms of emotional intelligence (see Chapter 15), it is the application of empathy, active listening and self-awareness that leads to relationship effectiveness, and setting people apart as inspirational (Goleman et al. 2002). People who do this are the ones you love to work with or want to work with. They speak to us from their heart with their values on show (Goleman 2013). Motivation can be associated with managerial steps to exercise control or support people to perform in their work environment, but inspiration is

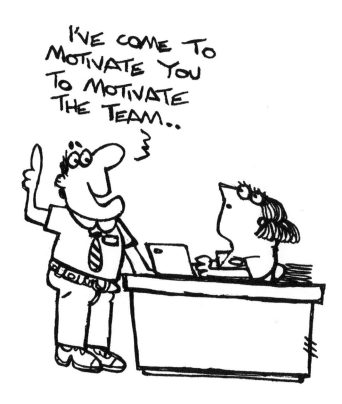

something that can lift people to achieve or create or contribute to an exceptional degree. Cleary et al. (2015, p. 317) suggest that it is 'moments of inspiration that keep us from becoming cynical about our professional lives' and help us focus on what is important to us.

Inspiration can come from anything (a person, a thing, nature, a song), and the impact will be different for different people. The key message here is that the actions of a clinical leader are often inspiring as well as motivational for people affected by or who witness to their actions. Part of the power of congruent leadership is that people are drawn to follow leaders who stand by their beliefs, values and principles, and this alone can support inspirational acts. Cleary et al. (2015) suggest that inspiration can come from even routine or standard activities such as clinical supervision, and from strong professional and supportive collegial networks. Therefore, focusing on our values of care can sometimes be a beacon for others to follow (Hungerford 2014).

I suspect that 'inspiration' is rarely the intent of any particular action, but clinical leaders should be aware that inspiration of their colleagues may indeed be the result of their engagement with congruent leadership and the embodiment of emotional intelligence (Goleman 2013). This supports the claim that demonstrating our values in our actions carries significant influence and may even negate the need to resort to titles, hierarchical positions and roles with control features in order to have an influence, motivate or genuinely inspire others.

Case Study 13.1   Amy and Ella Meek

Amy and Ella Meek are teenage sisters from Nottingham, England. They were relatively unknown until winning the 'Pride of Britain 2021 Award', and they provide an example of how leadership is not just the domain of the famous, the powerful or the domineering – leadership can be displayed by anybody who has the requisite skills and determination and can be achieved in many different ways. Read this brief account of Amy and Ella's achievements and consider the challenge that follows.

Amy and Ella founded a youth social action group in 2016 when they were very young teenagers. The group, 'Kids Against Plastic', has gone on to become a registered charity and has three main aims:

- Raise awareness and understanding of the problems caused by plastic misuse
- Encourage and support others to become 'Plastic Clever' and reduce single-use plastics
- Empower children and young people to believe they can make a difference

They campaign for communities to take action that reduces plastic pollution by campaigning at the micro, meso, and macro levels. They encourage individuals, schools, businesses, councils and festivals to avoid the use of single-use plastics wherever possible and to be 'plastic clever'. They have also given online TED talks, spoken with aviation industry leaders about how they can reduce their plastic footprint, addressed politicians in Westminster, London, and they have presented at the United Nations' Young Activist Summit (December 2019). They have also published a book, 'Be Plastic Clever'. To date, over 1000 schools and 50 cafes, businesses, festivals and councils have committed to reducing plastic pollution.

Their campaigning also takes the form of positive action, with both girls collecting nearly 100 000 pieces of rubbish so far on formal litter picks and in their everyday lives. They also run a programme to highlight the work of other activists who do the same in other parts of the country.

Challenge: Amy and Ella are teenagers with little leverage, so what underpins their success? How have they been successful in achieving tangible impacts? To what extent does this case study relate to clinical leadership? Are clinical leaders in positions of leading without managerial authority? Have you ever led when you have been in a position of little or no authority? How can healthcare professionals succeed as clinical leaders when they are newly qualified? How can 'quiet' leaders succeed in leading colleagues towards and implementing change? How can you stand up for your values and employ values-based leadership?

Summary

- Understand what sits underneath motivation, or a lack of motivation, and the impact it can have on the workplace and the individual. Recall that intrinsic factors (from within) often hold greater meaning than extrinsic factors (from outside).

- Consider models or concepts of motivation to support the development of motivation. Explore beyond the models offered.
- Self-awareness is vital, so understand what motivates you. Be prepared to examine your own performance and make changes.
- As a clinical leader, in order to facilitate the inspiration and motivation of colleagues, you need to demonstrate the desired behaviour yourself. You do not need to hold a managerial role to influence, inspire and motivate or lead others.
- Failure can be a motivational force, as long as it is seen as something that can be learnt from and responded to optimistically.
- Inspiration is that something that can lift people to achieve, create or contribute to an exceptional degree, and it is very much associated with congruent leadership.
- Positive behaviour can be contagious. As a clinical leader, learn to let go a little, be prepared to be wrong, allow ideas to be tested, and encourage and enable colleagues to try them out, and take a step away so that others can step forward. Find ways to renew your energy so that you can be motivational and inspirational to others.

Mind Press-Ups

Exercise 13.1

Answer the following questions – and be honest with yourself. Take 15 minutes to complete this, then discuss your answers with another person.
- Describe your level of autonomy now in the workplace.
- If you could make changes to increase your level of autonomy, what would they be?
- What would you like to gain greater mastery at?
- What steps would you need to take to achieve this mastery?
- How does your current purpose at work align with your values?
- What steps could you take to ensure your values align?

Exercise 13.2

Visual motivation: Select a picture or photograph (magazines can be useful or your own photo collection) and create an inspirational statement to accompany your image. If the result really resonates with you, place it somewhere you can see it so that you can be regularly inspired and motivated.

Exercise 13.3

Think of a time you have failed. How did you respond? Did you give up? Why? What might have happened if you had regrouped and tried again or tried a new approach to the issue? Can you see that failure is not a full stop but a comma? It is a pause and an opportunity to have a new go, a chance to learn! Think of a failure that you have learnt from. Why did you think differently about this failure?

References

Abbiati, M., Savoldelli, G.L., Baroffio, A., and Bajwa, N.M. (2019). 'Motivational factors influencing student intentions to practice in underserved areas. *Medical Education* 54: 356–363.

Amabile, T.M. (1993). Motivational synergy: toward new conceptualizations of intrinsic and extrinsic motivation in the workplace. *Human Resource Management Review* 3 (3): 185–201.

Bengtsson, M. and Ohlsson, B. (2010). The nursing and medical student's motivation to attain knowledge. *Nurse Education Today* 30 (2): 150–156.

Blanchard, K., Lacinak, T., Tompkins, C., and Ballard, J. (2003). *Whale Done: The Power of Positive Relationships*. London: Nicholas Brealey.

Cantwell, J. (2015). *Leadership in Action: Lessons from the Real World from a Real Leader*. Melbourne, VIC: Melbourne University Press.

Cleary, M., Thomas, S.P., and Hungerford, C. (2015). Inspiration and leadership in mental health nursing. *Issues in Mental Health Nursing* 36 (5): 317–319.

Daft, R.L. and Pirola-Merlo, A. (2009). *The Leadership Experience: Asia Pacific*, 1e. South Melbourne, VIC: Cengage Learning.

Health Direct (2021). *Motivation: How to get started and staying motivated*. www.healthdirect. gov.au/motivation-how-to-get-started-and-staying-motivated.

Germain, P.B. and Cummings, G.G. (2010). The influence of nursing leadership on nurse performance: a systematic literature review. *Journal of Nursing Management* 18: 425–439.

Giugni, S. (2004). Nurturing imagination: fostering creativity in your organisation. In: *Innovation and Imagination at Work* (ed. C. Barker and R. Coy), 256. North Ryde, NSW: McGraw-Hill.

Goleman, D. (2013). *Focus: The Hidden Driver of Excellence*. London: Bloomsbury.

Goleman, D., Boyatzis, R., and McKee, A. (2002). *Primal Leadership: Learning to Lead with Emotional Intelligence*. Boston, MA: Harvard Business School Press.

Hackman, J.R. and Oldman, G.R. (1976). Motivation through the design of work: test of a theory. *Organizational Behavior and Human Performance* 16: 250–279.

Handy, C. (1999). *Understanding Organizations*, 4e. London: Penguin.

Heller, R. (1998). *Motivating People*. London: Dorling Kindersley.

Holdford, D. and Lovelace-Elmore, B. (2001). Applying the principles of human motivation to pharmaceutical education. *Journal of Pharmacy Teaching* 8 (1): 1–18.

Hungerford, C. (2014). Recovery as a model of care? Insights from an Australian case study. *Issues in Mental Health Nursing* 35: 1–9.

Johns, G. and Saks, A.M. (2008). *Organisational Behaviour: Understanding and Managing Life at Work*, 7e. Upper Saddle River, NJ: Pearson Education.

Kpanake, L., Dounamou, T., Sorum, P.C., and Mullet, E. (2019). 'What motivates individuals to volunteer in Ebola epidemic response? A structural approach in Guinea. *Human Resources for Health* vol. 17 (81): 1–9.

Kudo, Y., Kido, S., Shahzah, M.T. et al. (2011). Work motivation for Japanese nursing assistants in small to medium-sized hospitals. *Tohoku Journal of Experimental Medicine* 225 (4): 293–300.

Lambrou, P., Kontodimopoulos, N., and Niakas, D. (2010). Motivation and job satisfaction among medical and nursing staff in a Cyprus public general hospital. *Human Resources in Health* 8: 26.

Lundin, S.C., Paul, H., and Christensen, J. (2000). *Fish! A Remarkable Way to Boost Morale and Improve Results*. London: Hodder and Stoughton.

Macdiarmid, R., Turner, R., Winnington, R. et al. (2021). 'What motivates people to commence a graduate entry nursing programme: a mixed method scoping review. *BMC Nursing* 20: 47.

MacKenzie, K. (2004). Surviving in the corporate jungle: strategies for becoming an innovative organisation. In: *Innovation and Imagination at Work* (ed. C. Barker and R. Coy), 256. North Ryde, NSW: McGraw-Hill.

Millar, R., Chen, Y., Wang, M. et al. (2017). 'It's all about the money? A qualitative study of healthcare worker motivation in urban China. *International Journal for Equity in Health* 16: 120.

Moghimian, M. and Karimi, T. (2012). The relationship between personality traits and academic motivation in nursing students. *Iran Journal of Nursing* 25 (75): 9–20.

Nguyen, V.A.T., Konings, K.D., Wright, E.P. et al. (2020). 'Why do graduates choose to work in less attractive specialty? A cross-sectional study on the role of personal values and expectations. *Human Resources for Health* 18: 32.

Pink, D.H. (2009). *Drive: The Surprising Truth About What Motivates Us*. New York: Canongate.

PRLog (2008). How to motivate others: Top tips on leadership. Press release, 19 April, http://www.prlog.org/10065474-how-to-motivate-others-top-tips-on-leadership.html (accessed 9 December 2010).

Robbins, S., Millet, B., and Waters-Marsh, T. (2004). *Organisational Behaviour*, 4e. Frenchs Forest, NSW: Pearson Education Australia.

Rose, S. (2011). Academic success of nursing students: does it matter? *Teaching and Learning in Nursing* 6: 181–184.

Rouse, A.G. (2004). Beyond Maslow's hierarchy of needs: what do people strive for? *Performance Improvement* 43 (10): 27.

Seligman, M. (2006). *Learned Optimism: How to Change Your Mind and Your Life* (Revised ed.). New York: Viking.

Sewdas, R., de Wind, A., van der Zwaan, L.G.L. et al. (2017). 'Why older workers work beyond the retirement age: a qualitative study. *BMC Public Health* 17: 672.

Shannon, E.A. (2019). 'Motivating the workforce: beyond the 'two-factor' model. *Australian Health Review* 43: 98–102.

Smith, G.P. and Williams, T.M. (2021). 'Harnessing motivation for sustainable practice change: from passive receivers to active co-creators. *Australian and New Zealand Journal of Psychiatry* 55 (5): 567–576.

Stanley, D. (2006a). In command of care: clinical nurse leadership explored. *Journal of Research in Nursing* 2 (1): 20–39.

Stanley, D. (2006b). In command of care: towards the theory of congruent leadership. *Journal of Research in Nursing* 2 (2): 134–144.

Stanley, D. (2008). Congruent leadership: values in action. *Journal of Nursing Management* 64: 84–95.

Stanley, D. (2010). Clinical leadership and innovation. *Connections* 13 (4): 27–28.

Stanley, D. (2011). *Clinical Leadership: Innovation into Action*. Melbourne, VIC: Palgrave Macmillan.

Stanley, D. (2012). Clinical leadership characteristics confirmed. *Journal of Research in Nursing* 19 (2): 118–128.

Stanley, D. and Stanley, K. (2019). 'Clinical leadership and rural and remote practice: a qualitative study. *Journal of Nursing Management* 27 (6): 1314–1324.

Stanley, D., Cuthbertson, J., and Latimer, K. (2012). Perceptions of clinical leadership in the St. John Ambulance Service in WA. Paramedics Australasia. *Response* 39 (1): 31–37.

Stanley, D., Latimer, K., and Atkinson, J. (2014). Perceptions of clinical leadership in an aged care residential facility in Perth, Western Australia. *Health Care: Current Reviews* 2 (2): http://www.esciencecentral.org/journals/perceptions-of-clinical-leadership-in-an-aged-care-residential-facility-in-perth-western-australia.hccr.1000122.php?aid=24341 (accessed 1 May 2016).

Stanley, D., Hutton, M. and McDonald, A. (2015). *Western Australian Allied Health Professionals' Perceptions of Clinical Leadership: A Research Report*, http://www.ochpo.health.wa.gov.au/docs/WA_Allied_Health_Prof_Perceptions_of_Clinical_Leadership_Research_Report.pdf (accessed 1 July 2016).

Sung, M.H. (2010). Correlations between motivation to achieve, clinical competence and satisfaction in clinical practice for diploma and baccalaureate nursing students. *Journal of Korean Academic Fundamentals in Nursing* 17 (1): 90–98.

Tan, C.-M. (2013). *Search Inside Yourself.* London: Collins.

Toode, K.P., Routasalo, P., and Suominen, T. (2010). Work motivation of nurses: a literature review. *International Journal of Nursing Studies* 48 (2): 246–257. https://doi.org/10.1016/j.ijnurstu.2010.09.013.

West, M. and Bailey, S. (2019). Five myths of compassionate Leadership. (The King's Fund). www.kingsfund.org.uk/blog/2019/05/five-myths-compassionate-leadership

14

Creating a Spirit of Enquiry (Enhancing Research)

Judith Anderson, Sarah Dineen-Griffin and David Stanley

> *Facts do not cease to exist because they are ignored.*
> Aldous Huxley, English critic and novelist, 1894–1963,
> in 'Note on dogma', 1928

Introduction: Is the Spirit with You?

The provision of evidence-based clinical care is now an essential aspect of modern healthcare (Richardson-Tench et al. 2018). The idea of evidence-based practice (EBP) feels intuitively sound: both professional intuition and clinical experience suggest that the client or patient is more likely to receive good-quality care if that care is based on sound evidence. However, the implementation of EBP remains a challenge with healthcare and policy decisions still being based on historical and unsystematic forms of clinical practice (Buckwalter et al. 2017). This chapter attempts to address this issue by discussing what constitutes EBP and how nurses and other health professionals can develop a spirit of enquiry. It also considers how clinical leaders can use evidence to support change and strengthen their practice by developing a nexus between research, clinical evidence, practice, and education to create a workplace that promotes critical thinking and new knowledge.

Two Keys

As with effective teamworking, there are two key strategies that will initiate a spirit of enquiry within a healthcare environment: support and challenge. A spirit of enquiry and critical thinking can be initiated by offering the challenge of a good question that makes health professionals think. Support is also vital, as it allows clinicians to take a chance and ask awkward, difficult or challenging questions. Not all clinicians will feel able to ask such questions. A good leader will provide them with the opportunity to do so (Bianchi

Clinical Leadership in Nursing and Healthcare, Third Edition.
Edited by David Stanley, Clare L. Bennett and Alison H. James.
© 2023 John Wiley & Sons Ltd. Published 2023 by John Wiley & Sons Ltd.

et al. 2018; Chawla and Learmonth 2018). Both support and challenge are central to creating a clinical environment where critical thinking, EBP and innovation can be fostered.

Evidence-based practice has become a core competency for healthcare practice internationally. It makes sense that people appreciate being shown evidence before they will accept changes (Bianchi et al. 2018). Although some authors (Waljee et al. 2018) indicate that this is specific to later generational groups (e.g. Generation Y) others suggest that differences exist within groups to such an extent that this is a myth (Jauregui et al. 2020). Data is now so available that people are taught to question, research and confirm the information they are given. Yet does the healthcare workplace welcome this and enhance their skills – or contrive to suppress their enthusiasm for knowing more?

Increasing research capacity in the healthcare environment requires strong leadership that generates a spirit of enquiry and a strategic approach (Monturo and Brockway 2019). Furthermore, the recognition of evidence that informs practice is captured under the umbrella of EBP, so it is wise to start by exploring this concept.

Evidence-Based Practice

EBP (in the form of evidence-based medicine) has its philosophical origins in early or mid-nineteenth century Paris (Sackett et al. 1996). The Cochrane Collection was the first attempt to collate international evidence of primary sources of research in order to inform practice. The Joanna Briggs Institute focuses on nursing research to synthesise and disseminate systematic reviews of evidence. Systematic reviews use rigorous methods to identify, appraise and synthesise information from several studies which attempt to answer the same research questions to inform best practice (Jordan et al. 2019). Evidence-based healthcare has come to represent the pinnacle of practice, with Jordan et al. (2019) defining it as 'clinical decision-making that considers the feasibility, appropriateness, meaningfulness and effectiveness of healthcare practices'. Feasibility encompasses the extent to which an intervention is practical in the context or situation. Appropriateness encompasses the fit of the intervention to the context or situation. Meaningfulness encompasses the meaning that the individual or group ascribes to the intervention, and effectiveness encompasses the degree to which the intervention achieves the desired result (Jordan et al. 2019). Together this results in a four-part formula for evidence-based healthcare (EBHC):

EBHC = feasibility + appropriateness + meaningfulness + effectiveness

The fundamental principle that supports EBP is the belief in a hierarchy of the reliability of evidence, based on research designs that minimise the effect of bias on the results obtained. Best research evidence is that which is derived from rigorous randomised controlled trials (RCTs) and lends itself to the development of criterion-referenced best-practice guidelines. As RCTs represent the so-called gold standard for biomedical research, there is an implicit assumption that guidelines derived from such studies carry greater validity than other studies (e.g. qualitative studies) (Schaefer and Welton 2018; Jordan et al. 2019).

One of the criticisms that has been levelled against EBP is that it encourages a 'recipe' approach to care or care devoid of its containing context. Furthermore, the narrow methodological perspective that RCTs represent limits the use and critical appraisal of research derived from other methodologies. However, part of the EBP formula, which includes clinical expertise, tacitly endorses the use of other sources of knowledge, such as personal experience, expert and reflective knowledge (Mugerauer 2021).

In the context of an EBP formula, two components act to mitigate the limits of treatment guidelines derived from (so-called) context-free studies, supported solely by RCTs. These include meaningfulness, since, if given equal weight in the EBP equation, it incorporates the meaning ascribed to the intervention by the patient, and appropriateness, which considers professional opinion about what is most suitable. As such, these components are free to interact with evidence-based guidelines in a manner that immediately contextualises a treatment regime and brings in consideration of clinical decision making (Jordan et al. 2019). Therefore, EBP refers to a synergistic relationship between the patient, the healthcare professional/clinical leader and the research evidence, and it is this interplay of the components of the formula that calls on the application of clinical leadership.

The key issue in adopting and applying EBP is not the presence or absence of context-free research evidence but rather the ability of the health professional to interpret research evidence (qualitative or quantitative) in the context of their clinical expertise and the preferences of the patient, and to apply their spirit of enquiry to the critical questions they face (Bianchi et al. 2018).

Another question is: 'How do we know that the evidence is sound?' If we adopt evidence for practice that is derived from systematic reviews that incorporate RCTs, the question becomes moot (or does it?), as RCTs are said to provide the strongest levels of evidence (Jordan et al. 2019). However, returning to the 'or does it' question, Wieringa et al. (2018) caution against limiting research strategies to a single experimental paradigm, especially in light of the desire to provide individualised, meaningful treatment. The focus of randomised control trials is on an average patient rather than an individual patient. From a percentage perspective, this means that a treatment that is effective for 80% of patients will not be effective for the remaining 20%. It is also possible that a statistically significant difference between a treatment and a control group does not actually indicate a clinically significant treatment. Even when the treatment is clinically effective, when variations in population are considered, the significance can be negated (Wieringa et al. 2018).

Having the best evidence is not always enough. Evidence alone, even if collected well and methodologically sound, may fail to move colleagues and others who choose to ignore it. Nurse practitioner (NP) roles have been legislated since 1998 in Australia; however, the general public are still unfamiliar with the (NP) role (Dwyer et al. 2021). Black and Dawood (2014), Fry et al. (2011) and Henderson et al. (2010) all suggested that there was ample evidence to show that the introduction of nurse practitioners (NPs) into emergency departments and other clinical environments facilitated more effective, more rapid patient care that is of a high standard. However, political forces driven by the powerful medical lobby and managers worried (incorrectly) about the perceived high costs of NPs have led to delays in introducing this approach to care in Australian health services. It wasn't until 2009 that privately practising nurse practitioners were given limited access to the Medicare Benefits Scheme and the Pharmaceutical Benefits Scheme, and even then they were required to be working in collaboration with a medical practitioner or an entity that employs medical practitioners (Chiarella et al. 2020).

This has been a short review of the nature of EBP. Inevitably, some issues have been omitted, as have some details and further discussion regarding the issues and ideas that have been presented.

How to Create a Spirit of Enquiry

There are a number of initiatives that can be employed to generate a spirit of enquiry and facilitate implementation of EBP in the clinical environment. As with most leadership strategies, some may be more applicable for your context than others, and, hopefully, combining several will encourage the process further.

Being Involved in Research

There is no point just talking about research or enquiry generation. Clinical leaders need to be involved and at the forefront of studies and quality improvement initiatives. Even small studies will keep clinical leaders engaged with the spirit of enquiry. Being seen as involved will allow greater role modelling, build research skills, foster a sense of pride in the ward or unit and offer useful clinical data. It will assist to create awareness of EBP and interest. This includes casual contact with team members in day-to-day conversation and more formal interactions such as in meetings. Enthusiasm and involvement generate interest in others, and a focus on improvement in patient care highlights possible positive outcomes. Linking these to organisational visions and values assists in engaging other stakeholders and gaining their support and resources. Other strategies for building interest and getting others involved include sharing information about EBP, journal articles, or professional conferences on notice boards. These assist to keep people up to date and encourage them to think about how things could be improved (Edie 2017).

Role Modelling Use of EBP

One approach is for clinical leaders to role model the practice and use of EBP. An academic can also be employed in the clinical area to job share or establish a joint appointment, so that clinical health professionals can be guided to develop critical clinical questions, establish quality initiatives, or research projects. Support could be offered to clinical 'champions' who actively engage in research or quality initiatives. Role modelling the use of EBP demonstrates to others what is expected, supported, and rewarded within the organisation and thereby encourages and supports others to follow that example. Behaviour influences the attitudes and behaviour of others, creating a 'trickle down' or cascading effect, thereby engaging others in a spirit of enquiry also (Guerrero et al. 2020).

Mentorship

A network of mentors to support and foster research and quality initiatives can be established. Mentors can assist in explaining EBP and the organisation. They can assist in the identification of barriers and how these can be overcome in a contextually specific manner. In this way, clinical leaders with research and enquiry skills can lead and guide novice practitioners and foster others to capture and practise with a spirit of enquiry, building an organisational culture of enquiry. Having a mentor increases the likelihood of success in implementing EBP (Edie 2017; Melnyk et al. 2017).

Understanding the Value of a Nexus

A nexus is the coming together of teaching, research and practice. It is recognised that the clinical environment is not just a place for practice, but one where education, research, enquiry and practice all merge and generate growth and value in the others. When research is based in the clinical environment, it addresses those issues that are important not only to the health professional but also the patient. Addressing these questions ensures that research is able to be implemented effectively and addresses any issues that need to be overcome in its implementation in practice. Valuing the nexus will foster a strategic approach to the development of enquiry (La Brooy and Kelaher 2017).

Encouraging Quality Improvement Initiatives

Research can sometimes be daunting. Therefore, it may be more productive to encourage enquiry through smaller quality initiatives (see Chapter 16). These should be local, small, focused on your immediate client group, founded in passion and enthusiasm for improving care or practice, and may be based on the ideas of clinical leaders. Managers and leaders should feed these ideas. Quality improvement initiatives lend themselves well to planning strategies for implementing EBP. Due to their smaller size they can allow data to be gathered in a manageable manner, identify strategies suitable for the local context, engage the entire team and build relationships that are essential to effective implementation and allow for continuous evaluation of the practice (Palinkas and Mendon 2019).

Fostering Innovation

Educate staff and colleagues to recognise the value of enquiry and research, facilitate new ideas, understand change management tools and processes and to apply them as the spirit of enquiry grows. Innovation can be difficult to quantify and thereby difficult to recognise and develop (Sørly et al. 2019). However, Sørly et al. (2019) in their study of implementing imposed innovation identify several factors that support its introduction: trust-based management, flexibility, continuity of care and an emphasis on competence. This stresses the value of leadership in implementing innovation. People need to feel sufficient trust to bring up issues and ideas that can lead to innovation. Innovation is unlikely to arise from a single person, leaders need to work with their teams to stay focussed on overall goals, but to consider all options and their possible impacts (Sørly et al. 2019).

Rewards

Rewarding innovation and ideas, with simple personal recognition of staff who foster a spirit of enquiry is often all that is needed for others to see its value and seek to engage. Set up awards for colleagues who have a genuine impact on the spirit of enquiry. Think creatively about how staff ingenuity can be celebrated, for example, with a poster competition (Beckett and Powell 2021). In their study on organisational commitment in healthcare, Berberoglu (2018) found that when employees perceive their supervisors to be trustworthy, and to listen to their ideas, the organisational climate improves and their commitment to the organisation increases. These intrinsic 'rewards' are inexpensive but very important in building a spirit of enquiry amongst a team.

Professional Development Opportunities

One of the best motivators is to provide support for staff on their professional and personal journey through ongoing professional development. Professional development enhances an individual's feeling of competence and personal growth, fostering engagement with their work and organisation. Readiness to use EBP and to undertake research or quality improvement activities is linked to educational level, but generally this is insufficient to ensure that they are utilised in practice. In particular, leaders have a significant role to play in suggesting and supporting people to learn research skills that can then be implemented in practice (Wiesmann 2017).

Collaboration

Collaboration with colleagues in other disciplines or wards may also help foster a wider range of research or quality improvement opportunities and expose clinical leaders to other people with research skills. Collaboration can also lead to the establishment of 'research buddies' or 'critical friends' who can encourage deeper engagement with research practice. Collaboration with a librarian can assist in gaining valuable access to up-to-date information. Each can raise the spirit of the other, bring different skill sets and share the work of building the research project (Edie 2017).

Clinical Leader Stories: 14 – Colleagues

An experience of clinical leadership I witnessed occurred while I was waiting for handover one morning. As we waited, we learned that a patient had just fallen over. The nurse about to give handover had asked the patient to wait as they were too exhausted to attend to them and deliver handover, and they had chosen to deliver the handover first. One of my co-worker colleagues saw what was happening and knew that the night duty nurse was clearly exhausted after working double shifts for the past four days. My colleague immediately stepped up and displayed clinical leadership: she reassured, comforted, and assessed the patient, and she clearly articulated and allocated tasks to other colleagues with appropriate skill sets. This clinical leader displayed an excellent representation of the congruent theory of clinical leadership. She did not judge the nurse on

---

(Continued)

duty or become frustrated with her, as she could see she was physically exhausted. She identified that she needed immediate help, and she took initiative by taking the lead without formal authority. She ensured patient-centred care was provided, and she clearly articulated and delegated specific tasks such as calling for the wards man and allocating other to various duties. As she did, it was clear that her values of compassion and kindness shone through as she reassured and comforted the patient. She showed support and advocacy for her night duty colleague, who was clearly burnt out from working very hard, and she even let management know the night nurse was simply exhausted and needed a break. In summary, she simply put her values about caring into action and saw the patient and her colleague's need for help addressed immediately. This experience was a positive example of clinical leadership because my co-worker colleague provided quality patient care, supported staff well-being and displayed professional unity. After reflecting on this experience – I feel it has empowered me to realise that by being confident with transferring my values into the professional clinical setting, that quality patient-centred care, unity among colleagues, a healthy work environment and a rewarding nursing career can be delivered and promoted.

Annie: RN and Post Graduate Student.

Journal Clubs

Clinical leaders can foster a spirit of enquiry by establishing journal clubs, tearoom talks or informal meetings about current research or practice trends. These informal activities can help raise the profile of enquiry and help colleagues contribute to the spirit of enquiry (Cooper and Brown 2018). Cooper and Brown (2018) recommend that when beginning a journal club for the first time that the first session should involve an outline of what a journal club is and what expectations would be of members. In addition, clinical leaders can join professional associations (such as the United Kingdom's Royal College of Nursing or the Australian College of Nursing) and take part in professional forums or in areas of specialist practice.

Making It Relevant to Practice

The most effective studies or research are those that relate to the practice and clinical focus of the clinical leaders involved (Schaefer and Welton 2018). Focus on improvements and enquiry in your own area of practice. Greater engagement will result if you are addressing the agenda of your personal spirit of enquiry. Start simple, start focused and start with a question from your own practice area.

Benefits of Evidence-Based Practice and a Spirit of Enquiry for Health Professionals

EBP aims to improve outcomes for patients, health professionals and organisations (Schaefer and Welton 2018; Wakibi et al. 2021). From a nursing and healthcare perspective, there can be several benefits to the integration of EBP into clinical practice. These include:

- Improved patient/client satisfaction with standards of care (Skela-Savič and Lobe 2021)
- Improved health professional/nurse satisfaction with their work (Skela-Savič and Lobe 2021)
- The development of more consistency in patient/client care and a stronger focus on patient/client outcomes (Schaefer and Welton 2018)
- The development of a process by which poor or ineffective practices are no longer used and innovation of new ways of working (Skela-Savič and Lobe 2021)
- Increased collaboration with other health professionals to provide patient care (Wakibi et al. 2021)
- The initiation of more research or quality improvement projects (Wakibi et al. 2021)
- A safer ward or clinical environment with fewer complaints and more empowered staff (Wakibi et al. 2021)

Barriers to the Development of a Spirit of Enquiry and the Use of Evidence-Based Practice

Implementation of EBP and a genuine spirit of enquiry remains variable. The major factors that have an impact on the implementation of EBP are related to the ability to recognise the need for EBP, quality of the evidence itself, the individual's mindset, the group norms of the profession, ability to access and interpret evidence-based practice, competence in EBP, the balance between confidence and critical reflection, and the support received from management (Schaefer and Welton 2018).

Schaefer and Welton (2018) acknowledge that nurses frequently welcome EBP but often do not have the knowledge and skills to implement it. Positive attitudes towards EBP are more likely to lead to implementation, but time constraints, a high workload and a lack of organisational support are barriers to its implementation (Schaefer and Welton 2018). Schaefer and Welton (2018) identify organisational constraints such as lack of autonomy to change practice, inadequate support from managers, insufficient resources and lack of time to devote to EBP as inhibiting its uptake by clinical nurses. Mugerauer (2021) particularly identifies that for research to meet the needs of practising nurses, the ideas for what should be researched need to come from them. This would make the research more valuable and more likely to be translated into practice. The barriers hindering nurses in the application of EBP are summarised as follows:

- A lack of skills in the use of EBP or a lack of insight into the benefits of enquiry (Schaefer and Welton 2018; Skela-Savič and Lobe 2021)
- Attitude and understanding (Schaefer and Welton 2018; Skela-Savič and Lobe 2021)
- A lack of time (Schaefer and Welton 2018; Skela-Savič and Lobe 2021)
- A lack of autonomy (Schaefer and Welton 2018)
- A lack of role models or facilitators (Skela-Savič and Lobe 2021)
- A lack of resources (Schaefer and Welton 2018)

- Organisational cultures that (continue) to fail in their recognition of the value of clinical-level professionals in the research/EBP process (Tayyib and Coyer 2017; Schaefer and Welton 2018; Skela-Savič and Lobe 2021)
- Organisational cultures that continue to fail in their recognition of the value of learning environments to support the integration of clinical practice and EBP (Schaefer and Welton 2018; Skela-Savič and Lobe 2021)
- Some professionals' resistance to adopting EBP practices (Schaefer and Welton 2018; Skela-Savič and Lobe 2021)
- Poor reading habits, with few clinical staff reading research and EBP-focused journals (Schaefer and Welton 2018)
- Bullying or managers who are too controlling
- A lack of understanding of the difference between research and quality initiatives (Skela-Savič and Lobe 2021)

Reflection Point

Speak to some senior colleagues. What are their attitudes to EBP in your clinical area or professional discipline? Repeat this with junior colleagues. Are their views about evidence different? Reflect on your own views on the use and accessibility of EBP. What is helping or preventing you from applying more EBP in your clinical setting?

Applying Evidence-Based Practice

Jordan et al. (2019) suggest that the process for applying EBP is to first generate evidence from research. This implies testing innovations, but it may also be wise to search the published literature for research that will support the proposed innovation without the need to re-create research. Second, evidence should then be synthesised. Jordan et al. (2019) propose a systematic search through websites such as the Cochrane (http://www.cochranelibrary.com) or the Joanna Briggs Institute (https://journals.lww.com/jbisrir). These, and other resources, can be the best place to commence the journey of EBP. The creation of evidence-based clinical guidelines can involve creating a clinically useful policy that balances the positive and negative aspects of the research with the realities of the clinical setting.

The net result is guidelines that support practitioners within their scope of practice and within a team structure, so that evidence can be seen to support clinical expertise and patient preference. Getting this balance right is often one of the key barriers to the implementation of EBP. Evidence-based policy should also be applied to practice. This implies getting the right person to practice, in the right way and at the right time. Many barriers may hamper this as when inexperienced practitioners or people who are unfamiliar with policies or procedures and persist with outdated or incorrect practices. Applying a new policy or practice necessitates a change that in itself may take time to institute (Schaefer and Welton 2018).

It may even be that in relation to some patients, this new practice is not relevant. This implies the need for the final step, using clinical decision making to apply the policy or procedure in each patient's individual case. Applying the patient's values and rights to the clinical situation might mean abandoning what may appear to be the best clinical approach to the problem. Then, even if patients are offered the prescribed EBP option, they will still need to follow the treatment plan themselves (Schaefer and Welton 2018).

Establishing EBP is fraught with difficulties, some relating to practitioners, their insights into research, resources, some to the organisation in which they are employed, or to the patients themselves. The process of establishing EBP requires considerable effort. Successfully developing EBP will not ensure that patients receive or accept optimal treatment. However, attempting to generate EBP in clinical decision making and policies will ensure that evidence finds its way into clinical practice, and it is incumbent on clinical leaders to understand, promote and articulate the value of EBP (Schaefer and Welton 2018).

Several authors (Schaefer and Welton 2018; Jordan et al. 2019) summarise these steps in EBP as (or similar to) the following:

- Ask a focused question
- Access the information available on the topic
- Appraise the evidence available
- Apply the evidence, considering the patient's values and preferences
- Audit the practice

Strategies for Breaching the Evidence/Practice Nexus

A number of models have been developed to support and facilitate the nexus between nursing or healthcare practice, clinical research and education. Some offer an overview of the research facilitation process from a practitioner's perspective (evidence-based practitioner models); some provide general guides for research use (embedded models); and others describe efforts to implement research in practice focusing on quality (organisational excellence models). Evidence-based practitioner models focus on the individual practitioner being responsible for access, appraisal and implementation of best practice. For instance, Harbman et al. 2017 proposes the use of advance practice nurses to promote EBP. Embedded models use policies, procedures, protocols, standards, and guidelines to direct practice, removing the need for practitioners to engage with evidence themselves. Organisational excellence models are often cyclical, frequently reviewing practice, making incremental changes, and adapting to different contexts. Advanced practice nurses are ideal to provide mentoring for research and quality improvement projects with the aim of improving organisational outcomes.

Current evidence does not allow an effective comparison of these different models (much less the examples within each group), but it is suggested that different models work in different contexts. Many models have limitations. Few adopt a holistic approach, may fail to consider all aspects of the process of research use and its impact on health outcomes, and not many assist both researchers and clinicians. Moreover, most focus on single professional groups and fail to recognise the multi-professional/interdisciplinary focus of healthcare (Schaefer and Welton 2018).

In contrast is the Ottawa Model of Research Use (OMRU), which was developed in 1995 (Kent and McCormack 2010; Tayyib and Coyer 2017) (see Box 14.1). It was originally designed as a tool to support the nexus between researchers and practitioners in central Canada. It has since proved very useful as a guide to the integration of research, practice and education. The model identifies six elements: evidence-based innovation, potential adopters, the practice environment, implementation of interventions, adoption of the innovation and outcomes resulting from that adoption. The first three elements involve assessing barriers and supports for the innovation (Kent and McCormack 2010; Tayyib and Coyer 2017).

Another model, the Critical Realism and Arts Research Utilisation Model (CRARUM), is built on OMRU (Kontos and Poland 2009). However, this model focuses on the links between organisational culture, leadership, the critical reflection of adopters and the context of the change or innovation. Its ontological conviction is that reality is greater than the domain of the empirical (recognising that knowledge transfer is never just a matter of having the best evidence). The context is seen as fluid with social and power relationships that influence the construct of the model. The CRARUM uses an arts-based approach to support knowledge transfer, as well as adoption strategies offering some very interesting ideas about role play, drama and theatre as tools for influencing change and innovation. It is more complex than OMRU, but it builds links to a sophisticated understanding of context (Kontos and Poland 2009).

Both models offer guidance about strategies for dealing with the nexus between nursing or healthcare practice, clinical research and education.

Rogers's (2003) decision-making process supports practical approaches to addressing nexus issues. This simple model requires the use of knowledge (awareness of innovation), persuasion (development of positive attitudes), decision (a cognitive decision to adopt the innovation), implementation (use of the innovation) and confirmation (continued use of the innovation) as strategies to enhance the relationship or connections between research,

---

Box 14.1   The Ottawa Model of Research Use (OMRU)

Practice environment	**Strategies for transfer**	**Adoption**
(e.g. belief system, setting, resources, structure, decision-making processes, workloads, supplies, social factors, personalities, champions)	(e.g. diffusion/ dissemination/ implementation)	(e.g. use of the innovation)
Potential adopters		
(e.g. patients, wider stakeholders, staff and their attitudes, knowledge, motives, skills)		
Evidence-based innovation		**Outcome**
(e.g. the innovation itself, risk/ benefit, time saved, process of implementation, cost factors)		(e.g. audit, assess, evaluate, 'social validation', what is the 'true value' of the innovation?)
With the constant application of assessment, monitoring and evaluation		

Source: Adapted from Logan (1998).

clinical practice and education. However, more detailed strategies are offered that relate to the diffusion, dissemination and implementation of relevant research information to facilitate nexus success. Using the 'transfer strategy' headings offered by the Ottawa model (Logan and Graham 1998), the following strategies are considered to be effective.

Diffusion: A Simple Form of Nexus Development

This can be done via publication and access to journals, the internet and textbooks.

Dissemination: More Involved with Wider Nexus Results

The aim here is to bring research from an abstract topic to a relevant practice-related concept. For instance:

- Sharing information at conferences
- Sharing with colleagues at meetings, e.g. curriculum development opportunities
- Sending targeted information to specific colleagues, e.g. clinical leaders
- Placing relevant research-related publications in course and professional development outlines or prospectuses
- Using relevant research papers in undergraduate and postgraduate programmes

Implementation: Key Nexus Activity Integration

The third approach is implementation. Using a model for research implementation, such as the OMRU, allows for the identification of strategies to support effective implementation (Tayyib and Coyer 2017). These strategies are key to nexus activity integration and involve more collaboration, and may include:

- Putting up posters, using postcards, advertising or promoting the research/innovation (social marketing)
- Using product representatives and drug companies to support education
- Accessing opinion or clinical leaders
- Supporting change and innovation with patient and staff feedback, research findings or audit results
- Supporting an organisational culture that promotes quality initiatives and supports staff in generating new ideas, adopting initiatives and engagement EBP (e.g. role modelling, identification of champions, and rewards)
- Accessing interest and lobby groups
- Developing skills in relation to change management models (to support the 'how' of change constructively) (Tayyib and Coyer 2017)
- Employing specific incentives (e.g. promotion, study leave, financial rewards, gifts, or conference attendance)
- Listening to patients (establish partnerships) and staff, focus on organisational goals and colleagues' needs (this will drive research and an educational agenda, as research is not all about the researchers' agenda or research goals) (Tayyib and Coyer 2017)
- Avoiding jargon – a nexus is impossible without clear understanding and communication

- Engaging in 'shared reciprocity' (mutual search for meaning) with a shared environment, language, humour, goals, perspectives, value for patients, critical thinking and knowledge transfer

The university sector prepares undergraduates for practice. Increasing their involvement in the clinical area can assist implementation through the provision of meaningful clinical practice to students, involving students in clinical research and developing clinical leadership capacity, skills and values. It not only prepares clinicians but is also driven to research. Implementation that involves academics can provide a synergy, where academics can further their research and clinicians can be supported to implement effective strategies. Encouraging the development of this nexus where academia meet clinician can be fruitful for all involved. It can enhance gathering data about the need for change; ensure that research is context specific; enhance staff development (of both academics and clinicians); provide support at conferences and for research proposals; develop research promoting policies; support the development of a research culture; access research funding and grant opportunities. Supporting the creating of clinical chairs of nursing between universities and health service providers is an ideal way to promote research and clinical links (Anderson et al. 2016; Harbman et al. 2017).

Many people have struggled with the problems and challenges of building a successful approach to enhancing the relationships among nursing practice, education, and clinical research. All implementation strategies work at least some of the time, but none work all of the time. It is also evident that multiple strategies appear more effective than single ones. Strategies that are nearer to the end users and integrated into the process of care delivery are also more likely to be effective (Logan and Graham 1998).

The implementation of strategies to enhance research evidence in clinical practice is likely to be dependent on tailoring the transfer strategies to the environment, barriers, potential adopters, champions, and supporters found in a particular setting. Transfer strategies are more likely to be successful when nursing practice determines the nursing knowledge and research to be undertaken (Mugerauer 2021). The key may be to harness the skills and enthusiasm of people, particularly clinical leaders, and facilitating them to lead change. This will bring the change and innovation into the domain of the clinical team, securing their investment in the nexus activity.

What Can Clinical Leaders Do to Promote Evidence-Based Practice and a Spirit of Enquiry?

As well as the strategies offered earlier in the chapter, Jordan et al. (2019) and Tayyib and Coyer (2017) suggest that as the implementation of EBP and the generation of enquiry relate to the organisation, the environment and the individual, an approach that addresses each area, often in combination, should be used. For clinical leaders to have a positive influence on the development and implementation of EBP and a spirit of enquiry, they need to role model the application of these in their daily clinical activities, seeking out and using evidence or taking part where possible in clinical trials or other research activities. They should become mentors or guides for other health professionals. They should develop research as part of the organisation's strategic plan (including financial resources) and build a commitment to use EBP and sound clinical guidelines or clinical policies. Clinical leaders can establish EBP and critical enquiry as clinical competencies, ensure that neophyte health professionals are exposed and become proficient. Managers can support clinical leaders by incorporating time for professional development in relation to EBP into the work life of the ward, unit or clinical environment (Tayyib and Coyer 2017) or enquiry can be initiated simply by reading more research-focused journals.

EBP and enquiry are about integrating individual clinical expertise with the best available evidence to influence and support best practice, but they (and the lessons from history) remind us that these alone are not enough. It is through the exercise of clinical leadership that evidence gains meaning and can be successfully applied in practice and with each individual client or patient. Barriers exist on many levels, but it is not enough simply to accept that the barriers are unassailable. If overcoming them in the short term proves difficult, it may be best if clinical leaders at least show a willingness to drive practice forward by using their initiative and acting to improve care based on the best available evidence. Recognising the problems hindering the implementation of EBP may be the first step, but effective clinical leaders need also to seek out and secure solutions that will foster more efficient use of evidence in clinical practice (Schaefer and Welton 2018).

Case Study 14.1   Florence Nightingale

Florence Nightingale is rightly remembered as a significant contributor to modern nursing. Ironically, she did very little genuine nursing, and although she contributed significantly to the science of statistics and to the laws for the poor and military reforms in Britain and India, it is for her pioneering work as the 'lady with the lamp' in the Crimean War for which she is predominantly remembered. She was born in 1820 in Florence (the city after which she was named) into a rich, upper-class, well-connected English family and lived there until August 1910. Her early years were spent between a number of stately homes and travelling across Europe. She was fortunate to have been well educated, and she developed a powerful mind and sound literary skills.

In Rome in 1847, Florence met Sidney Herbert (who was to become the British Secretary of War during the Crimean War) and established a strong friendship. At this stage of her life, she was struggling to find direction and purpose that involved more than just marriage and the social circuit. She was courted by Richard Monckton Milnes, a politician and poet, but after a long holiday travelling through Greece and Egypt in 1850, Florence rejected Milnes's marriage proposal (against her mother's wishes) to concentrate on working towards a 'career' caring for the sick and deprived. She spent a few months at the Lutheran religious community at Kaiserswerth-am-Rhein in Germany in 1850, where she undertook some nursing training and participated in elements of nursing care. It was here that she found some direction and began the process of dedicating her life to her chosen career.

On her return from Germany, Florence faced opposition from her sister and mother, who both felt her career choice unwise and inappropriate for a young woman of her

(Continued)

class. Undaunted, Florence finally secured a post as superintendent of the Institute for the Care of Sick Gentlewomen in London. It took some time to negotiate the terms of her contract, and she began work, principally as the organisation's manager, in 1853. Her father supplemented her salary and supported her career choice, albeit reluctantly.

The Crimean War broke out the following year, and Florence and 38 other 'nurses' (many were nuns) travelled (at the request of Sidney Herbert) to support the military medical service already established in the theatre of war. She was based at Scutari Barracks Hospital (over 500 km from the fighting on the Crimean Peninsula) and after some time many other nurses followed (a fact that Florence resented at first), so that soon a number of other hospitals were under her managerial influence. From the outset she clashed with the military medical personnel and supply departments. Her advantage was that she had the support of the *Times* newspaper and a huge monetary fund that was raised in Britain to aid her work. Seeking to avoid disputes, she held her nurses back from involvement with care until she was asked to help, and only then did the 'Nightingale' nurses intervene.

It was assumed that the female nurses had a positive impact on the death rates at Scutari, but this is not the case. The cramped unsanitary conditions, poor diet and medical neglect meant that death rates rose into 1855, and only fell after the Sanitary Commission supervised the flushing of the sewers under the hospital. Following this and the onset of spring, the death rates dropped from 42 to 2% quite rapidly, data supported by Florence's own statistics. Florence was, in effect, the manager of the women's medical service and – contrary to popular belief – did little or no actual nursing. Even her nightly rounds with her famous lamp were related more to catching nurses occupied in nocturnal shenanigans than offering care and comfort, although this may have been the net result.

Florence became very ill during her time in the Crimea, possibly as a result of brucellosis, which became a chronic condition limiting her activity – but not her influence and energy – for the rest of her life. She returned to Britain after the war (under an assumed name) and shunned publicity where she could. However, the legacy of her war work was a huge reputation and a considerable fund that was used to establish the Nightingale Nurse Training School at St Thomas' Hospital in London. This was established in 1860, and by 1865 Florence had supported other nursing endeavours, for example, helping to set up the Liverpool Workhouse Infirmary. In 1859, she published the book *Notes on Nursing*, following an earlier publication *Notes on Hospitals*. She also worked hard to evaluate the impact of the Crimean War on the army and, although not its official author, laboured behind the scenes to produce a statistically stunning assessment of the military's treatment of enlisted men that was to have a profound impact on future military medical services. Mainly bedridden, Florence still found time to influence Britain's foreign policy on India.

Nurses trained in Nightingale schools spread around the world to America, Japan and Australia. In 1883, Florence was awarded the Royal Red Cross by Queen Victoria and became the first woman to be honoured with the Order of Merit in 1907. In 1908, she was given the freedom of the city of London, and her birthday (12 May) is celebrated as International Nurses Day. She remained active in influencing nursing training

(Continued)

Case Study 14.1 (Continued)

throughout the remaining years of her life and contributed greatly to issues of social and welfare reform with her prodigious writing. Although well known for her contribution to nursing, she should be equally well known for her passion for statistics. From an early age she is said to have excelled at mathematics, and later in life she used this knowledge to expand her use of statistics. In 1869, she was the first female member of the Royal Statistical Society.

Florence Nightingale's influence on nursing was profound, and her contributions to social welfare helped advance Victorian society and improve the plight of the poor and the military rank and file. In many respects her lamp still burns (although in reality she carried a lantern), mainly because of her contribution to the care of the sick and injured soldiers during the Crimean War and her legacy within the nursing world. While her achievements in the Crimea were remarkable, it was not nursing that she did there, and to a significant degree her influence can be attributed to very effective propaganda back in Britain. What she achieved in the 50 years before her death in 1910, even though ill and often bedridden, is also testament to her influence and determination to make a difference and follow her life's path.

Challenge: Find out as much as you can about Florence Nightingale's involvement with statistics and how she used to them to record issues, gather evidence and change practice. Furthermore, think about how you use and apply evidence and statistics. How do you access knowledge that will help inform decision making and practice?

Summary

- EBP is based on a combination of research evidence, clinical experience and patient preference.
- Clinical expertise tacitly endorses the use of other sources of knowledge, such as personal experience, expert and reflective knowledge.
- The key issue in adopting and applying EBP is the ability of health professionals to interpret the research evidence in the context of their clinical expertise and the preferences of the patient. This application can be described as a function of a clinical leader.
- Evidence alone is often not enough to change practice habits.
- There are many barriers to the application of EBP. These should be considered and assessed carefully when seeking to implement clinical practice changes. Some relate to the practitioners, their resources, or insights into research, some to the organisation in which they are employed and others to the patients themselves.

Mind Press-Ups

Exercise 14.1

Are you able to define EBP? Try to put it in your own words. Imagine that you are explaining it to a neophyte health professional in your area. What will you say?

Exercise 14.2

Can you name three areas of your practice that are supported by EBP? Can you name any areas that are not?

Exercise 14.3

What might be the barriers to the successful implementation of EBP in your clinical area or area of professional practice? Are the barriers and issues likely to be resolved? If they have been, how was this achieved where you work?

References

Anderson, J., Bruce, B., Edwards, M., and Podham, M. (2016). Engaging rural nurses in the policy development process. *Contemporary Nurse: A Journal for the Australian Nursing Profession* 52 (6): 677–685. http://doi.org/10.1080/10376178.2016.1221323.

Beckett, C.D. and Powell, J. (2021). Dissemination of evidence-based practice projects: key strategies for successful poster presentations. *Worldviews on Evidence-Based Nursing* 18 (3): 158–160. http://doi.org/10.1111/wvn.12502.

Berberoglu, A. (2018). Impact of organizational climate on organizational commitment and perceived organizational performance: empirical evidence from public hospitals. *BMC Health Services Research* 18 (1): 390–399. http://doi.org/10.1186/s12913-018-3149-z.

Bianchi, M., Bagnasco, A., Bressan, V. et al. (2018). A review of the role of nurse leadership in promoting and sustaining evidence-based practice. *Journal of Nursing Management* 26: 918–932. http://doi.org/10.1111/jónm.12638.

Black, A. and Dawood, M. (2014). A comparison in independent nurse prescribing and patient group directions by nurse practitioners in the emergency department: a cross sectional review. *International Emergency Nursing* 22 (1): 10–17. http://doi.org/10.1016/j.ienj.2013.03.009.

Buckwalter, K.C., Cullen, L., Hanrahan, K. et al. (2017). Iowa model of evidence-based practice: revisions and validation. *Worldviews on Evidence-Based Nursing* 14 (3): 175–182. http://doi.org/10.1111/wvn.12223.

Chawla, G. and Learmonth, M. (2018). The wicked problem of leadership in the NHS. In: *The Management of Wicked Problems in Health and Social Care*, 1e (ed. W. Thomas, A. Hujala, S. Laulainen and R. McMurray). Florida: Routledge.

Chiarella, M., Currie, J., and Wand, T. (2020). Liability and collaborative arrangements for nurse practitioner practice in Australia. *Australian Health Review* 44 (2): 172–177. http://doi.org/10.1071/AH19072.

Cooper, A.L. and Brown, J.A. (2018). Journal clubs: engaging clinical nurses and midwives in research. *The Journal of Continuing Education in Nursing* 49 (3): 141–144. http://doi.org/10.3928/00220124-20180219-09.

Dwyer, T., Craswell, A., and Browne, M. (2021). Predictive factors of the general public's willingness to be seen and seek treatment from a nurse practitioner in Australia: a cross-sectional national survey. *Human Resources for Health* 19 (1): 10–21. http://doi.org/10.1186/s12960-021-00562-7.

Edie, A.H. (2017). Organizing an evidence-based practice implementation plan. In: *Evidence-Based Practice in Nursing: Foundations, Skills, and Roles*, 1e (ed. T.L. Christenbery). New York: Springer Publishing Company.

Fry, M., Fong, J., Asha, S., and Arendts, G. (2011). A 12-month evaluation of the impact of transitional emergency nurse practitioners in one metropolitan emergency department. *Australasian Emergency Nursing Journal* 14 (1): 4–8. http://doi.org/10.1016/j.aenj.2010.10.001.

Guerrero, E.G., Frimpong, J., Kong, Y. et al. (2020). Advancing theory on the multilevel role of leadership in the implementation of evidence-based health care practices. *Health Care Management Review* 45 (2): 151–161. http://doi.org/10.1097/HMR.0000000000000213.

Harbman, P., Bryant-Lukosius, D., Martin-Misener, R. et al. (2017). Partners in research: building academic-practice partnerships to educate and mentor advanced practice nurses. *Journal of Evaluation in Clinical Practice* 23 (2): 382–390. http://doi.org/10.1111/jep.12630.

Henderson, S.O., Ahern, T., Williams, D. et al. (2010). Emergency department ultrasound by nurse practitioners. *Journal of the American Academy of Nurse Practitioners* 22 (7): 352–355. http://doi.org/10.1111/j.1745-7599.2010.00518.x.

Jauregui, J., Watsjold, B., Welsh, L. et al. (2020). Generational "othering": the myth of the millennial learner. *Medical Education* 54 (1): 60–65. http://doi.org/10.1111/medu.13795.

Jordan, Z., Lockwood, C., Munn, Z., and Aromataris, E. (2019). The updated Joanna Briggs institute model of evidence-based healthcare. *International Journal of Evidence-Based Healthcare* 17 (1): 58–71. http://doi.org/10.1097/XEB.0000000000000155.

Kent, B. and McCormack, B. (2010). *Clinical Context for Evidence-Based Nursing Practice*. Chichester, West Sussex: Wiley-Blackwell.

Kontos, P.C. and Poland, B.D. (2009). Mapping new theoretical and methodological terrain for knowledge translation: contributions from critical realism and the arts. *Implementation Science* 4 (1): http://doi.org/10.1186/1748-5908-4-1.

La Brooy, C. and Kelaher, M. (2017). The research-policy-deliberation nexus: a case study approach. *Health Research Policy and Systems* 15 (1): 65–75. http://doi.org/10.1186/s12961-017-0239-z.

Logan, J.O. and Graham, I.D. (1998). Toward a comprehensive interdisciplinary model of health care research use. *Science Communication* 20 (2): 227–246. http://doi.org/10.1177/1075547098020002004.

Melnyk, B.M., Fineout-Overholt, E., Giggleman, M., and Choy, K. (2017). A test of the ARCC© model improves implementation of evidence-based practice, healthcare culture, and patient outcomes. *Worldviews on Evidence-Based Nursing* 14 (1): 5–9. http://doi.org/10.1111/wvn.12188.

Monturo, C.A. and Brockway, C. (2019). Micro-learning: an innovative strategy to cultivate a spirit of inquiry, step zero. *Worldviews on Evidence-Based Nursing* 16 (5): 416–417. http://doi.org/10.1111/wvn.12373.

Mugerauer, R. (2021). Professional judgement in clinical practice (part 1): recovering original, moderate evidence-based health care. *Journal of Evaluation in Clinical Practice* 27 (3): 592–602. http://doi.org/10.1111/jep.13513.

Palinkas, L.A. and Mendon, S.J. (2019). Translation of evidence-based practices in health. In: *Handbook of Health Social Work*, vol. 3 (ed. S. Gehlert and T.A. Browne). New Jersey: Wiley.

Richardson-Tench, M., Nicholson, P., Taylor, B., and Kermode, S. (2018). *Research in Nursing, Midwifery and Allied Health: Evidence for Best Practice*, 6e. Melbourne, Victoria: Cengage Learning.

Rogers, E.M. (2003). *Diffusion of Innovations*, 5e. New York: Free Publishing.

Sackett, D.L., Rosenberg, W.M.C., Gray, J.A.M. et al. (1996). Evidence based medicine: what it is and what it isn't. *British Medical Journal* 312 (7023): 71–72. http://doi.org/10.1136/bmj.312.7023.71.

Schaefer, J.D. and Welton, J.M. (2018). Evidence based practice readiness: a concept analysis. *Journal of Nursing Management* 26 (6): 621–629. http://doi.org/10.1111/jonm.12599.

Skela-Savič, B. and Lobe, B. (2021). Differences in beliefs on and implementation of evidence-based practice according to type of health care institution—a national cross-sectional study among Slovenian nurses. *Journal of Nursing Management* 29 (5): 971–981. http://doi.org/10.1111/jonm.13234.

Sørly, R., Krane, M.S., Bye, G., and Ellingsen, M.-B. (2019). "There Is a Lot of Community Spirit Going On." Middle Managers' stories of innovation in home care services. *SAGE Open Nursing* 5: 2377960819844367. http://doi.org/10.1177/2377960819844367.

Tayyib, N. and Coyer, F. (2017). Translating pressure ulcer prevention into intensive care nursing practice: overlaying a care bundle approach with a model for research implementation. *Journal of Nursing Care Quality* 32 (1): 6–14. http://doi.org/10.1097/NCQ.0000000000000199.

Wakibi, S., Ferguson, L., Berry, L. et al. (2021). Teaching evidence-based nursing practice: a systematic review and convergent qualitative synthesis. *Journal of Professional Nursing* 37 (1): 135–148. http://doi.org/10.1016/j.profnurs.2020.06.005.

Waljee, J.F., Chopra, V., and Saint, S. (2018). Mentoring millennials. *The Journal of the American Medical Association* 319 (15): 1547–1548. http://doi.org/10.1001/jama.2018.3804.

Wieringa, S., Engebretsen, E., Heggen, K., and Greenhalgh, T. (2018). How knowledge is constructed and exchanged in virtual communities of physicians: qualitative study of mindlines online. *Journal of Medical Internet Research* 20 (2): 441–465. http://doi.org/10.2196/jmir.8325.

Wiesmann, U. (2017). Well-being in health professionals: positive psychology at work. In: *The Wiley Blackwell Handbook of the Psychology of Positivity and Strengths-Based Approaches at Work* (ed. L.G. Oades), 439–465. Chichester, West Sussex, UK: Wiley Blackwell.

15

Reflection and Emotional Intelligence

David Stanley

We do not learn from experience – we learn from reflecting on experience –

John Dewey
(https://thelearnersway.net/ideas/2019/11/24/
if-we-learn-from-reflecting-on-experience)

Introduction: The Noblest Way to Wisdom

This chapter discusses how clinical leaders can develop emotional intelligence and reflective practice skills to support leadership, innovation and the development of values. It will address the concepts of emotional intelligence and reflection, what they are and when they can be used. Finally, it will explore how emotional intelligence and reflection can be used as strategies to sustain clinical leaders and assist them with personal and professional development and learning. Kahraman and Hicdurmaz (2016) indicated, in a study of Turkish clinical nurses, that while age, gender or other sociodemographic factors had limited impact on the demonstration or application of emotional intelligence, higher emotional intelligence was associated with longer exposure to clinical practice and greater professional development. Artioli et al. (2021) supported this by suggesting that reflective writing also enhanced the learning of advanced clinical skills. This makes emotional intelligence and the practice of reflection a feature of how clinical leaders may be recognised and points to the importance of clinical leaders understanding and applying emotionally intelligent techniques and reflection.

What Is Reflection?

Reflection invites us to look in the mirror and remove our individual mask, so that we can look beneath what we see on the surface. As health professionals move from novice to expert, each action or omission to act needs to be carefully considered, and the process of doing this is based on reflection. This is achieved by exploring our previous thoughts,

Clinical Leadership in Nursing and Healthcare, Third Edition.
Edited by David Stanley, Clare L. Bennett and Alison H. James.
© 2023 John Wiley & Sons Ltd. Published 2023 by John Wiley & Sons Ltd.

emotions and behaviours, which leads to useful insights for future experiences and increases the potential for congruence in leadership and professionally appropriate interventions (Barksby et al. 2015; Dosser 2016). According to Johns (2006, p. 3) 'reflection is being mindful of self, either within or after experience, as if a window through which the practitioner can view and focus self within the context of a particular experience'. Johns (2006) further suggests that reflection enables us to confront, understand and move towards resolving a contradiction between our vision or values and those of our actual practice. This means that we are not only able to learn through reflection, we are also able to meet our objectives by linking theory to our everyday behaviour.

Reflection and Learning

Dewey first introduced the idea of reflective practice in 1933. His belief was that reflection involved the whole person, in an open-minded and wholehearted endeavour, and that it was a rational, intellectual act (Ruth-Sahd 2003). Reflective thinking should be purposeful, encouraging the individual to confront their values and beliefs, which includes examining their emotions as a holistic activity (Horton-Deutsch and Sherwood 2008; Dosser 2016).

Brockbank and McGill's (2000) exploration suggests that our learning activity is very much influenced by our values and philosophies; it is because of this that reflecting on our practice can indeed close the gap between theory and practice. Chang and Daly (2012) add that being reflective also encourages us to think critically and to problem solve. They contend that critical thinkers are autonomous, because they are able to analyse issues and challenge beliefs. Critical reflection, as with critical thinking, assists us in thinking about and distinguishing between our beliefs, as well as in questioning our existing assumptions and perspectives. Therefore, combining critical thinking with critical reflection enables us to learn through our experiences, which helps create the opportunity for us to form new knowledge and insights and change our behaviours appropriately (Jarvis 2013; Dosser 2016). Acquiring the ability to analyse assumptions and become more critically aware could certainly assist individuals, as well as leaders, by enabling each to speculate more imaginatively (Bishop 2009).

Reflection can be done:

- Before action (before an event)
- In action (during the event)
- On action (following the event, looking back) (Schon 1983)

As well, reflection can be about:

- describing an experience
- understanding your reactions to the experience
- critically analysing situations
- developing new perspectives
- evaluating the learning process

Benefits of Reflection for Clinical Leaders

There are a number of benefits to be found from the application of reflection, as follows.

Better Self-Knowledge/Increased Self-Awareness

Socrates is reported to have said, 'To find yourself, think for yourself'. As a philosopher, he clearly knew the value of reflection, because he believed that it would help individuals move towards understanding themselves more fully. According to Bishop (2009), understanding the 'self' is an attribute that enables leaders to become more transformational, especially through their actions, and through those actions they are capable of inspiring and motivating others to achieve desirable outcomes and develop innovative practices.

Identification of Your Values

Individuals tend to align themselves with others they view as like-minded and who demonstrate the same values and beliefs that they hold. The application of these values and beliefs is something that leaders share with others because they work closely and frequently with their team (Dosser 2016). According to Stanley (2011, 2017), they are role models who provide direction and guidance for the quality of care and the interactions that take place between individuals and teams. Congruent leaders and values-based leaders in particular are followed, in the main, for their values and beliefs. This is because they are viewed as having specific clinical knowledge, and therefore in the eyes of the follower this makes the leader a credible individual.

Connection to Caring

Reflection, according to Benner and Wrubel (1989), can also assist the individual in reconnecting to caring, especially when there is a loss of caring due to burnout. Clinical leaders may have a better understanding of this phenomenon because they are linked more closely with the values of caring than are managers, who may be more interested in the outcomes of care delivery rather than the process of care.

More Effective Working Relationships/Stronger Teams

Dosser (2016, p. 37) suggests that 'effective working relationships rely on shared and mutually respectful perceptions of who we are'. Therefore, reflection is central to ensuring the healthcare team is able to meet patient needs and support a common purpose while learning with and from each other. Schmutz and Walter (2017) agree and found that shared reflection promoted greater learning and a stronger collective competence, in the teams they worked with

Empowerment

Chang and Daly (2012) state that reflection can be both emancipatory and empowering, because it can be used as a tool to assist with self-knowledge, thereby freeing leaders to explore future scenarios that support others while improving clinical practice. Although it can be common for leaders to hold power, congruent leaders do not necessarily use this power to inspire and empower others. This is because there is a shared understanding and alignment of a congruent leader's values and beliefs with regard to therapy or care that is visible through the leader's consistent actions (Stanley 2017). This said, reflection can, and is, sometimes associated with 'judging', and this can make being open and honest a challenge when practice is not ideal or when mistakes have been made. As Dosser (2016, p. 38) states, 'openness and honesty are integral to nursing (and all health professions) and are promoted and expected as part of national and international codes of ethics and standards of practice'.

Learning from Mistakes

Protecting the public sits at the heart of standards of practice and codes of ethics for all health professionals. But it would be foolish to expect that mistakes will not occur. However, the value of reflection is in taking a step back, critically analysing and moving forward with a view to not repeating the same mistake. This works because the process of introspection and analysis enables professionals to critically examine what was right and wrong in a particular situation and to take responsibility for the choices they made or actions they omitted. Mistakes are part of the human experience, and this is no different for leaders. However, the way in which leaders deal with their mistakes gives others an insight into their integrity. If leaders want to gain respect and loyalty, they must be trustworthy. Trust comes before loyalty, and once loyalty is established commitment follows (Chang and Daly 2012).

Models to Support Reflection

A multitude of models have been developed over the years to support reflective thinking and learning. These include the following models (although there may be others not on this list):

- Mezirow (1981/1997)   Mezirow's Model of Transformative Learning
- Boud et al. (1985)   Reflective Learning
- Schon (1987)   Reflection in and on Action
- Gibbs (1988)   The Gibbs Reflective Cycle.
- Atkins and Murphy (1993)   The Cyclical Model
- Kolb (1984)   Kolb's Learning Cycle
- Freshwater et al. (2001)   Rolfe, Freshwater and Jasper's Framework of Reflective Practice
- Johns (2006)   Johns' Model of Structured Reflection
- Bain et al. (2002)   The 5R's Model of reflection.

None is highlighted over any others (although if pressed, I quite like Gibbs (1988) model). The 5R's model has been adapted, and I have seen a 4R's model and a 3R's model as various R's get dropped. The preceding models list is intended to give readers a starting point, and it is hoped that you feel encouraged to seek out or consider all of them and identify one or a combination of reflective models that best supports your application of reflection. Each offers a template to support your development of a reflective habit, and any model that is more easily remembered or applied might suit best. As the next section indicates, the application of reflective models is very much a personal choice.

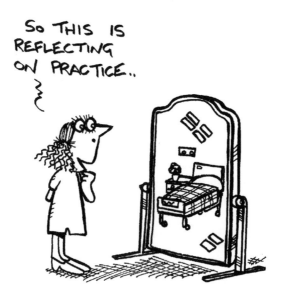

Using Reflective Models

Reflection can have many layers (Johns and Freshwater 2005), and key theorists such as Mezirow (1981), Boud et al. (1985), Casement (1985), Schon (1987) and Freshwater et al. (2001) all discuss the different levels of reflection, viewing it as more of an intuitive, holistic way to view the self from within. Mezirow's (1981) model can be used for promoting critical reflection (Freshwater et al. 2001), whereas other models such as those of Gibbs (1988) and Schon (1987) offer a more linear approach, with prompts to guide the reflector through the reflective process. However, contemporary thought is that reflective models can be combined to provide deeper reflection. The value of combining models and modifying them is that this type of layering approach can maximise reflection and facilitate greater learning, so that the reflector can explore a situation more fully.

Reflection Point

Think back to a significant personal or professional situation that you found challenging. Identify a reflective model with which you feel comfortable and explore this situation using the model's prompts. While reflecting on the events that took place, think about the emotions associated with them and how this affected your reactions and the outcome to the situation. Not all models will encourage this, which points again to the value of finding a model that you are most comfortable with.

Approaches to Reflection

There are a range of views about reflective writing, with a common question being whether the reflection needs to follow a prescriptive, structured or formal approach. All of the models already discussed offer a systematic, structured approach to reflection; however, some reflective writing techniques can provide the individual with the intellectual space to 'stop and think', without structuring the reflection. Two approaches in particular can be used:

- **Reflective diaries journals and portfolios:** Horton-Deutsch and Sherwood (2008) discuss the value of reflective diaries as a way to retain an account and historical record of our own developments, whether they are personal or professional. Maintaining a diary, journal or portfolio enables us to undertake personal reflection and keep our thoughts private. Artioli et al. (2021) emphasise that regardless of the approach taken, any form of creative, critical, reflective writing will have benefits for human and professional development.
- **Clinical supervision:** Some reflection can be more beneficial if undertaken verbally, as this may provide the opportunity to seek clarification and advice on specific issues. Clinical supervision offers an individual space to reflect with a supervisor/mentor who can be an expert or clinical guide. In group supervision, individuals may also benefit from the reflections shared by others, as this provides additional insights and support when they are a group of professionals reflecting on their practices (Chang and Daly 2012). In clinical supervision, the supervisor/mentor is able to assist the supervisee(s) to recall events and guide them through the process of reflection, which can be achieved by utilising a reflective model or a combination of models to promote deeper levels of reflection (Latimer 2007; Jarvis 2013).

Utilising either of these approaches can be beneficial, as reflection can be viewed as a learning strategy that assists with the development of economically competent leaders (Horton-Deutsch and Sherwood 2008; Jarvis 2013).

Clinical Leader Stories: 15 – Visiting Times

One of the research interviews in the initial research study relates to an account of a junior registered nurse (RN) who was faced with an anxious husband whose wife had that day undergone emergency surgery. The husband wanted to visit his wife and be at her side, but he needed to work when the ward had visiting times. The ward enforced strict visiting times (14:00–16:00 and 18:00–20:00) for all relatives and other visitors, and although the ward was 'open' for a number of hours, this particular man was unable to attend at these times due to working evening and afternoon shifts. The junior RN, knowing she was acting against the specific instructions of the ward manager and senior RN, allowed the man onto the ward at 10:30 to visit his wife. The junior RN undertook to do this because she believed that had this been her husband or had she been the wife, this was the action she would have wanted the nurse to follow.

  The nurse knew that she could have incurred disapproval or a reprimand from the ward manager and senior RN, but she undertook to support the husband and defended her stance against the more senior nursing staff. The incident caused some discomfort for the more junior nurse, and the fall-out from her action was that she was indeed reprimanded. This initiated debate at the regular ward meeting that ultimately resulted in many of her colleagues agreeing that they would have liked to have done the same, and this, in time, led to a revision in the ward's visiting processes and procedures.

(Continued)

The junior RN employed no long-term strategy in admitting the husband outside of the permitted visiting times and had not set out to disrupt the ward visiting-time procedures. However, by following her beliefs about respecting the needs of patients and in this case their relatives too, the nurse initiated what developed into a slow revolution that resulted in significant change and an improvement in relatives' access to their ill, worried and isolated friends and family. Clinical leaders who display congruent leadership match their values and beliefs to their actions, and in this example the junior RN took a risk in following her beliefs. Nevertheless, her colleagues recognised this action as part of the qualities and characteristics associated with a clinical leader. As the junior RN was visible and present in the clinical area and through her commitment and passion for the core values of nursing, she was (even unintentionally) able to motivate and inspire others to follow. The more senior nurses who had developed the visiting policy were not as present on the ward, did not deal as regularly with dissatisfied or upset relatives and friends and were not as commonly in the position of having their nursing and caring values and beliefs challenged.

Sue: Senior Nurse

What Is Emotional Intelligence?

Emotional intelligence is described as the ability to monitor one's own and others' feelings and emotions, to discriminate among them and to use this information to guide one's thinking and actions (Salovey and Mayer 1990). Goleman (1998) describes emotional intelligence as the capacity for recognising our own feelings and those of others, for motivating ourselves and for effectively dealing with our own and others' emotions. Ellis (2017a) adds that emotional intelligence requires people to be self-aware and understand the reasons behind our emotions and use an emotionally measured and literate response.

Goleman (1998) reminds us that our emotions are instrumental in our lives, and goes as far as saying that they are elemental in our development on a personal and professional level. Emotions are a human factor and are also an essential part of who we are. Expressing emotions at the right time and in the right place is a concern for most of us. Emotional intelligence means judging when to deal with emotions or when, as Brockbank and McGill (2000) state, to 'park' them. Many people react to life events with their emotions, claiming that they are not able to control them adequately. Anger, fear, jealousy, regret, feelings of betrayal or of hurt at being let down are some of the common emotions we experience, as well as the more positive ones of joy and relief. Emotional intelligence is about exercising control over these emotions so that our response is tempered by a conscious acknowledgement of the feelings we are experiencing.

The Five Building Blocks of Emotional Intelligence

According to Goleman (2005), the five building blocks of emotional intelligence are:

- **Self-awareness (of your own feelings):** This is the ability to gauge and understand your emotions and recognise how they will influence your work performance and relationships. It is also about recognising and being realistic regarding your strengths and weaknesses (Ellis 2017a; Mansel and Einion 2019).

- **Self-management or self-regulation (of your emotions):** This is self-control. It involves the ability to keep disruptive emotions and impulses in check. It requires you to be conscious of your emotions (Ellis 2017b).
- **Social awareness or empathy (to recognise the feelings of others):** This is about recognising and sensing the emotions of others, understanding their perspective and employing empathy. It is an essential skill for networking and navigating through relationships.
- **Social skills (to manage emotions in others):** This is a set of skills that build on communication, listening and conflict management. These are skills that build bonds and cooperation.
- **Motivation:** This is the drive to go beyond superficial motivations (money or status) and see the 'bigger picture' in building successful and meaningful personal and professional relationships. It captures ideas of optimism and a willingness to be committed to more than just yourself.

So emotional intelligence is about exercising self-control and applying zeal and persistence in motivating ourselves in the face of frustrations. It is also connected to delaying gratification, monitoring and regulating our mood and keeping distress away from our ability to think (Mansel and Einion 2019). Emotions are essential aspects of the human condition, but they are meant to serve us and not control us, so emotional intelligence helps us recognise that emotions can promote our well-being, but only if they are employed appropriately or in a controlled way. Instead of trying to avoid emotions, especially at work, leaders have an important role in regulating emotions within groups and within themselves by providing support and guidance that harness the energy of emotional interactions positively (Rajah et al. 2011; Taylor et al. 2015). Goleman et al. (2013) suggest that when it comes to shaping our decisions and actions, feelings count every bit as much as our thoughts, if not more so.

Self-awareness is key to the development of emotional intelligence, as it allows us to recognise the feelings we have and become aware of our mood and the thoughts that are driving our mood (Mansel and Einion 2019). Being attuned to our emotions also helps us recognise the emotions of others. So much so, that in a study by Lewis et al. (2017) of radiographers in Australia, it was clear that emotional intelligence was significantly enhanced as practitioners advanced through their careers. This leads to the next key in the development of emotional intelligence: the development of empathy and our ability to recognise the often subtle social signals that help us understand another person's needs or wants. Once developed, emotional intelligence can help us to manage relationships well, which leads to more effective interpersonal and professional relationships, more effective leadership and a greater ability to manage conflict successfully (Antonakis et al. 2009; Taylor et al. 2015; Taylor 2017).

Developing and employing an emotionally intelligent approach in your work and personal life can have the following benefits:

- Knowing your feelings and using them to make life decisions you can accept
- Being better informed about your level of self-awareness

- Knowing what triggers or 'pushes' your buttons
- Not being overwhelmed by worry or anger
- Persisting in pursuing your academic, professional and personal goals despite occasional setbacks (Por et al. 2011)
- Handling feelings and relationships with skill and maturity (Taylor et al. 2015)
- Moderating the impact of stressful situations on your mental health (Benson et al. 2010)
- Fostering effective interprofessional communication that influences the quality of care and patient safety (Bulmer Smith et al. 2009)
- Managing clear communication in a crisis, which may be central to clarifying and resolving disputes – remaining calm and in control will have immediate effects!
- Improving your communication and conflict management styles, helping you build rapport and get the job done better (Taylor et al. 2015)

Chang and Daly (2012) indicate that emotional intelligence can be critical even when an individual is not in a leadership role, as it assists with identifying and developing skills of self-regulation, empathy, social skills and motivation across the five building blocks. In effect, emotionally intelligent people are 'people-people', or people who understand people (Ellis 2017b). This can lead to the effective management of emotions in a variety of situations. No person is an island, and emotional intelligence does not concern being nice to ourselves and others; it concerns making choices about how we feel, identifying emotions in others and providing the support they need. This can have a dramatic impact on the success of our work and personal relationships and ultimately on our ability to advance in our career or grow as a person (Taylor et al. 2015). It is often said that a great resume will get you the job, but it is effective emotional intelligence that will keep you in the job. The good news is that emotional intelligence can be learnt and developed over time (Goleman 2005).

Reflection on Reflection and Emotional Intelligence

Chang and Daly (2012) assert that the ability to reflect on evidence – and more importantly to reflect critically – has become an essential skill for the clinician of the future. Clinical leaders can benefit from this process by challenging their thoughts, feelings and behaviours and therefore creating new realities (Jarvis 2013). Boud and Walker (1991) say that if professionals accept positions of responsibility, they need to learn from experience. Reflection on experience helps us understand and gain insights into previous situations. While critical thinking is important to support decision making, reflection enables us to view situations from different perspectives and can be transformative (Schutz 2007; Beauvais et al. 2011; Jarvis 2013). The benefits of emotional intelligence are also optimal when we willingly engage purposefully in the self-awareness process. Taylor (2017) goes further and suggests that leaders who apply emotional intelligence practices retain staff, and report higher job satisfaction and productivity. Reflection can be a vital tool for bringing our values and beliefs to consciousness, which enables us to respond and behave in ways that are ethical and professional. Reflection is one way in which we can access preconceived ideas, by challenging ourselves in an emotionally safe capacity and applying new knowledge and insights to the next interaction or situation. The outcome of this new knowledge and insight is facilitation of our own learning and maximising of personal and professional development (Chang and Daly 2012; Jarvis 2013).

A final note on the link between congruent leaders and emotional intelligence is the concept that a leader's values and beliefs are deemed to be more visible when they are demonstrated in practice.

Leaders who are congruent in their actions foster constructive emotional responses that are conducive and effective in a variety of interactions and situations. Emotionally competent leaders are able to regulate their emotions confidently and can motivate others by sharing collective values and beliefs that have positive impacts in all environments (Bulmer Smith et al. 2009; Heckemann et al. 2015). Goleman et al. (2013) refer to this as the 'primal' emotional task of a leader, because it is both original and the most important act of leadership. Congruent leaders are therefore capable through their actions of inspiring and motivating others to achieve desirable outcomes and develop innovative practices.

Case Study 15.1   Malala Yousafzai

Malala Yousafzai grew up in the Swat Valley in north-western Pakistan. She spoke up for the rights of women to be educated and nearly paid with her life. Many of the 'rights' taken for granted in Western society have been hard won and have not been entrenched for long. Women still receive lower wages on average than men in comparable jobs and their right to an education was not something most women could expect as a given only 100 years ago. Malala was born in 1997, in a part of the world were women and girls were expected to be wives and mothers and therefore an education was not encouraged. Malala though wanted to learn, and she actively promoted women's rights to learn and attend school. The dominant religious group in her area were the Taliban, and they placed restrictions on girls and women being educated.

Malala protested about these restrictions, and when she was between the ages of 11 and 12, she wrote a blog detailing her life under the Taliban. This was brought to the attention of a wider international community, and in 2012 the *New York Times* produced a documentary about her life as a woman seeking to gain an education. The documentary made her out to be an advocate for human rights and women's rights, and she spoke out about the restriction placed on women being educated by the Taliban.

This was not viewed favourably by the Taliban, and in the same year she and two girls were attacked in an assassination attempt as they rode on a bus in northern Pakistan. Malala was critically injured after being shot in the head, and she was eventually transferred, with international support, to the Queen Elizabeth Hospital in Birmingham, UK. She slowly recovered and eventually made a full physical recovery before settling down to live in the UK.

The attempt on her life made international news and highlighted the difficult situation faced by girls and women in the areas controlled by the Taliban. In spite of the international support, the Taliban continued to threaten her life, and Malala remained in the UK. There, she set up a non-profit organisation and co-authored a book: *I am Malala,* with the aim of continuing to speak out about the repression of women and to advocate for the rights of women and girls to be educated. In 2014, she was a

(Continued)

co-recipient of the Nobel Peace Prize, making her one of the most recognised and influential women in the fight for women's equality.

She went on to study at Oxford, UK, and in spite of the *fatwa* against her, she continues to speak out for women's rights, and she remains a prominent activist and advocate for the rights of women. Malala put her life on the line by remaining true to what she believes.

Challenge: I have no idea of the courage it would take to stand up to an oppressive and violent regime. I have grown up in a settled and stable country were the rule of law and the power of the free press is evident (even though it feels like it is constantly under threat). I take access to education and access to the internet for granted. Reflect about what you have 'taken for granted', what 'rights' would you be willing to stand up for? Think too about the tenuous nature of what we have now and how quickly it could all be snatched away if we are not vigilant and practice ways to hold and strengthen the advances and gifts we have. Reflect for a moment about what Malala risked.

Try to capture your thoughts by writing them down or recording them. Constant 'doing' will get things done, but reflection might mean that you find new ways to do things or have an opportunity to do things better.

Summary

- Reflection encourages and supports critical thinking, problem-solving and decision-making skills.
- Reflection assists with linking theory to practice.
- Both reflection and emotional intelligence help with the development of insight and self-awareness.
- Models of reflection can be utilised to provide a framework for more critical reflective practice.
- Clinical supervision, reflective diaries, journals, portfolios or a reflective companion can support the reflective process.
- Emotional intelligence may be developed through emotional awareness and can promote personal and professional growth.
- Emotional intelligence is more evident as professionals grow and develop in their clinical role, linking effective clinical leaders with the application of emotional intelligence.

Mind Press-Ups

Exercise 15.1

Decide on two methods of reflection, such as writing a journal or verbalising your thoughts with a reflective companion and compare them to assess what the more effective reflective method is for you.

Exercise 15.2

Watch the animated film *Inside Out*. What does it say about emotional intelligence and about the emotional internal dialogue that might be going on inside all of us?

Exercise 15.3

Think about a recent conversation with a friend or work colleague. Did you practice emotional intelligence? Do you think they left the conversation feeling enhanced or diminished by the dialogue? How did you feel?

References

Antonakis, J., Ashkanasy, N., and Dasborough, M. (2009). Does leadership need emotional intelligence? *The Leadership Quarterly* 20: 247–261.

Artioli, G., Deiana, L., De Vincenzio, F. et al. (2021). Health professionals and students' experiences of reflective writing in learning: a qualitative meta-synthesis. *BMC Medical Education* 21: 395.

Atkins, S. and Murphy, K. (1993). Reflection: a review of literature. *Journal of Advanced Nursing* 18: 1188–1192.

Bain, J.D., Ballantyne, R., Mills, C., and Lester, N.C. (2002). *Reflecting on Practice: Student teacher's Perspectives*. Flaxton, QLD: Post Pressed.

Barksby, J., Butcher, N., and Whysall, A. (2015). A new model of reflection for clinical practice. *Nursing Times* 111 (34/35): 21–23.

Beauvais, A., Brady, N., O'Shea, E., and Quinn Griffin, M. (2011). Emotional intelligence and nursing performance among nursing students. *Nurse Education Today* 31: 396–401.

Benner, P. and Wrubel, J. (1989). *The Primacy of Caring*. Menlo Park, CA: Addison-Wesley.

Benson, G., Ploeg, J., and Brown, B. (2010). A cross-sectional study of emotional intelligence in baccalaureate nursing students. *Nurse Education Today* 30: 49–53.

Bishop, V. (2009). *Leadership for Nursing and Allied Health Care Professions*. Maidenhead: Open University Press/McGraw-Hill Education.

Boud, D. and Walker, D. (1991). *Experiencing and Learning: Reflection at Work*. Geelong, VIC: Deakin University Press.

Boud, D., Keogh, R., and Walker, D. (1985). *Promoting Reflection in Learning: A Model in Reflection: Turning Experience into Learning*. London: Kogan Page.

Brockbank, A. and McGill, I. (2000). *Facilitating Reflective Learning in Higher Education*. Buckingham: Open University Press.

Bulmer Smith, K., Profetto-McGrath, J., and Cummings, G. (2009). Emotional intelligence and nursing: an integrative literature review. *International Journal of Nursing Studies* 46: 1624–1636.

Casement, P. (1985). *On Learning from the Patient*. London: Routledge.

Chang, E. and Daly, J. (2012). *Transitions in Nursing: Preparing for Professional Practice*, 3e. London: Churchill Livingstone.

Dewey, J. (1933). *How We Think: A Restatement of the Relation of Reflective Thinking to the Educative Process*, 2e. New York: Heath.

Dosser, I. (2016). Understanding reflective practice. *Nursing Standard* 30 (36): 34–40.

Ellis, P. (2017a). What emotional intelligence is and is not. *Wounds UK* 13 (3): 62–63.

Ellis, P. (2017b). Learning emotional intelligence and what it can do for you. *Wounds UK* 13 (4): 66–68.

Freshwater, D., Rolfe, G., and Jasper, M. (2001). *Critical Reflection for Nursing and the Helping Professions: A User's Guide*. Basingstoke: Palgrave Macmillan.

Gibbs, G. (1988). *Learning by Doing: A Guide to Teaching and Learning Methods*. Oxford: Further Education Unit, Oxford Brookes University.

Goleman, D. (1998). *Working with Emotional Intelligence*. New York: Bantam.

Goleman, D. (2005). *Emotional Intelligence*. New York: Random House.

Goleman, D., Boyatzis, R., and McKee, A. (2013). *Primal Leadership: Unleashing the Power of Emotional Intelligence*. Boston, MA: Harvard Business School Press.

Heckemann, B., Schols, J., and Halfens, R. (2015). A reflective framework to foster emotionally intelligent leadership in nursing. *Journal of Nursing Management* 23: 744–753.

Horton-Deutsch, S. and Sherwood, G. (2008). Reflection: an educational strategy to develop emotionally-competent nurse leaders. *Journal of Nursing Management* 16 (8): 946–954.

Jarvis, M. (2013). *Beginning Reflective Practice*, 2e. Andover: Cengage Learning.

Johns, C. (2006). *Engaging Reflection in Practice: A Narrative Approach*. Oxford: Blackwell.

Johns, C. and Freshwater, D. (2005). *Transforming Nursing through Reflective Practice*, 2e. Oxford: Blackwell.

Kahraman, N. and Hicdurmaz, D. (2016). Identifying emotional intelligence skills of Turkish clinical nurses according to sociodemographic and professional variables. *Journal of Clinical Practice* 25: 1006–1015.

Kolb, D.A. (1984). *Experiential learning: Experience as the source of learning and development*, vol. 1. Englewood Cliffs, NJ: Prentice-Hall.

Latimer, K. (2007). Clinical supervision for pre-registration student nurses. In: *Reflective Practice*, 2e (ed. T. Gaye and S. Lillyman), 91–95. Oxford: Blackwell Science.

Lewis, S.J., Mackay, S.T., Eccles, G.R., and Robinson, J. (2017). Emotional intelligence throughout the life cycle of Australian radiographers. *Radiology Technology* 89 (1): 12–19.

Mansel, B. and Einion, A. (2019). "'It's the relationship you develop with them": emotional intelligence in nurse leadership. A qualitative study. *British Journal of Nursing* 28 (21): 1400–1408.

Mezirow, J. (1981). A critical theory of adult learning and education. *Adult Education* 32 (1): 3–24.

Por, J., Barriball, L., Fitzpatrick, J., and Roberts, J. (2011). Emotional intelligence: its relationship to stress, coping, well-being and professional performance in nursing students. *Nurse Education Today* 31: 855–860.

Rajah, R., Song, Z., and Arvey, R. (2011). Emotionality and leadership: taking stock of the past decade of research. *The Leadership Quarterly* 22: 1107–1119.

Ruth-Sahd, L. (2003). Reflective practice: a critical analysis of data-based studies and implications for nursing education. *Journal of Nursing Education* 42 (11): 488.

Salovey, P. and Mayer, J. (1990). Emotional intelligence. *Imagination, Cognition and Personality* 9: 185–211.

Schmutz, J.B. and Walter, E.J. (2017). Promoting learning and patient care through shared reflection: a conceptual framework for team reflexivity in health care. *Academic Medicine* 92 (11): 1555–1563.

Schon, D.A. (1983). *The Reflective Practitioner: How Professionals Think in Action*. London: Temple Smith.

Schon, D.A. (1987). *Educating the Reflective Practitioner*. San Francisco, CA: Jossey-Bass.

Schutz, S. (2007). Reflection and reflective practice. *Community Practitioner* 80 (9): 26–30.

Stanley, D. (2011). *Clinical Leadership: Innovation into Action*. South Yarra, VIC: Palgrave Macmillan.

Stanley, D. (2017). *Clinical Leadership in Healthcare: Values into Action*, 2e. Oxford: Wiley Blackwell.

Taylor, G. (2017). Nurse managers: why emotionally-intelligent leadership matters. *Australian Nursing and Midwifery Journal* 25 (2): 20.

Taylor, B., Roberts, S., and Smyth, T. (2015). Nurse managers' strategies for feeling less drained by their work: an action research and reflection project for developing emotional intelligence. *Journal of Nursing Management* 23: 879–887.

16

Quality Improvement

Clare L. Bennett and Alison H. James

> *Drop a pebble in the water:*
> *just a splash, and it is gone;*
> *But there's half-a-hundred ripples*
> *Circling on and on and on,*
> *Spreading, spreading from the center,*
> *flowing on out to the sea.*
> *And there is no way of telling*
> *where the end is going to be.*

James W. Foley (1874–1939)

Introduction: What Does Good Quality Healthcare Look Like?

In healthcare, definitions of quality often reflect differing stakeholder positions, with patients, providers, managers and funders often having quite different perceptions. However, the Institute of Medicine's (2001) six dimensions of quality have been widely adopted internationally. The framework outlines six aims for healthcare systems, asserting that they should be:

- **Safe:** the avoidance of unnecessary harm to patients
- **Effective:** the provision of evidence-based and appropriate healthcare
- **Patient-centred:** care that reflects individual patient preferences, needs and values
- **Timely:** care delivery at the right time, minimising potentially harmful delays
- **Efficient:** avoidance of waste
- **Equitable:** an equal chance of the same outcomes regardless of gender, ethnicity, geography and socioeconomic status

In reality, many patients will not have experienced healthcare that meets each of these pillars of quality. Healthcare is paradoxical; despite constant attempts at change, performance has flatlined over the last three decades with just 60% (approximately) of care delivery aligning with evidence- or consensus-based guidelines, around 30% being of low value and approximately 10% being identified as harmful (Braithwaite et al. 2020). This is known as the 60-30-10 Challenge (Braithwaite et al. 2020).

This chapter addresses two concerns central to the effectiveness of clinical leaders and how they can have a positive impact on the health service. It is in the domain of quality initiatives that clinical leaders can and do often shine. When initiating, leading and following up on quality initiatives, clinical leaders can have a dramatic influence on quality, innovation and change in the health service. Part of taking quality initiatives forward involves planning for change so that it has the greatest opportunity to succeed. The most effective way to initiate change is with a clear plan of how the quality project can be developed, accompanied by the application of knowledge, skills, tools and techniques to meet the project requirements. This chapter therefore focuses on the relationship of clinical leaders to quality initiatives and project management.

Reflection Point

Before reading on, think through what 'quality' means to you. Consider what quality indicators you might look for if purchasing a car or a choosing a holiday. Now, consider what the various dimensions of healthcare quality might be.

Systems Thinking

Braithwaite et al. (2020) argues that improving health services can be challenging because healthcare is a complex adaptive system, characterised by numerous funding models, multiple components, patients with diverse needs, multiple treatment options, unpredictable demand, numerous sub-systems and nested systems and many stakeholders with differing priorities. Effective improvement is, therefore, underpinned by 'systems thinking', which takes account of all the interacting systems that are relevant to the intended improvement, rather than just taking into account factors at the team or unit level.

In contrast to change, which is often an isolated event, quality improvement is concerned with making sustainable improvements that positively affect the wider healthcare system (Lenoci-Edwards 2018). A system is a set of two or more interrelated elements with the following properties:

1) Each element has an effect on the functioning of the whole.
2) Each element is affected by at least one other element in the system.
3) All subgroups of the elements also have the above two properties (Ackoff 1981).

A 'system' might be a computer system, the body's respiratory system, the global financial system, an ecological system or a healthcare system. Regardless of the type of system, it 'embodies the idea of a set of elements connected together which form a whole, this showing properties which are properties of the whole, rather than properties of its component part' (Checkland 1981, p. 3). A system is composed of parts which must all be related (directly or indirectly), otherwise there are two or more distinct systems. As we see in healthcare, a system can be nested inside another system, for example, a phlebotomy system might be nested inside a hospital system or a primary care system. A system also consists of intangible elements, such as norms and assumptions, and these are essential factors in understanding how a system works.

'Systems thinking' is an approach to problem solving, by viewing 'problems' as parts of an overall system, rather than reacting to an isolated issue, outcome or event. It is based on the belief that the component parts of a system can best be understood in the context of relationships with each other and with other systems, rather than in isolation. In our experience, clinical leaders find systems thinking advantageous because it supports them in tackling problems scientifically and holistically with sustainable outcomes, with many finding the prominence that is given to the human element particularly useful.

So, when considering quality improvement, clinical leaders need to consider the bigger picture. For example, a seemingly small improvement at the ward level regarding timings of drug administration is likely to have unintended consequences for other areas of the system. For example, pharmacy staff, if drugs need to be prepared for different times, and the multi-disciplinary team, if nurses and patients are no longer free for established ward rounds and team meetings. To help see the bigger picture it can be useful to consider a conceptual framework for quality in healthcare, known as the Donabedian model (Agency for Healthcare Research and Quality 2021), whereby structures, processes and outcomes of care are considered. Examples are provided below:

- Structure: The context in which healthcare is provided, e.g. the skill mix and educational background of healthcare professionals and resources
- Process: Adherence to guidelines/evidence, safety considerations, timeliness of diagnosis and interventions
- Outcomes: Changes in patients' health status as a result of the care received

Although it is acknowledged that this model does not incorporate antecedents such as patient characteristics and environmental factors, these prompts can be useful as a starting point in examining the various facets involved in quality improvement.

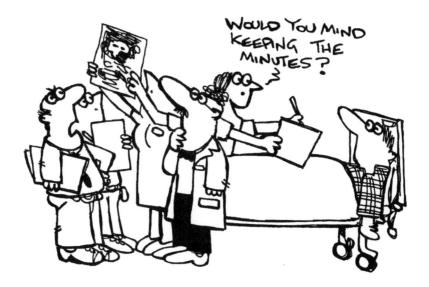

Reflection Point

Consider how health systems could be improved to address the 60-30-10 Challenge.

The Quality Cycle – A Quality Management System

Welsh Government (2021) argue that healthcare quality is intrinsically linked to healthcare leadership, highlighting how failings in specific services are often linked to wider organisational weaknesses. Conversely, they assert that organisations which are quality driven are more likely to prioritise quality improvement as an integral part of their long-term planning, use data to inform improvement (as opposed to only using data for assurance or control) and engage staff and patients in quality improvement as part of a dominant culture of openness, continuous improvement and effective clinical leadership.

A quality management system incorporates a constant cycle of quality planning, quality improvement and quality control, with quality assurance being integral to each of these aspects and a learning environment at its heart, as depicted in Figure 16.1. This is also known as The Juran Trilogy (DeFeo 2019).

Quality Planning involves a design process which focuses on enabling innovation through the design of services, information and products (DeFeo 2019). Health Improvement Scotland (2021) calls this stage 'Planning for Quality' and advocate:

- the prioritisation of improvement through user need
- analysis of quality control issues
- a focus on issues which will have the greatest impact

Quality improvement is a formal approach to the analysis of performance and systematic efforts to improve it. It is proactive, positive and focuses on the entire system, thus fostering

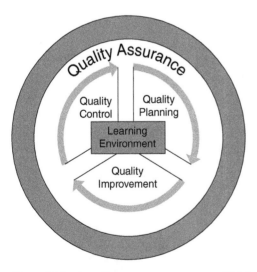

Figure 16.1 A quality management system. (Welsh Government 2021).

system change. To improve a system, you need a good understanding of it; you need to understand where it is failing, identify what is wrong and make sure that you are focusing on the right element of the system. Then you can implement a change to the system. Quality improvement is a method that aims to ensure that all the activities required to design, develop and implement a product or service are both effective and efficient in relation to the system and its performance. Typical questions that quality improvement aims to address in healthcare include:

- How can we make [a process, e.g. patient flow in the Emergency Department, paramedic response times, rehabilitation] more efficient?
- Why have patients developed pressure ulcers on this ward?
- How can we ensure that all patients are seen by [a specific healthcare professional] within *x* hours of admission?

Quality control is concerned with maintaining quality through process control with the goal of achieving compliance to certain standards (DeFeo 2019). Health Improvement Scotland (2021) argues that quality control should largely be conducted by teams themselves through data (qualitative and quantitative) gathering and analysis, so that they can continuously assess their performance and spot when things are slipping. If quality control is integral to each 'microsystem', a culture where everyone within the organisation is cognisant of quality is more likely to be created.

A quality management system is underpinned by effective clinical leadership and a learning system which enables staff to share and learn about specific issues which, in turn, builds knowledge and increases the speed of improvements (Health Improvement Scotland 2021).

Reflection Point

Identify a quality improvement that is required in your clinical area. How would you go about developing a service improvement to address this need?

Clinical Leader Stories 16: Water

Prior to planning the research interviews for the initial clinical leadership research in the UK, I had a conversation with friend working in an aged-care facility in Australia about what they thought clinical leadership looked like. She told this story: She explained that, as in many aged-care facilities, like the one she was currently working in, they were plagued with the problem of residents with chronic constipation. As such, the use and cost of laxatives had skyrocketed, and many of the residents were suffering with debilitating constipation. This hampered the residents' ability to mobilise or engage with social or rehabilitation activities and by all accounts the situation was a real 'bummer'. She went on to explain that where she worked, they had employed a new senior nurse, and her solution to the problem was to initiate a two-hourly fluid round. There was some initial resistance, but eventually after some explanation and a

(Continued)

Clinical Leader Stories 16: (Continued)

projected cost–benefit analysis, a trial was initiated. This meant that during the day, a healthcare assistant would make a point of offering every resident a cup of tea, or coffee or water or a flavoured water or even a high-energy drink, so for that one staff member, their main role was hydrating all the residents. The senior registered nurse (RN) knew that one of the main causes of constipation in the elderly client group was dehydration and that focusing on addressing this rather than the use of laxatives might provide a better solution.

The program was evaluated after six weeks. They found that while they were paying one health care assistant to mainly deal with the fluid round, they were saving 15% of their pharmacy bill each week, and this more than offset the cost of the fluid round. As well, residents were more active, felt better and could engage more confidently with social and therapy interventions. The point of the example was that she saw the RN who initiated the fluid round as a clinical leader, who applied what she knew about human physiology to address a cost-effective and quality driven program to resolve a problem that had plagued the aged-care facility for a long time. Sometimes the solution to a problem seems both simple and obtuse, but often when clinical leaders think outside the box, quality care can be achieved.

The most widely known approach to quality improvement is the Model for Improvement by Langley et al. (2009). It commences with three key questions:

1) What are we trying to accomplish?
2) How will we know that the change will be an improvement?
3) What change can we make that will result in an improvement?

In our experience, the second question is pivotal and is the one that is most commonly overlooked!

The next stage is implementation of the Plan–Do–Study–Act (PDSA) cycle:

- Plan: Agree on objectives, predict outcomes, plan the who/what/when/where/how and plan data collection.
- Do: Carry out the change, document all observations, collect and record data.
- Study: Conduct data analysis, compare results to predictions, compile a summary of insights and knowledge gained.
- Act: Identify what changes need to be made for the next PDSA cycle.

As the last bullet point above indicates, the PDSA model is an ongoing cycle to ensure that improvement is a continuous process.

There are numerous other models that can be applied to quality improvement, such as LEAN, Six Sigma, Root Cause Analysis, Ishikawa situational analysis and process flowcharting. Clearly, the employment of a model can help structure approaches to changing practice and implementing quality initiatives in a structured and planned way. Health services employ quality assurance departments, undertake audits and collect data on a wide range of quality indicators. They also seek to comply with government or industry- driven standards and institute key performance indicators (KPIs) and others for measuring performance and quality.

Reflection Point
Consider how you might lead a quality improvement initiative.

There can be numerous barriers to quality improvement such as resistance to change, a lack of resources (particularly time) and limited knowledge across teams regarding improvement science. However, Lenoci-Edwards (2018) proposes the following tips for leading quality improvement:

- Work with others across the healthcare team and gain the support of patients and senior clinical leaders to enable you to see beyond an individual change to systems improvement.
- Ensure that you understand all of the relevant data so that you can use this information to identify which areas should be prioritised for improvement.
- Build the quality improvement skills of your team.

Quality Initiative Stories

Clinical leaders can and do make a real and tangible difference to the quality of care and the quality of life of clients and patients every day by suggesting, inventing, initiating and leading new ways to do things. Indeed, a key feature of the literature on quality initiatives is that it is leadership and clinically focused leaders who make the most significant difference in influencing the success or failure of quality initiatives (Pexton 2016). Juran (1993, p. 38) goes as far as stating that 'the most decisive element' in the success or failure of a quality initiative relates to leadership. Box 16.1 offers one example.

Box 16.1   Bedside Diary in ICU
Having read about the idea of placing a diary at the bedside of unconscious patients in the intensive care unit (ICU), one of the RNs doing a clinical leadership course that David Stanley was running undertook to make this initiative her 'change project'. As such, she sought permission to run a trial where each unconscious patient in the ICU where she worked was provided with a spiral-bound notebook. This was placed on the bedside locker, and relatives and visitors, nurses and medical staff were encouraged to make notes, draw pictures and record their thoughts about the client's situation, care and progress.
The idea came about originally because ICU nurses were aware that when they recovered from their serious medical or surgical condition, clients often awoke with no recollection of what had happened to them when ventilated or unconscious. Many described a gap in their life and memory. The idea of the bedside diary was to help fill

(Continued)

Box 16.1   (Continued)

the gap. The patient could read it once they recovered and at least part of their story would be available to them.

The quality initiative required some preparation, with consent and ethical hurdles to be overcome, including devising clear guidelines about how the diary was to be used and by whom. The purchase of the notebooks also needed to be arranged. A force-field analysis was conducted that demonstrated the benefits of the activity and the ward manager was persuaded to fund a pilot project. The results were evaluated, and the viability and effectiveness of the project were soon proved.

The clients' relatives quickly took to the idea, and a range of health professionals soon felt comfortable adding short diary entries. There was an issue with taking photos that sat outside the ethical parameters of the project, and photos were initially not permitted to be used. However, relatives saw them as valuable, and soon further ethical permission was sought so that they could be added with the consent of the patient's immediate relative.

The patients who survived their ICU experience, and had diaries to take with them, provided feedback that they were very grateful for the notebooks and often added that they wished these offered even more information.

This is an example of a clinical leader, operating from a clinically driven focus, using her knowledge of change tools to institute and follow through a change and quality initiative. The pilot soon became a formal programme on this ICU and was part of the activities that helped others see this unit as a progressive and quality-driven clinical area and the RN as a practitioner driven by a focus on quality.

Reflection Point

Can you think of any quality initiatives that you have been involved in, suggested, proposed or seen in action? What were they? Did they work? Was there any resistance? How was this overcome? What sort of response was there from clients or patients to the initiative?

Project Management

This part of the chapter explores project management, what it is and how using the stages of project management *correctly* can have a positive impact on change and innovation in health services, while enhancing quality (Abdallah 2014).

Health professionals are not usually instructed in the formal practice of project management, despite being expected to act as change agents and managers of both small and large projects. The processes for making changes in health services are no different from such processes in any industry. If managed correctly, a change follows a process, and this is often known as 'project management' (Kloppenborg 2019).

Project Management Explored

What Is a Project?

A project is defined as 'a temporary endeavour undertaken to create a unique product, service or result' (Project Management Institute 2017, p. 32). As such, every project has a beginning and an end. The end is when the project is terminated, when the objectives of the project have been reached or it is clear that they never will be. In the definition here, 'temporary' does not mean of short duration, since some projects can span many years. Each project is characteristically unique because even if projects appear similar, they are all different in some way (Kloppenborg 2019), in terms of factors such as time frame, location, budget, suppliers and so on. Even the presence of repetitive elements does not change the reality that each project is unique.

A key attribute of a project is that it is progressive; that is, it advances in steps. Projects are commonly a means of handling activities that cannot be addressed within an organisation's normal operating limits.

What Is Project Management?

Project management is the application of knowledge, skills, tools and techniques to project activities to meet the project's requirements (Project Management Institute 2017). Most project management is applied though the integration of the steps of initiating, planning, executing, monitoring and controlling, then closing the project (Kloppenborg 2019). Project management is often closely associated with engineering projects, which typically have a complex set of components that need to be completed and assembled in a set fashion in order to create a functioning product (Project Management Institute 2017; Kloppenborg 2019). It is a methodical approach to planning and guiding project processes from start to finish through five stages: definition, initiation (or selecting), planning, executing (or controlling) and closing (Project Management Institute 2017). Project management can be applied to almost any type of project and is widely used to manage the complex processes involved in any developmental project.

Another view is that project management is an endeavour in which human/machine/material or financial resources are arranged in a unique way, to undertake a novel set of work, of a given specification, within constraints of cost, time or resources, so as to deliver beneficial change defined by quantitative and qualitative methods (Kloppenborg 2019). Project management uses specific techniques to plan and control the scope of the work in order to deliver a product to satisfy the clients' and stakeholders' needs and expectations. As such, project management involves planning and arrangement of an organisation's resources in order to move a specific task, event or duty towards completion (Project Management Institute 2017). It typically involves a one-time project rather than an ongoing activity, and the resources managed include both human and financial capital.

Reflection Point

Given this description, have you ever been involved in project management? If so, what was your role and how was the project managed? Was what you were involved with seen in the same way that project management is described here?

What Is the Role of a Project Manager?

A project manager will help define the goals and objectives of the project, determine when the various project components are to be completed and by whom, and create quality control checks to ensure that completed components meet a certain standard. Project managers use tools including visual representations of workflow, such as Gantt and Program Evaluation Review Technique (PERT) charts, to determine which tasks are to be completed by which departments and people. These tools are not restricted to business, engineering or construction and they fit well with health projects and processes.

The project manager is the person who holds responsibility for managing the project, identifying resources, establishing clear lines of communication and distinct objectives, as well as balancing the competing demands for quality, scope, time and cost, the needs of various stakeholders and adapting the plans as required. These responsibilities may be shared with a project team, but it is essential that within the team clear responsibilities are identified (Kloppenborg 2019). As project management is a methodical approach to planning and guiding project processes from start to finish, it is the project manager who leads and monitors the overall process.

Reflection Point

Have you had a project manager role? If so, what did you do? How did it feel and what was your experience? Did things go well? How did you set the project up? Were you ever trained in project management principles, or were you just left to get on with things? Talk to others who may have led projects. What was their experience of leading projects to fruition?

How Is Project Management Structured?

The information in this section outlines how change projects using a project management approach are structured. Figure 16.2 outlines the general structure employed to take a project from initiation to product delivery, often referred to as 'phases' (Kloppenborg 2019). All projects, regardless of their scope and size, have a similar profile.

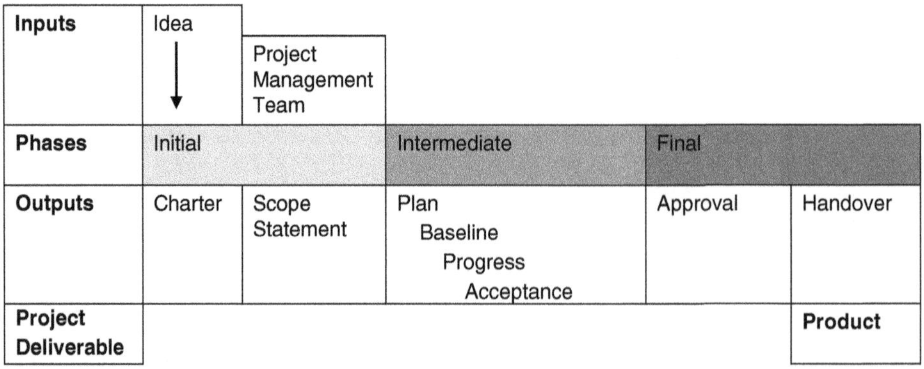

Inputs	Idea				
		Project Management Team			
Phases	Initial		Intermediate	Final	
Outputs	Charter	Scope Statement	Plan Baseline Progress Acceptance	Approval	Handover
Project Deliverable					Product

Figure 16.2 Phases of a project plan. Image by David Stanley.

Phase 1: The Initial Phase

A project's life cycle begins with an idea. This could be anything, such as a plan to change a handover system, a new staffing model, a new workload plan, the initiation of a new clinical service, or the building of a new hospital. The initial phase starts with 'inputs' or a general outline that something needs to be developed, built or changed. Developing the inputs requires the establishment of the project team. The initial phase also requires a number of 'outputs'. These require the consideration of a number of critical components: time, money, scope and the creation of the project charter as a scoping exercise.

Project Management Team

The project management team can be one person, but usually includes a number of people led by the project manager. Having the right team and team membership can enhance the overall competence of the team, improve team engagement and heighten project performance (Project Management Institute 2017). Team building should start with establishing team ground rules, encouraging participation, maintaining team cohesion and ensuring confidentiality. Managing misunderstandings and handling conflict appropriately so that trust is built and maintained are also vital (Stanley and Anderson 2015). In addition, project managers need to manage meetings well, establish team roles, maintain time lines and team focus and, crucially, make decisions promptly. These actions make up the inputs for the initial phase of the project.

Time, Money and Scope

Frequently, project management is referred to as having three components: time, money and scope. Reducing or increasing any one of the three will have an impact on the other two. If a health service reduces the amount of time it can spend on a project, that will affect the scope (what can be included in the project) as well as the cost (since additional people or resources may be required to meet the abbreviated schedule). All these have an impact on the initial phase of the project (Kloppenborg 2019).

Charter

The charter is the formal agreement of project responsibilities. This is where the business case is set up and links are established between the project and the work of the organisation and the parties involved. It sets out contracts if required, works out a project statement and defines organisational or individual responsibilities (Project Management Institute 2017).

Scope Statement

The scope statement outlines the project's deliverable requirements; in other words, what will be achieved or delivered and when. It could involve the boundaries of the project, methods to be used and, if various multi-level projects are involved, how they will relate to each other and the scope of each level of the project. Issues about the general scope of the project need to be discussed and agreed from the outset (Project Management Institute 2017; Kloppenborg 2019). Once the idea is established and the project management team set up, they meet to work out the charter and the scope statement for the project. Project teams commonly use a SMART framework (S = Specific, M = Manageable, A = Achievable, R = Realistic and T = Time framed) to help establish what the specific goals are (general goals may also be important at this stage, but the objectives are more focused and specific). Developing the scope statement for, say, the introduction of a new waste disposal system will require the involvement of the project leader, project team and significant stakeholders and should result in a set of clear objectives for each stage of the project. Having achieved these steps, the project can move on to the next phase.

Phase 2: The Intermediate Phase

This phase is made up only of outputs, and it represents the principal and most significant part of the project. It is here that the project is brought to life and eventually to fruition. The outputs involve a plan of action, baseline, progress and acceptance (Kloppenborg 2019).

Planning the Project

The project manager defines what the project is and what the users hope to achieve by undertaking it. It also includes a list of project deliverables, that is, the proposed outcome of a specific set of activities. The project manager works with the business sponsor or clinical leader who wants to have the project implemented and with other stakeholders, who have a vested interest in the outcome. If the project is setting up a new mobile public health service, for example, the project manager would need to be clear as to what is to be achieved, by when and with what resources, and specific outcomes would need to be established by the project team. It is also at this time that all the project's activities are defined. The project manager lists all activities or tasks, how the tasks are related, how long each task will take and how each task is tied to a specific deadline.

Models exist that are used to design and execute the project effectively and to guide the project management process from initial feasibility study through to maintenance of the complete application. Current approaches or methodologies include Prince 2, Agile and PMBOK (Project Management Body of Knowledge). Applying one of these models in this phase allows the project manager to define the relationships between tasks, so that, for example, if one task is x number of days late, the project tasks related to it will also reflect a comparable delay. Likewise, the project manager can set 'milestones' or dates by which important aspects of the project need to be met.

Baseline

Here the minimum requirements for completing the project are defined and the project manager identifies how many people (often referred to as 'resources') and how much expense ('cost') are involved in the project, as well as any other requirements that are necessary for project completion. The project manager will manage assumptions and risks related to the project and will identify project constraints, typically relating to schedule, resources, budget and scope. A change in one constraint will typically affect the other constraints; for example, if the project involves supporting or planning a new ward, or new staffing structures or staffing levels in an emergency department, and this implies that additional resources will be needed, these features are added as part of the project scope, which will have possible impacts on scheduling, other resources and the budget.

Progress or Executing the Project

Once the project team is established and the project manager knows what resources are available and how much is in the budget, those resources and budget are then allocated to various tasks in the project. Key to this is the act of delegation and the manager's communication skills (Stanley 2011). For example, if the project involves the introduction of new medical or nursing equipment, the project manager might allocate the testing or training required to others in the project team. This phase is about doing what is planned and putting the plan into practice (Kloppenborg 2019).

Acceptance or Controlling the Project

The project manager is in charge of updating the project plans to reflect the actual time elapsed for each task. By keeping up with the details of progress, the project manager is able to understand how well the project is progressing overall. Gone are the days of pen-and-paper mapping exercises, and with the advent of greater information technology and computer software, health professionals are able to lead projects of increasing size and complexity. Specific products (such as Microsoft Project®) can be used to facilitate the administrative aspects of project management. However, basic Excel® spreadsheets can offer a suitable tool for less-complex projects.

Phase 3: The Final Phase

This phase is where the project is concluded and, if required, the product or service is handed over. Prior to final handover, formal approval, sometimes called the 'signoff', has to be implemented. Reports are exchanged, responsibilities are handed over and the project team is closed down.

Closure of the Project

The project manager and business owner (or other levels of management) bring together the project team and those who had an interest in the outcome of the project (stakeholders) to analyse its final outcome and successes, and consider whether things could have been improved or done differently.

Key Issues

The key features of project management include making sure that there are predetermined start and finish dates, a planned potential life cycle and an assigned budget (Kloppenborg 2019). It is important that non-repetitive (unique) tasks, resources from various allocations, a single point of responsibility and team roles and relationships are established from the outset. In addition, no matter what the type of project, project management typically follows the same pattern of definition, planning, execution, control and closure.

The Components of Project Management

The following is a summary of the key components of project management. Underpinning all of these should be consideration of the particular organisational culture you are working within.

- **Scope:** What does the project cover? How is it going to be conducted? Why is it necessary? What work needs to be done?
- **Objectives:** Use a SMART framework. What specifically are your goals? (General goals may also be important at this stage but the objectives are more focused and specific.)
- **Strategy:** This is your master plan. How will you meet your objectives?
- **Budget:** What can you spend? What might be your costs?
- **Schedule:** What is the timeline? What are the milestones for the project?
- **Customer or client:** Who are you working for?
- **Stakeholders:** Who else is involved in this project or will be affected by it?
- **Methodologies:** What project management methodology and/or charting methods are you planning to use?
- **Quality:** What are your standards? What are the criteria for success?
- **Environment:** What impact will the environment (internal and external) have on your project?
- **Risks:** What could go wrong? How will you foresee such events happening and plan to avoid them?
- **Resources:** What can you lay your hands on? What is available? What do you need? Can you afford it?
- **The end:** How will you measure success?

Final Project Management Issues

Recent trends in project management include project portfolio management (PPM), which is a move by organisations to maintain control over numerous projects by evaluating how well each project aligns with the overall strategic goals and quantifying its value (Project Management Institute 2017). An organisation will typically be working on multiple projects, each resulting in potentially differing amounts of return or value. The company or agency may decide to eliminate those projects with a lower return in order to dedicate greater resources to the remaining projects or in order to preserve those with the highest return or value.

Implications for Clinical Leaders

Project management is a valid and well-known approach to dealing with change in a structured way, yet we have found that it remains peripheral to health professional education. Few health professionals are aware of what project management is or are prepared for the phases required to initiate and successfully implement it. Gaining greater understanding of project management in health services may streamline or facilitate more effective change management at all levels of healthcare and have positive impacts on health service quality.

This may allow clinically focused health professionals to play a greater part in initiating and/or leading projects at a range of levels across the health services and to manage them with confidence and competence.

Therefore, instruction in the use and application of project management, and tools to support effective project management, should be introduced into education programmes for healthcare professionals. A specific recommendation is to include project management as a fundamental component of education for clinical leaders. This may help bring the voice and values of clinically focused health professionals to a greater range of projects, innovative change activities and healthcare initiatives.

Case Study 16.1   Sahar Hashemi

Sahar Hashemi is best known as the co-founder of the coffee shop chain Coffee Republic and the confectionery brand Skinny Candy in the UK. The book she wrote with her brother Bobby, *Anyone Can Do It: Building Coffee Republic from our Kitchen Table*, outlines how their coffee shop project moved from an idea to a high-street brand that for a time rivalled the big US coffee chains. Read this brief biography and consider the challenge that follows.

Sahar attended the City of London School for Girls and then studied law in Bristol. She worked for a very successful law firm for a few years, and in 1995 she and her brother, Bobby, set out plans to open a US-style coffee shop in London. The brand proved very successful, and by 2001 there were 108 stores across the UK. This was the year Sahar left Coffee Republic to focus on other ventures.

The coffee shop soon went into decline, and by 2009, after a number of shops had been closed, the business was sold to an investment firm and now operates under the name Coffee Republic Trading.

Sahar went on to write two books about her business management style and became more involved in charity work, including with The Prince's Trust, the National Society for the Prevention of Cruelty to Children (NSPCC) Corporate Development Board and as a patron of the charity Child Bereavement UK. In 2005, she started a new business, Skinny Candy, which offers low-fat sweets and chocolates, although in 2007 she sold 50% of the business to a partner. She has been a strong advocate for women in business and frequently speaks about innovation, entrepreneurship and women's business issues. In 2012, she was appointed an Officer of the Order of the British Empire (OBE) and has received a number of other awards.

Challenge: Can 'anyone do it', as Sahar's book suggests? Do you have to go to a privileged school, win a scholarship or have an elite career path? Is success about being 'switched on', as she suggests in her second book? Sahar's view is that we all have the capacity to do great things, we just need to turn on our risk-taking switch and have a go. What do you think about these ideas? Are you 'just a nurse' or 'just a physio' or 'just a whatever'? Is what we are or who we are important in terms of us dreaming or trying for our dreams? Could mastery of project management skills help in terms of making a smoother transition for us all in terms of realising our dreams or reaching our career goals? Reflect on these questions as you consider what Sahar Hashemi achieved 'from her kitchen table'.

Summary

- Systems thinking is essential when considering quality initiatives.
- A quality management system incorporates a constant cycle of quality planning, quality improvement and quality control, with quality assurance being integral to each of these aspects and a learning environment at its heart.
- Improvement can best be achieved through a structured approach, such as following the patterns of quality improvement models and project management.
- Project management allows clinical leaders to initiate change in a controlled, measured and systematic way.
- Success in implementing a project will be dependent on good planning, effective communication with all people involved, understanding and anticipating the risks and putting plans in place to manage them.
- Once the project has been implemented and is complete, this is not the end of the cycle. Continuous monitoring and evaluation are required and, often, the full quality improvement cycle needs to be implemented.

Mind Press-Ups

Exercise 16.1

Now that you have an idea of what constitutes project management, imagine you have a birthday party to deliver. Undertake the following task:

- **Plan a birthday party:** Budget $2000.
- **Customer specifications:** The party should be in your community.

Think about drinks, gifts, food, entertainment, music, dancing, guests and all the aspects of a really good party. Consider all the information offered in this chapter as you plan your project.

Exercise 16.2

Does managing a project mean taking total control? What are the other skills (some are outlined in this book) that you think might be used to support the job of managing a project successfully?

Exercise 16.3

Can clinical leaders really change the quality on offer to clients in the health service? Have you seen it happen? Look around your clinical area. What can you see in practice that has come about because of the initiative, courage and involvement of clinically focused health professionals?

References

Abdallah, A. (2014). Implementing quality initiatives in healthcare organisations: drivers and challenges. *International Journal of Health Care Quality Assurance* 27 (3): 166–181.

Ackoff, R.L. (1981). *Creating the Corporate Future*. New York: Wiley.

Agency for Healthcare Research and Quality (2021). Types of Health Care Quality Measures. https://www.ahrq.gov/talkingquality/measures/types.html (accessed 17 October 2021).

Braithwaite, J., Glasziou, P., and Westbrook, J. (2020). The three numbers you need to know about healthcare: the 60-30-10 challenge. *BMC Medicine* 18 (102): https://doi.org/10.1186/s12916-020-01563-4.

Checkland, P. (1981). *Systems Thinking, Systems Practice*. New York: Wiley.

DeFeo, J.A. (2019). *The Juran Trilogy: Quality Planning*. https://www.juran.com/blog/the-juran-trilogy-quality-planning (accessed 17 October 2021).

Health Improvement Scotland (2021). *Quality Management System Portfolio*. https://ihub.scot/improvement-programmes/quality-management-system-portfolio (accessed 17 October 2021).

Institute of Medicine (2001). *Crossing the Quality Chasm: A New Health System for the 21st Century*. Washington, D.C: National Academy Press.

Juran, J.M. (1993). Why quality initiatives fail. *Journal of Business Strategy* 14 (4): 35–38.

Kloppenborg, T.J. (2019). *Contemporary Project Management*, 4e. Sydney, NSW: Cengage Learning.

Langley, G.J., Moen, R.D., Nolan, K.M. et al. (2009). *The Improvement Guide: A Practical Approach to Enhancing Organizational Performance*, 2e. London: Wiley.

Lenoci-Edwards, J. (2018). *The Difference Between Change and Improvement*. http://www.ihi.org/communities/blogs/the-difference-between-change-and-improvement (accessed 17 October 2021).

Pexton, C. (2016). Healthcare quality initiatives: The role of leadership. *iSixSigma* (March 12). https://www.isixsigma.com/implementation/change-management-implementation/healthcare-quality-initiatives-role-leadership (accessed 17 October 2021).

Project Management Institute (2017). *A Guide to the Project Management Body of Knowledge (PMBOK® Guide)*, 6e. Newtown Square, PA: Project Management Institute.

Stanley, D. (2011). *Clinical Leadership: Innovation into Action*. South Yarra, VIC: Palgrave Macmillan.

Stanley, D. and Anderson, J. (2015). Advice for running a successful research team. *Nurse Researcher* 23 (2): 34–38.

Welsh Government (2021). Quality and Safety Framework: Learning and Improving. https://eur03.safelinks.protection.outlook.com/?url=https%3A%2F%2Fgov.wales%2Fnhs-quality-and-safety-framework&data=04%7C01%7Cjamesa43%40cardiff.ac.uk%7C8b028b5bb1df40b200b508d979ff4d6b%7Cbdb74b3095684856bdbf06759778fcbc%7C1%7C0%7C637674959944209387%7CUnknown%7CTWFpbGZsb3d8eyJWIjoiMC4wLjAwMDAiLCJQIjoiV2luMzIiLCJBTiI6Ik1haWwiLCJXVCI6Mn0%3D%7C2000&sdata=mxaJKt8J%2BTFY1mg3p34TPxrhhmrbfe9pP5dIg9OZuBs%3D&reserved=0 (accessed 17 October 2021)

Part III

Clinical Leadership Issues: The Context of Values-Based Leadership

In politics if you want anything said, ask a man; if you want anything done, ask a woman.

Margaret Thatcher 1925–2013, prime minister of the UK 1979–1990

The final part of this book places clinical leadership issues in context. Part I dealt with who clinical leaders are, their characteristics and the theories and details of leadership, in order to support an understanding of how health professionals can be seen as leaders in the clinical arena. Part II offered a range of tools that offer insights into how health professionals can effectively manage values to help bring about innovation, change and improvements in quality. Part III considers matters that affect the context within which nurses and other health professionals work.

Chapter 17 outlines the impact of gender and generational differences on how leadership is perceived and applied. How these two factors are viewed within organisations and by health practitioners can have a significant influence on the clinically focused leader's ability to express their values and may indeed affect the expression of their values. Chapter 18 discusses the impact of power and politics on how health professionals lead. Power, influence and politics are defined, the types and styles of power are outlined and critical social theory is used as a vehicle to explore the impact of politics on healthcare. The chapter also offers some practical advice about dealing with the media and becoming politically active or being 'influenced'. Chapter 19 addresses issues of empowerment and oppression. These are defined and explored in relation to their impact on nursing in particular, and health professional activity in general. A number of personal reflections are offered as examples throughout the chapter, and empowerment is explained as 'the walk and the choice about which path to take'. The characteristics of an oppressed group are outlined and strategies for dealing with oppression are offered. Chapter 20 discusses how leadership may be conceptualised when leading through a crisis. Finally, Chapter 21 offers a summary of the main points covered in the book through a discussion of congruent leadership and clinical leadership. It offers further examples of congruent leadership and how this leadership theory influences a clinical leader's values and capacity to initiate change and promote innovation and quality in clinical practice.

Clinical Leadership in Nursing and Healthcare, Third Edition.
Edited by David Stanley, Clare L. Bennett and Alison H. James.
© 2023 John Wiley & Sons Ltd. Published 2023 by John Wiley & Sons Ltd.

17

Gender, Generational Groups and Leadership

Julie Reis and Denise Blanchard

We are here to claim our right as women, not only to be free, but to fight for freedom. That it is our right as well as our duty.
Christabel Pankhurst, 1880–1958, British suffragette, in 'Votes for Women', 31 March 1911

Introduction: The Impact of Gender and Generations

This chapter addresses the issues of gender and its relationship to leadership for health professionals and how different generational groups may or may not influence leadership. It begins by asking whether there is a difference between the leadership styles of men and women. The challenges women face in achieving leadership recognition are outlined and factors that hinder women from attaining leadership roles. The chapter also considers the potential causes of gender differences and the barriers women may face in reaching their leadership potential, offering recommendations to help women overcome the challenges. The theory of congruent leadership is linked to a female perspective on leadership to demonstrate that clinical leaders (male or female) may be advantageous by applying a congruent leadership approach to their clinical leadership role. The discussion then moves to the issue of generational differences and considers whether such differences affect how health service leaders lead or manage. The chapter concludes by exploring what can be done to address the impact of generational differences.

Is There a Difference?

Over the past 25 years, much has been written regarding the relationship between gender and leadership from various disciplines, including healthcare, education, management, economics, political science, sociology and psychology. Despite this, the literature remains fragmented and incomplete (Abdallah and Jibai 2020; Shen and Joseph 2021). Discussions about the different leadership styles between men and women continue due to the

Clinical Leadership in Nursing and Healthcare, Third Edition.
Edited by David Stanley, Clare L. Bennett and Alison H. James.
© 2023 John Wiley & Sons Ltd. Published 2023 by John Wiley & Sons Ltd.

recognition that women remain underrepresented in leadership positions (Seo et al. 2017; Badura et al. 2018; Madsen and Andrade 2018; Smith et al. 2021).

The Case for a Difference

Several studies have supported the hypothesis that gender differences in leadership styles exist (Eagly and Carli 2007; Rincón et al. 2017; Faizan et al. 2018). Vinnicombe (1999) and Sandberg (2015) support that both male and female managers agree that gender-based differences in management styles exist. Nielsen and Huse (2010) undertook research that supported this notion and proposed that while men and women do not differ in their ability to perform operational tasks, there is a difference in their perspectives on strategic decision making because of their different sensitivity to the needs of others. Women's leadership competencies are superior in taking the initiative, self-development, integrity, honesty and driving for results (Zenger and Folkman 2012; O'Reilly 2015). In terms of leadership styles, Eagly and Johnson's (1990) study and another by Eagly and Carli (2007) suggested statistical differences in the perceived leadership roles and effectiveness of male and female leaders. These studies demonstrated that female leaders preferred a more democratic/participative style and were less directive/autocratic (Sahoo and Das 2012; Abdallah and Jibai 2020). Women leaders were also more transformational (Vinnicombe 1999; Nash et al. 2017), people-orientated and participative (Faizan et al. 2018). In contrast, male leaders were more likely to show a preference for autocratic, transactional reward and punishment and laissez-faire styles of leadership (Vinnicombe 1999; Faizan et al. 2018). Women were demonstrated to be less hierarchical, more cooperative and collaborative, place more emphasis on communication affiliation and nurturing, and be more attuned to the self-esteem of others (a feature of emotional intelligence; see Chapter 15).

The McKinsey and Company (2021) study, which surveyed 423 companies and over 65 000 employees in the United States and Canada, supported these views and added that women in senior positions showed styles that supported their teams' well-being and promoted diversity equity and inclusion. Similarly, in Australia, Griffiths et al. (2019) investigated gender stereotypes and desired leadership attributes in 1,885 participants from 25 companies and found that women were generally more closely associated with communal qualities than men. They were more focused on building relationships, collaborating and developing others. These were leadership attributes and qualities that participants preferred in their leaders (Griffiths et al. 2019). This finding aligns with Sahoo and Das (2012), who proposed that female entrepreneurs (leaders) in the twenty-first century succeeded because they gave more attention to intellectual capital, the creation of self-organising networks, clear organisational goals, transparency, consensus building and collaboration and demonstrated a more 'connected' style of leadership. Women's leadership can be described as people-focused, role modelling and focused on clear expectations and rewards. Appelbaum et al. (2003) call these feminine values and see them as having traction in rebalancing the traditional masculine values of competitiveness and authoritarianism. They see the feminine values as heightened communication skills, advanced conflict resolution skills, well-developed interpersonal skills and a softer approach to handling people, including empathy. They add that rebalancing values towards more feminine approaches is increasingly identified as key to business success.

The Case for No Difference

Vinnicombe (1999) believes that gender in leadership terms is a 'red herring', citing other factors such as the organisational culture, the leadership style of the 'boss' and office attitudes as having a more influential role. Gender is proposed as only one feature of the maze of issues that determine excellent or effective managers or leaders, and both men and women can be good and bad as leaders. This view that it is more a case of individual attributes is supported by Appelbaum et al. (2003). They claim that leadership style is based on an analysis of the context or situation rather than an inherent gender-based predisposition.

Issues of socialisation appear to drive leadership styles, and the dominant theme in leadership has been the masculine model. This is being rebalanced with a more flexible emotional approach used to offset the traditional rational approach to understanding leadership. Effective leadership is not the exclusive domain of either gender, and both can learn from the other (Appelbaum et al. 2003). Andersen and Hansson (2011) found minimal evidence supporting how gender differences affected leadership styles. Moran (1992) suggested that while some slight differences may be found, these may result from differences in socialisation. Leaders are instead simply people with divergent abilities regardless of their gender. Moran (1992) also identified that male and female leaders could learn from each other,

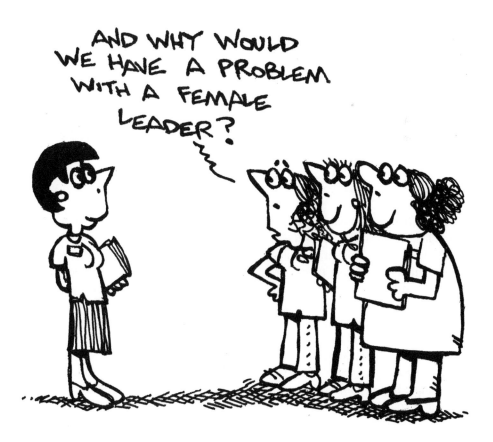

adding strength to their organisations and helping each other to produce a win-win situation for both genders.

A recent study by Shen and Joseph (2021) proposes that the body of literature has focused on the role of gender rather than on the nature and nuanced criterion of leadership behaviour and job performance and could not capture the unique implications and interconnection of gender and leadership outcome. When they applied Campbell et al.'s (1993) theory and model of job performance to the literature, they discerned a highly complex relationship that demonstrated that leader gender appeared to influence leadership processes directly, indirectly, and had a moderating effect on the leadership process. Significantly, they found that female leaders engaged in more effective leadership behaviours than men.

While there is little agreement on evidence supporting gender differences in leadership styles, there are clear differences in the challenges women face when seeking leadership or senior management positions. These are explored in the following section.

Challenges for Women in Leadership

Gender inequality remains evident in leadership roles worldwide. While Catalyst (2020) reports that the proportion of women in senior management roles grew in 2019 to 29%, the highest number on record, men were still likely to dominate senior executive roles globally. Although women have made substantial gains in representation in leadership roles, women leaders face challenges from personal, professional, and global circumstances (Patel 2013). In Europe, the United States, Canada, and Australia, women only represented approximately 30–36% of all management positions while accounting for almost half of the labour force. In healthcare services, women represent 71% of the global workforce, and the sector is advancing women into leadership roles faster than other sectors (Cassells and Duncan 2020; Mousa et al. 2021). This situation creates a compelling case for unlocking the full potential of women leaders. The first case supporting a proposition to include more women as leaders is that greater leadership diversity leads to more significant competitive advantage, with a more flexible approach to products and services that ultimately leads organisations to better meeting service users' needs (Hanna 2012; Cassells and Duncan 2020).

Evidence that women have a positive effect on corporate performance or on the business bottom line is offered by Catalyst (2007), an American non-profit organisation devoted to the advancement of women in business, who compared Fortune 500 companies on the representation of women on their boards and their corporate performance. They noted that companies with a higher representation of female leaders had a return on equity increase of 53%, a profit margin increase of 42% and an increased return on invested capital of 66%. Management consultancy McKinsey (2007) confirmed the relationship between high levels of female leadership by indicating that the greater the gender diversity at the higher levels of an organisation, the greater the returns on equity and the better the operating results, which led to a more robust stock price growth of up to 70%. Wilson and Atlantar (2009) found that having at least one woman on the board of directors decreased bankruptcy by a complete 20%, and Franke (1997) suggested that companies with women on their boards employed more ethical behaviour and better corporate governance. Further, based on an analysis of more than 150 companies, Post et al. (2021) found that women on management teams were able to change perspectives relating to innovation and, in so doing, were able to enable firms to consider a wider range of strategies for creating value. Specifically, firms moved from merger and acquisition strategies to more investment into internal research and development, resulting in an average 1.1% increase. Additionally, firms began to exhibit higher levels of both openness to change and aversion to risk (Post et al. 2021).

Despite these advantages, from a global perspective women do not seem to advance quickly into leadership or decision-making roles and even when they do, there is still a considerable disparity in salaries compared to men in similar management positions (Tsui 1998; Marshall 2021). Women do not seem to receive equal access to education and are not being employed at equal rates to their male counterparts, and in some countries women still face legislative barriers, have limited access to credit or mentorship and there may even be laws denying them access to collateral. Women are universally under-represented on business boards in Europe and across the globe (European Commission 2020). In the United States, women make up 16% of board members; in Australia and Canada, female representation is at about 11%; in India, female board members account for 5% (European Commission 2020); in the Asia-Pacific region, female board members are 14.8%, and in the Middle East, board members constitute only 3.7% of leadership teams (Corporate Women Directors International 2020).

Globally, women are also less represented in primary and secondary education, although more women are being educated at the tertiary level. This is not reflected in the employment figures, though, as women in many parts of the world have lower participation in the workforce than men, with rates below 25% in Egypt, India, Pakistan, Saudi Arabia and Morocco; below 45% in Italy, Greece and Rwanda; below 50% in South Africa, Belgium and Chile; and 60% in the UK, United States and Germany (World Bank 2021).

The COVID-19 pandemic decreased advancement opportunities for women, and it has taken a toll on women's leadership roles especially, with stress and burnout outcomes (McKinsey and Company 2021; EgonZehnder 2021). Mercer (2020) analysed over 1,100 organisations across the world and found that the representation of women in leadership was decreasing. The COVID-19 pandemic has affected women's participation in the labour force and has exacerbated the pay gap between women and men (Catalyst 2021). Women have experienced unprecedented job losses across the world. Employment and income trends in China, Italy, Japan, South Korea, the United Kingdom, and the United States have found that women are 24% more likely to lose their jobs permanently than men (Catalyst 2021).

Women also face personal issues not attributed to male workers, such as the 'double burden', where they retain a high proportion of responsibility for domestic and care-giving duties and searching for paid employment and professional opportunities. Also known as the 'double burden syndrome', this is more pronounced in Asian and African communities, although women in Europe and other developed parts of the world are also responsible for twice as many domestic duties as men (McKinsey 2007). Research by Artabane et al. (2017) suggests that midcareer women with children were almost six times more likely to be the primary parent, and in addition, 61% of midcareer women have a spouse or partner pursuing a more intense or equally intense career versus 38% of midcareer men. This impacts the ability of women to advance their career.

Women may face a crisis of confidence, and in environments expected to be dominated by male behaviour, women lack belief in their abilities and the capacity to communicate confidence (Eagly 2003). Finally, women also suffer from gender bias and stereotyping, with many unfortunate assumptions made about their ambitions and potential, and women having to work harder to be perceived as equally competent to men in many leadership and management areas (Lyness and Heilman 2006; Evans and Maley 2021). All these factors impact women's capacity to reach or participate in attaining higher-level leadership roles.

The Causes of Gender Differences in Leadership

Several factors may lead to perceptions that men and women lead differently or seek leadership position roles because of their gender. Patel (2013) separates these into personal differences and professional differences.

Personal Differences

- **Confidence:** Generally, men can be characterised as more confident than women (Bengtsson et al. 2005). Research by Artabane et al. (2017) indicates that lower confidence levels can serve to undermine the willingness of women to seek out opportunities for leadership positions, voice opinions to which others may not agree, or make a decision that may be risky, especially if they suspect that their supervisor might not be fully supportive.
- **Apologetic:** Women are more apologetic than men (Schumann and Ross 2010).
- **Bluffing:** Guidice et al. (2009) found that men show a greater capacity to bluff, or at least they believed that they were better at bluffing than women (Holm 2005). Holm's (2005) study also found that both genders were more likely to lie to women than to men.
- **Social risk:** While women are considered more risk averse than men, they are more risk ready because they have greater social sensitivity and can handle social uncertainty better. As such, they will take social risks (Harris et al. 2006).
- **Emotional and facial recognition:** Women are better at recognising subtle facial expressions (Hoffman et al. 2010), helping them more effectively 'read' someone else's intentions and state of mind (Enticott et al. 2008). This supports their capacity to take more social risks.
- **Communication styles:** Marquis and Huston (2012) uphold the view that men and women communicate differently, with men often focusing on business issues while women bring social and personal issues into the business domain.
- **Emotions and actions:** Cunningham and Roberts (2012) indicate that men and women differ in their impulsive base reaction, where women are more likely to respond through feelings and men to respond through action. Thus, men's immediate reaction to a stimulus is to act or look for a solution, while women tend to feel. Patel (2013, p. 15) concludes that men are generally 'more overconfident and optimistic, whereas women have a higher social sensitivity and react by feeling'.
- **Conscientiousness:** Huszczo and Endres (2017) found that women's conscientiousness levels were significantly higher than men. Their study found that conscientiousness is an

important predictor of leadership self-efficacy in that conscientious individuals have higher confidence in their ability to lead as they are more organised, proactive and responsible.

- **Openness to experience:** Characterised by creativity and an appreciation for new experiences, openness is reported to play an essential role in leadership self-efficacy (Huszczo and Endres 2017). In their study, Huszczo and Endres (2017) found that women were more open to experiences than men.

Professional Differences

- **Risk aversion:** Generally, women are reported as more risk-averse than men (Weber et al. 2002; Eckel and Grossman 2008). Higher levels of testosterone in men have been correlated with higher levels of risk-taking (Sapienza et al. 2009).
- **Competitive environments:** Niederle and Versterlund (2007) found that women have a lower preference for competitive environments and, as Appelbaum et al. (2003) established, these environments make women feel less welcome and possibly even threatened.
- **Response to uncertainty:** Women are said to respond to uncertainty with fear, while men are reported to respond with anger (Grossman and Wood 1993). This is significant, as these emotions trigger different risk perception and risk-taking responses, with fear diminishing risk-taking and anger increasing it (Lerner and Keltner 2001). When confronted with stress, according to Lighthall et al. (2012), women decide more slowly and tend towards less risk-taking, while men veer in the opposite direction (Lighthall et al. 2012).
- **Context:** In a 2009 study, women were reported to react to the environment more emotionally and are generally more perceptive, being more likely to be affected by the context (Croson and Gneezy 2009).
- **Evolution:** From an evolutionary perspective, men were hunters and women were gatherers. These traditional roles may have evolved into preferences for certain behaviours (Buss 2012), with hunting skills more associated with leadership roles. Risk-taking is also thought to be associated with status: taking greater risks increases status and may lead to more opportunities for leadership.
- **Team relationships:** Grossman and Valiga (2021) suggest that men see issues as black and white, while women see more grey issues; men also often deal with teams from a purely business focus, while women bring broader personal or social issues into their team relationships, possibly enabling women to establish more effective team relationships.
- **Cultural norms in the workplace:** Workplaces are impacted by cultural norms in the workplace, which are shaped by both conscious and unconscious bias. According to Artabane et al. (2017), bias impacts the experiences one has in the workplace. For women, such bias can limit a woman's opportunities to take on challenging projects. Results cited from Artabane et al. (2017) found that in comparison to midcareer men, 41% of midcareer women were more likely to believe that they do not have the same opportunities for advancement, 20% more likely to not feel inspired and motivated by their work and 38% more likely to believe that the volume and pace of work expected to advance is not reasonable.

Professional differences focus on the different approaches that men and women have to risk taking. Patel (2013) also emphasises biological differences in the structure and function of the brain. It is claimed that whereas men favour right-brain functions (logic, detail, linear tasks), women's brains do not favour the left brain (holistic, intuitive, abstract) but instead operate on a higher interconnectedness between the right and left hemispheres. This interconnectedness may explain women's greater social risk-taking, better facial recognition skills and higher ability to process emotional information (Cunningham and Roberts 2012).

Potential Barriers that Female Leaders Face

There is considerable agreement that women face more barriers to becoming leaders and more pressure from their roles than men do, especially for leadership roles in male-dominated professions or industries (Gardiner and Tiggemann 1999; Eagly and Johannesen-Schmidt 2001). They remain a minority on corporate boards and organisations (Roberts and Brown 2019; Cassells and Duncan 2020) and underrepresented in healthcare leadership (Kalaitzi et al. 2017; Mousa et al. 2021). Women can exhibit styles that allow them to work effectively as leaders, but several barriers keep them from fulfilling senior leadership or mid-level management roles remain. In their systematic review of women leadership barriers in healthcare, academia and business, Kalaitzi et al. (2017) found 26 barriers to women's leadership. Some or all of these barriers affected all of the discipline areas and included:

1) **Lack of career advancement opportunities:** These were affected by rigid criteria for promotion and recognition, lack of funding, further compounded by unequal access to research positions, publishing and awards.
2) **Culture:** This was related to cultural and institutional barriers that generated both indirect and direct discrimination
3) **Family** (espousal) support: Support cited included partners, other family members, and childcare.
4) **Gender bias** (discrimination): The perception that some professions were classed as female or male. As outlined in the previous section, women are subject to bias based on their approach to leadership. Heilman and Parks-Stamm (2007) showed that female leaders were likely to be viewed negatively when adopting masculine leadership characteristics. However, if female leaders demonstrate feminine traits but perform a 'male role', they are seen as too emotional and lacking in assertiveness (Eagly and Carli 2007). These stereotypical views of women as less capable leaders than men persist (Appelbaum et al. 2003).
5) **Gender gap:** Referred to the under-representation of women in hierarchical positions even when they represented the majority of the workforce.
6) **Gender pay gap:** Unequal pay for work of equal value.
7) **Glass ceiling:** Referred to the 'invisible barriers' based on prejudice that limited the advancement of women to higher positions in their career paths.
8) **Glass cliff:** Related to those women assigned to risky, precarious positions, with little material and social resources and support.

9) **Isolation:** Exacerbated by the predominance of 'old boys clubs', inflexible corporate cultures and male dominated leadership teams.

10) **Lack of a flexible work environment:** Referred to organisational features that reflected men's lives and situations.

11) **Lack of confidence:** This was impacted by self-doubt and underestimating personal capabilities. Women continue to under-rate their ability to perform effectively in senior or mid-level management or leadership positions (Eagly 2003). A lack of confidence manifests in women leaders seeking or accepting less in terms of money, rewards and praise for their leadership skills (Appelbaum et al. 2003).

12) **Lack of mentoring:** This related to the availability of and access to mentors.

13) **Lack of networking:** Impacted career trajectories, access to jobs and the ability to channel information and referrals to create influence and reputation. It also impacted upon emotional support, feedback and advice. Although women are more skilled at social engagement, their networking skills are not as well-honed as those of men in the workplace. Ely et al. (2011) have found that women are reluctant to use networking as it is perceived as inauthentic and embroiled in stereotypical male-orientated social activities. Forret and Dougherty (2004) recommend that women adopt different strategies to become more visible in the organisation to have their leadership skills recognised.

14) **Leadership skills:** Access to leadership programs to enable the transition to more senior roles is not available.

15) **Personal health:** Served to devalue and marginalise women.

16) **Race discrimination:** Described how minority and underrepresented groups had a competitive disadvantage.

17) **Sexual harassment: Being subjected to unwelcome or unwanted sexual advances or harassment creating feelings of disempowerment / discomfort / being objectified and abused.**

18) **Lack of social support**: Resistance to female leadership and adoption of new cultures and social norms.

19) **Stereotypes (male-dominated culture, negative organisation environment):** This referred to the habitual privileging of stereotyped 'maleness' as the only credible context for leadership, created a heavily-gendered work environment.

20) **Work/life balance:** The need to successfully reconcile professional and family obligations.

21) **Negotiation:** Cialdini (2001) found that while women can negotiate as well as men, they enter negotiations with lower expectations.

22) **Work environment:** Some women experience work environments where they feel less welcome and even threatened by what they may perceive as a self-serving or domineering organisational culture. Some organisations favour masculine values and masculine attributes propagated by traditional structures or the 'old boy network' and there may be a lack of value placed on 'feminine' characteristics (Appelbaum et al. 2003).

23) **Authority and leadership identity:** Women find it more challenging to claim authority over their leadership roles (Lagace 2003). Thus, when leadership roles are associated with decisiveness, assertiveness and independence, women, who are

commonly assumed to be friendly, caring and selfless, suffer from a form of gender bias that interferes with developing an appropriate leader identity. The leadership identity constructed is often overly masculine, causing women to avoid taking up leadership roles or feel that they fit better with men. Although men make up a minority in the nursing workforce, this phenomenon may explain why they are more evident in higher numbers in the management and middle-management ranks.

24) **Role models and mentors:** Successful and effective female leadership role models are few. They do exist, but in relatively small numbers (Ely et al. 2011). To avoid disapproval, women will role model modest behaviours, seeking to avoid attention, and making it difficult for women aspiring to management or leadership positions to recognise or locate mentors or role models (see the Female Leader role models offered at the end of each chapter).

25) **Career paths:** Women are more likely to have non-linear career paths. Taking time out with family commitments and avoiding jobs that feature travel led McKinsey (2007) to conclude that many organisations are intolerant of women's career paths and needs.

26) **Scrutiny:** While female leaders are noted as adopting modest behaviours to avoid attention, once a female leader is identified they are commonly subjected to increased scrutiny, watched more closely and assessed with greater attention than many of their male counterparts. The net effect of this may be an increase in risk aversion, preventing their performance from being as competent as it might otherwise be.

The organisational structure and policies that serve to normalise gender stereotypes within workplaces have also created challenges and barriers for women. Unconscious bias and affinity bias remain a significant challenge for women who aspire to leadership positions (Evans and Maley 2021). In their study, Evans and Maley (2021) highlight that organisational regimes serve to reinforce men's dominance within the workplace in that they are perceived as more competent. This perception contributes to feelings of disillusionment due to lack of opportunity and scarcity of role models (Artabane et al. 2017). Additionally, unconscious bias has contributed to power imbalances and negative work environments that have enabled bullying, harassment, discrimination, a culture of silence and microaggressions and have had a negative effect on leadership aspirations and also the treatment of women in the workplace (Hillstrom 2018).

For almost 20 years, American activist Tarana Burke has worked with women and children who have experienced sexual assault and abuse within structures that support gendered violence and permit this violence, for example, workplace policies (Rose 2021). In a workshop led by Burke in 2006, she encouraged the girls to write the phrase 'me too' on a sticky note to identify if they had been victims of sexual assault (Stevens 2021) and discovered there was a significant issue with over half the class identifying *#MeToo*.

In 2017, the *#MeToo* became an online social movement where many women shared experiences of sexual assault or harassment using *#MeToo* on social media (Suk et al. 2019), where the American actress Alyssa Milano posted on Twitter, 'If you've been sexually harassed or assaulted write "me too" as a reply to this tweet'. The response was unparalleled, with the hashtag 'MeToo' used half a million times in the first 12 hours of Milano's post (Kaufman et al. 2019; Suk et al. 2019). Due to this movement, clearer policies on sexual harassment are evident (Rose 2021).

It remains a vexed question of how existing structures can change due to this movement challenging the structural violence and the required changes needed to impact the behaviours and actions highlighted through the *#MeToo* movement (Kaufman et al. 2019). French et al. (2021) findings indicate that 32% (n = 1847) of women identify that work relations between males and females are different now than in the previous two years, with female employees not getting the mentoring necessary for advancement opportunities in their career. The #MeToo movement highlights the need to create safe work environments in mentoring and growing female leadership opportunities for the future (Kaufman et al. 2019; French et al. 2021).

Reflection Point

Reflect on gender differences and then speak with a female colleague whom you see as an excellent leader. Ask them if they have felt they have been disadvantaged because of their gender, or if they have found any advantages in being a woman as they sought to secure a leadership position? What advice could they offer to aspiring female leaders? Also reflect on any work or social gender bias you may have faced yourself.

Recommendations and Strategies to Address Gender Differences Manage Gender Bias

Women are becoming more prominent in senior leadership and middle management positions in a range of organisations. They are also placed into environments that are built upon gender bias. Women in clinical leadership positions thus require skills and strategies to overcome challenges mentioned in this chapter. These points are offered as advice for female leaders to diminish gender differences and overcome the challenges that women may face when seeking leadership and management roles. Whilst it is acknowledged that the following recommendations are aimed at women taking personal responsibility for their goals and aspirations. These strategies are not suggested in place of the need to also pay attention to the inherent systemic gender bias in organisations and visibly increasing women's presence in leadership roles within society as a whole.

- **Become a role model:** If you are in a leadership position or aspire to one, be visible and approachable. Be there for others to come to and make time to share your own leadership journey with other women (EgonZehnder 2021).
- **Make health a priority:** EgonZehnder (2021) suggest that physical, mental and emotional health are important for balancing both work and personal life.
- **Join or start networks** (see Chapter 11): Professional and industry organisations offer many networking opportunities, although it may be that more local and specific networks can support colleagues. Establish mixed-gender professional and business networks (even beyond your own professional group) to establish relationships, widen perspectives and create opportunities.

- **Build your skills:** Become talent ready. Learn skills that will enhance your leadership potential and push your comfort zone of develop IT competence and people or communication skills. Take responsibility for growing your own career, skills and talents.
- **Be open:** As found by Huszczo and Endres (2017), the ability to be curious, flexible and open to experiences is a good predictor of leadership self-efficacy and ability.
- **Mentorship:** Find and connect with a quality mentor or life coach. Do not be afraid to ask for advice and show gratitude for any help or advice offered. Provide yourself available as a resource for others and seek out key individuals with whom you can build a trusting and symbiotic relationship (Rowe 2009; EgonZehnder 2021). As indicated by Evans and Maley (2021), confidence is an important success factor and confidence is attained by having a mentor who 'believes in you'.
- **Align your style with your values and beliefs:** Women's predominant leadership style may match well with congruent leadership as their values and beliefs are in line with or match their actions (Stanley 2011; Huszczo and Endres 2017). Gender congruency suggests that in maintaining a genuine and authentic approach to leadership, credibility will be enhanced, and trust will be fostered within the team. Sahoo and Das (2012) also recommend a 'connective' leadership style that allows women to perceive common ground and possibilities for handling division and difference.
- **Build technical and cultural competence:** The modern workplace means that leaders (male and female) need to be at ease with modern technology, as this facilitates communication strategies and networks. The complexity of any work environment also results in a need for leaders to become competent in dealing with the work culture, employing cultural, social and emotional intelligence. A work culture based on a patriarchal model presents specific challenges for female leaders. Investing in personal skills around emotional intelligence and social intelligence is vital to meeting your career goals.
- **Develop your confidence:** McKinsey (2007), Artabane et al. (2017) and Huszczo and Endres (2017) suggest confidence and self-belief increases aspiration. Thus, for female leaders to succeed they need to develop their confidence. This means making your achievements visible and being assertive. This can be achieved by ensuring that your manager knows your achievements (by sending on reports, telling your manager about your work and presenting your team's results), seeking the credit for work you have done, looking for feedback on your performance and asking for promotion (Catalyst 2011). Recent research by Carney et al. (2010) also recommends taking on a posture of confidence (called 'Power Poses') that will support your own confidence and show others your 'power'. These poses include physically taking up more space and keeping limbs open, or at least avoiding a subservient and powerless posture such as slumping and hunching your shoulders. Confidence is an attitude you can own.
- **Communication:** Speak directly and do not apologise. Speak as though you know you will be believed (Feldt 2012). Remain authentic and find a communication style that maximises your feeling of being genuine and that will diminish any miscommunication or misunderstanding based on stereotypical bias.
- **Be yourself:** Many women succeed as leaders and they often achieve great success without having to take on or infuse 'male' or masculine approaches to leadership. Do not adopt a leadership style that is unnatural or uncomfortable just to get ahead. Maybe the organisational culture is at fault or that an 'old boy network' dominates. Just be yourself.

Gender and Congruent Leadership

All leaders are different and use different styles or approaches depending on the situation, socialisation approach, relationships they have with their followers and their power. Gender is one factor in establishing these differences, although it need not be a barrier to successful leadership in the health service. Deuskat (1994) feels that organisations based on traditional masculine approaches are less inclined to promote or value transformational leadership approaches common to women's styles.

As the health service seeks to promote change and leadership that drives a values-based change agenda, maybe this favours female leaders, who are more likely to demonstrate a transformational or congruent style. But as Moran (1992) suggests, the core differences between male and female leadership styles are minor, and the similarities may be more substantial. Sharing or building on the styles and talents of both male and female leaders may provide a situation that allows both genders to flourish.

From a clinical leadership perspective, recent research supports that clinical leaders show the same attributes regardless of gender (Stanley 2014, 2019). In the studies that support this book, male and female paramedics and nurses mentioned identical characteristics when asked to describe the attributes of clinical leaders. Both genders suggested that clinical leaders need to have integrity and be approachable, clinically skilled, visible good communicators and supportive. Both groups suggested that they would be least likely to follow clinical leaders who were 'controlling' or who demonstrated strong 'management' skills, again linking the attributes of clinical leaders with a congruent approach to leadership. Both genders supported leaders who lived out their values and beliefs in their actions (Stanley 2011, 2014, 2019). Gender did not seem to be a feature that prevented clinical leaders from demonstrating practical congruent leadership skills.

Reflection Point

Men in nursing have been described as being on the 'glass elevator', while the 'glass ceiling has disadvantaged women seeking to advance'. Is this the case for other health professions where men are in the minority? If it is the case, how much of this phenomenon is down to gender, and how much is governed by other, non-gender-specific issues? What might these other issues be and how can they be overcome? Why does the elevator only carry men?

Generational Differences and Leadership

Generational cohorts allow for a way of understanding how formative life experiences interact to shape people's views of the world and offer suggestions as to why generational groups express different characteristics or are motivated and driven to express different values (De Meuse and Mlodzik 2010; Cahill and Cima 2016; Dimock 2019). Different generational groups are engaged in the workforce, and it is widely acknowledged that generational issues may affect how leaders emerge or are followed (Kogan 2001), because different generational groups are motivated and follow leaders for varying reasons (Nelsey and Brownie 2012). There are several generational groups to consider, described in the following sections.

Builders

Also known as Veterans, Traditionalists, the Silents, the Forgotten Generation and the War Generation, this includes people born before 1946. They make up few, if any, of the current workforce, although some will still be found in the ranks of volunteers serving generously in hospitals and community service organisations. They have a wealth of experience and continue to contribute because they believe in lifetime employment and they generally value hierarchies. They also appreciate dedication, rules and loyalty and believe that hard work will produce rewards. They prefer command-and-control management/leadership structures. Their core values are hard work, respect for authority, law and order, duty, honour, dedication and sacrifice (McCrindle 2021a).

Baby Boomers

This generation includes people born after World War II (between 1946 and 1964), who were raised in an era of optimism, opportunity and progress. Generally, 'Boomers' had secure jobs, access to good education and relative prosperity. As such, they question the status quo, embrace the 'big picture' and recognise the world as a smaller place. They value optimism, personal growth, equal rights, health and wellness and involvement (Weingarten 2009; McCrindle 2016). Baby Boomers are still evident in the health professional workforce and can be found in many senior and leadership positions, making them ideal mentors and preceptors (Nelsey and Brownie 2012). Their work ethic is strong. They value flexibility, they want to know that their ideas matter; for many, their work or career matters greatly and often defines them (Cahill and Cima 2016; McCrindle 2016).

Generation X

People born between 1965 and 1979 entered an age of rapid change, with changing social and economic factors affecting their education and social development. Many grew up in two-career families, faced high divorce rates, industrial downsizing and rapid developments in technology and communication. Those in this generation focus on personal development and actively oppose authority, the status quo and the belief that job security is a given. They value thinking globally, work/ life balance, technological and communication literacy and global diversity (Gursory et al. 2008; Weingarten 2009; Cahill and Cima 2016). At work, they want independence, informality, and time to pursue their own interests and to have fun (McCrindle 2016).

Generation Y

Also known as the 'nexters', 'internet generation' or 'Millennials', Generation Y includes people born between 1980 and 1994 (McCrindle 2021a). They are more numerous, more affluent, better educated and more ethnically diverse than any previous generation. By 2020, they made up over 50% of the workforce (Cran 2016). They display a range of positive social habits and are clear about the value of belonging to a group. Social media, constant connectivity and on-demand entertainment and communication are innovations in technology that Generation Y subscribe to. They are technologically savvy, good at multitasking and are keen to participate or collaborate in decisions. They like team- orientated workplaces, they expect to be treated with respect and they want to feel positive about themselves (Cahill and Cima 2016; McCrindle 2016). Their core values are optimism, civic duty, confidence, diversity, modesty, achievement, morality and teamwork. The focus of Generation Y in the workforce is to find an employer for which they *want* to work, and not to work because they *need* to (Cran 2016).

Generation Z

Describes those born between 1995 and 2009 (McCrindle 2021a). Gen Z are described as 'true digital natives' as they have been exposed to and been consumers of social, visual and network technology since birth (Francis and Hoefel 2018). Its members are well connected, well-educated and sophisticated and are commonly described as early adopters, brand influencers, social media drivers and pop-culture leaders. Gen Z has recognised that education is essential, and to survive in a competitive environment, they need to up-skill and retrain and cannot rely on work stability. Thus, lifelong learning is their mindset (Francis and Hoefel 2018; McCrindle 2021a). This generational group is developing during a time of crisis, with global recessions, acts of global terrorism and, significantly, the impact of climate change and COVID-19. Economically and socially, they have adapted and become more resilient. Concerning their participation in the workforce, O'Hara et al. (2019) have suggested that they expect to work in safe, collaborative, flexible, and motivating environments. Gen Z eschews traditional hierarchy, preferring a coach over a boss.

Generation Alpha

Generation Alpha is the generation emerging from 2010. This generation is set to conclude in 2024, and they are immersed in technology in a way that no previous generation has been. However, they are a generation faced with major issues that will require adaptability and acceptance, for example, being climate conscious and learning to address more climate uncertainty in the world. COVID-19 will also impact upon their formative years through home education and disruptions to face-to-face personal connections. Their leadership is likely to be accepting diversity and view diversity as a strength (McCrindle 2021b, c)

It is worth adding that the peer-reviewed literature concludes there are very few meaningful differences between generational groups (De Meuse and Mlodzik 2010) and that leaders (and organisations) would be better served by focusing on individuals and their intrapersonal/interpersonal issues rather than generational groups (Cahill and Cima 2016). However, health professionals, and nurses enter the workforce at a range of ages (Keepnews and Shin 2010; Stevanin et al. 2020), implying that the health workforce will comprise a wide range of generational groups. While recognising that each person, leader or manager is an individual, it is still good to understand each generational group. As found in Stevanin et al.'s (2020) study, leadership practices in clinical setting need to be flexible and tailored to meet the needs of each generation. This may allow leaders and managers in the health service to come to terms with what may drive or motivate each group and to work more collaboratively and keep staff engaged, valued and respected (Hayes et al. 2010; Stanley 2010; Stevanin et al. 2020). Dealing with employees across the generational spectrum is vital if employers are to retain their workforce, motivate staff and lead or be led by professional colleagues. Engaging with multiple generational groups will help develop a more diverse workforce and support strategies for dealing with conflict based on generational differences or consequent differences in values. It may also allow employers to prepare for the impending shift as Baby Boomers leave the workforce and Generations X, Y and Z move into more prominent positions (De Meuse and Mlodzik 2010; Stevanin et al. 2020).

Case Study 17.1   Greta Thunberg 'The Greta Effect'

Greta Thunberg rose to prominence in August 2018, when, at age 15, she skipped school and staged a solo protest outside of the Swedish parliament calling for action on climate change. She inadvertently started a global movement. Read her story and consider the challenge that follows.

Greta Thunberg was born in Sweden in 2003. Her mother, Malenda Ernman, was an internationally acclaimed opera singer, and her father, Svante Thunberg, was an actor (Watts 2019). She is also the granddaughter of actor and director Olof Thunberg Ernman. Greta has a younger sister named Beata.

Greta was an exceptionally bright child, but introverted. She felt she was never like her classmates, 'I have always been that girl in the back who doesn't say anything' (in Watts 2019), and she felt that she had the propensity to overthink things.

> I overthink. Some people can just let things go, but I can't, especially if there's something that worries me or makes me sad. I remember when I was younger, and in school, our teachers showed us films of plastic in the ocean, starving polar bears and so on. I cried through all the movies. My classmates were concerned when they watched the film, but when it stopped, they started thinking about other things. I couldn't do that. Those pictures were stuck in my head. (Watts 2019)

At age 8, Greta's class was shown documentaries about climate change and global warming and Greta recalled thinking that 'it was very strange that humans...could be capable of changing the Earth's climate' (Thunberg 2018). Further, Greta could not understand the inaction around the burning of fossil fuels. She was shocked that adults did not appear to take the issue seriously.

> If burning fossil fuels was so bad that it threatened our very existence, how could we just continue like before? Why were there no restrictions? Why wasn't it made illegal? To me, that did not add up. It was too unreal. (TEDx Stockholm 2018)

Greta reports that that after learning about global warming, she was profoundly affected and could not continue as normal. As quoted in Watts (2019) 'I kept thinking

---

Case Study 17.1   (Continued)

---

about it and I just wondered if I am going to have a future. And I kept that to myself because I'm not very much of a talker, and that wasn't healthy'.

This situation contributed to being diagnosed with depression. At age 11, Greta became ill and in her own words,

> I stopped talking, and I stopped eating. In two months, I lost about ten kilos of weight. Later on, I was diagnosed with Asperger syndrome, obsessive-compulsive disorder and selective mutism (TEDx Stockholm 2018).

During this period of depression, Greta did not attend school, and her parents took care of her at home. She shared her concerns about the climate crisis and the environment with her parents: 'It felt good to just get that off my chest'. She recognised that by talking about her worries, she could influence others and make a difference. She persuaded her parents to adopt lifestyle choices that reduced their own carbon footprint and overall impact on the environment. She used various means of influence including showing films, sharing pictures, graphs, articles and reports. She also expressed that 'they were stealing my future'. Her family became vegetarian, commenced upcycling, and gave up flying. For her mother, this meant relinquishing her international career (Watts 2019).

In May 2018, Greta entered and won a writing competition focused on the environment held by Swedish newspaper *Svenska Dagbladet*. Her essay was titled 'We know – and we can do something now'. After the paper published her essay, Greta was contacted by Bo Thorén, an activist with the environmental group Fossil Free Dalsland. Fossil Free Dalsland was a group interested in acting on climate change. In a meeting with Thorén, the idea about school children striking for climate change was discussed. This idea was inspired by the students at Marjory Stoneman Douglas High School in Parkland, Florida, who after their school shooting in 2018 started striking to change the gun laws in the United States. This idea resonated with Greta, who 'liked the idea of a school strike' (Whiting 2019). Greta attempted to get others to participate but was unsuccessful. Her parents also tried to dissuade her. She decided to strike alone.

On August 20, 2018, 15-year-old Greta skipped school and sat down outside the Swedish parliament in Stockholm. She had with her a piece of wood on which she had painted 'Skolstrejk for Klimatet' (School Strike for Climate (n.d.)). She sat there for the entire school day, handing out flyers on which she had written a list of facts about global warming and climate change. During the day, she started posting photos on Twitter and Instagram. Her message started to gain traction. The following day Greta returned to the Swedish parliament, striking again. However, other people joined her. By the end of the first week, her strike had drawn coverage from Sweden's biggest newspapers. As the media attention grew, she handed out flyers bearing the message 'You grownups don't give a shit about my future', and supporters dropped by to join the protest on their lunch breaks. For three weeks, Greta picketed outside the Swedish parliament. Her demands were simple: for the Swedish government to commit to

(Continued)

Case Study 17.1   (Continued)

---

reducing carbon emission to the levels agreed by the Paris Agreement of 2016 (Haynes 2019; Watts 2019; Whiting 2019).

After Sweden's general election day occurred on the September 9, 2018, and following three weeks of protest, Greta returned to School – from Monday to Thursday. She continued to protest on Fridays. After her first solo protest, Greta was asked to make a speech at a People's Climate March rally to be held on September 13, 2018. This would involve an audience of thousands. Her selective mutism meant that she sometimes could not speak in certain situations. Her parents were reluctant and attempted to talk her out of this speech as they felt she might struggle to speak out at such a public event. Greta was determined that she needed to speak out about the climate crisis, and that her selective mutism would not prevent that: 'In some cases where I am really passionate, I will not change my mind' (Watts 2019; Whiting 2019). Greta delivered her speech flawlessly and fluently in English. The crowd filmed her, and the videos spread through social media.

Greta made several other small speeches, before speaking at the TEDx event in Stockholm in November 2019. In her speech, Greta spoke of her selective mutism, 'This basically means, I only speak, when I think it is necessary. Now is one of those moments'. Further she describes her diagnosis of Asperger's Syndrome as a 'superpower' as it provides her with the ability to be direct and speak her mind. It drives her strong sense of social justice.

> "For those of us, who are on the spectrum, almost everything is black or white. We aren't very good at lying and we usually don't enjoy participating in the social games that the rest of you seem so fond of. I think, in many ways, that we autistic are the normal ones and the rest of the people are pretty strange" (TEDx Stockholm 2018).

In December 2018, Greta addressed the United Nations Climate Change Conference held in Katowice, Poland (COP 24). It was here that the world began to listen. Her brutal honesty shamed the room of much older statesmen and dignitaries,

> You only talk about moving forward with the same bad ideas that got us into this mess, even when the only sensible thing to do is pull the emergency brake. You're not mature enough to tell it like it is. Even that burden, you leave to us children. You say you love your children above all else, and yet you're stealing their future in front of their very eyes.

Her speech at this conference went viral and a global movement emerged. Within three months of her initial protest, tens of thousands of students in nearly 300 towns and cities across the world joined her #FridaysForFuture protest. Her protest actions spread to other school children of her age on social media, and they held similar protests in their own communities. In Belgium, at the end of January, over 30 000 students had walked out of class (Aronoff 2019). In March 2019 a global school strike was held;

Case Study 17.1   (Continued)

1.6 million people participated in the strike and included 2,233 cities in 128 countries. It was the biggest single day of climate action that had ever occurred

Since then, Greta has continued to fight for her cause on the world stage. Her well-researched and sobering speeches have contributed to her rise as a spokesperson for environmental issues and for mobilsing people worldwide. Her ability to inspire others globally is now known as the 'Greta effect' (Watts 2019). She has received numerous honours and awards, including *Time* Person of the Year (2019), inclusion in the *Forbes* list of The World's 100 Most Powerful Women (2019), three nominations for the Nobel Peace Prize in 2019, 2020, and 2021, Swedish Woman of the Year (2019), The Geddes Environment Medal (2019) with Honorary Fellowship of the Royal Scottish Geographical Society and an honorary doctorate conferred by the University of Mons (Belgian) for 'contribution to raising awareness on sustainable development' (2019).

Greta's rise to fame, however, has not been without criticism. As summarised by Adams (2019),

> They've attacked her because she is young and, therefore...can't possibly understand the so-called complexities of the science or of world affairs... They've attacked her because she has Asperger's syndrome, attempting to exploit society's ignorance of the autism spectrum by claiming she is a 'deeply disturbed', 'unstable', 'mentally ill' teenager.... They've attacked her appearance by comparing her trademark pigtail hairstyle to that of Nazi propaganda that featured young girls with the same hairstyle and by claiming she was 'too emotional to see things clearly'.

Greta's response to her critics demonstrates maturity beyond her years:

> "When haters go after your looks and differences, it means they have nowhere left to go. And then you know you're winning! I have Aspergers and that means I'm sometimes a bit different from the norm. And – given the right circumstances – being different is a superpower." #aspiepower

Challenge: Greta Thunberg's story exemplifies several challenges to leadership, including age, gender, intergenerational conflicts and mental health diagnoses. Despite this, she has become a leading spokesperson on environmental issues. What are the leadership characteristics that she embodies? How has Greta been able to assert her message and advocate for change? What do you consider her strengths and weaknesses to be? How can you identify your weaknesses and enhance your strengths? Chapter 15 on reflection and emotional intelligence offers several tools and advice to help with reflection. Or you could start with a simple list of strengths and weaknesses and then consider strategies to deal with each. How can you help yourself be a 'better version of yourself each day'? How can you bring what is most wonderful about you as a person to the fore?

Summary

- This chapter has addressed the issue of gender and leadership, asking whether there is a difference between the leadership styles of men and women.
- It has described a number of challenges that women face in achieving leadership recognition, including lower than average salaries, under-representation in leadership roles, gender bias and a lack of confidence.
- Greater leadership diversity has been identified as leading to greater competitive advantage, with a more flexible approach to products and services that ultimately leads organisations to be better able to meet service users' needs.
- This chapter has suggested that past studies have reported there are several reasons for the gender disparity in leadership roles, with women being seen as having a lack of confidence, to be more apologetic, poorer at bluffing, more risk averse, more emotional and to employ different communication skills, while they also have higher social sensitivity and react by feeling.
- Women face several barriers in reaching their leadership potential, which include gender bias, a lack of confidence, lower expectations in negotiation, being less comfortable in some work environments, being less identified as leaders, a lack of role models and mentors, having career interruptions, not networking as effectively as some men and being subjected to greater performance scrutiny.
- To overcome these barriers, women could employ strategies of becoming or finding a role model, starting a network of their own, building their leadership skills, aligning their leadership style with their values and beliefs, building technical and cultural competence and developing their confidence and communication skills.
- The chapter also links the theory of congruent leadership and a feminine perspective on leadership to demonstrate that clinical leaders (male or female) may hold an advantage by applying a congruent leadership approach to their clinical leadership role.
- The main generational groups are outlined: Builders, Baby Boomers, Generation X, Generation Y, Generation Z and the Alpha Generation.
- Leaders and managers within the health service need to recognise the motivators and drivers within each generation and incorporate these into their management and leadership approaches to make the most of the core values of each generational group.

Mind Press-Ups

Exercise 17.1

There is a common perception that many men in nursing (or healthcare in general) are focused on seeking a career in management. Do male health professionals have any advantages over their female counterparts in progressing more effectively through to more senior levels? Why might this be?

Exercise 17.2

Do generational differences exist in your workplace? Talk to your colleagues about this question. Are the main differences generational or are there other, less 'global' issues that cause conflict or sit between people? If there are generational issues, how do you plan to overcome them so values can be more easily understood and shared?

References

Abdallah, J. and Jibai, S. (2020). 'Women in leadership: gender personality traits and skills. *Business Excellence and Management* 10 (1): 5–15.

Adams, M. (2019). Greta Thunberg is a true leader by every definition. The Sydney Morning Herald. www.smh.com.au/national/greta-thunberg-is-a-true-leader-by-every-definition-20190925-p52uqd.html (accessed 12/11/21).

Andersen, J.A. and Hansson, P.H. (2011). At the end of the road? On differences between women and men in leadership behavior. *Leadership and Organisations Development Journal* 32 (5): 428–441.

Appelbaum, S.H., Audet, L., and Miller, J.C. (2003). Gender and leadership? Leadership and gender? A journey through the landscape of theories. *Leadership and Organisational Development Journal* 24 (1): 43–51.

Aronoff, K. (2019). How Greta Thunberg's Lone Strike Against Climate Change Became a Global Movement. *Rolling Stone*. https://www.rollingstone.com/politics/politics-features/greta-thunberg-fridays-for-future-climate-change-800675 (accessed 12/11/21).

Artabane M., Coffman, J. & Darnell, D. (2017), Charting the course: getting women to the top. Bain & Company, https://www.bain.com/insights/charting-the-course-women-on-the-top (accessed 29/11/21).

Badura, K.L., Grijalva, E., Newman, D.A. et al. (2018). 'Gender and leadership emergence: a meta-analysis and explanatory model. *Personnel Psychology* 71 (3): 335–367.

Bengtsson, C., Persson, M., and Willenhag, P. (2005). Gender and overconfidence. *Economics Letters* 86: 199–203.

Buss, D.M. (2012). *Evolutionary Psychology: The New Science of Mind*. Boston, MA: Pearson Education.

Cahill, T.F. and Cima, L.E. (2016). *On Common Ground: Addressing Generational Issues in Nursing Services*. Washington, DC: Catholic Health Association of the United States https://www.chausa.org/publications/health-progress/article/january-february-2016/on-common-ground-addressing- generational-issues-in-nursing-services (accessed 2 May 2016).

Campbell, J.P., McCloy, R.A., Oppler, S.H., and Sager, C.E. (1993). A theory of performance. In: *Personnel Selection in Organizations* (ed. N. Schmitt and W.C. Borman), 35–70. San Francisco, CA: Jossey-Bass.

Carney, D.R., Cuddy, A.J., and Yap, A.J. (2010). Power posing: brief nonverbal displays affect neuroendocrine levels and risk tolerance. *Psychological Science* 20 (10): 1–5.

Cassells, R. and Duncan, A. (2020). *Gender Equity Insights 2020: Delivering the Business Outcomes*. BCEC|WGEA Gender Equity Series, Issue #5 March 2020, https://bcec.edu.au/

publications/gender-equity-insights-2020-delivering-the-business-outcomes (accessed 23/11/21).

Catalyst (2007). The Bottom Line: Corporate Performance and Women's Representation on Boards (Report). https://www.catalyst.org/research/the-bottom-line-corporate-performance-and-womens-representation-on-boards (accessed 23/11/21).

Catalyst (2011). *The Myth of the Ideal Worker: Does Doing All the Right Things Really Get Women Ahead?* New York: Catalyst http://www.catalyst.org/system/files/The_Myth_of_the_Ideal_Worker_Does_Doing_All_the_Right_Things_Really_Get_Women_Ahead.pdf (accessed 4 April 2014).

Catalyst (2020). Women in Management (Quick Take). https://www.catalyst.org/research/women-in-management (accessed 23/11/21).

Catalyst (2021). Women in the workforce: Global (Quick Take). https://www.catalyst.org/research/women-in-the-workforce-global (accessed 23/11/21).

Cialdini, R.B. (2001). *Influence: Science and Practice.* Needham Heights, MA: Allyn & Bacon.

Corporate Women Directors International (2020). *Regional Comparison of Women on Boards.* Washington: Globewomen Research and Education Institute https://globewomen.org/CWDINet/wp-content/uploads/2020/05/Regional-Comparison-Chart-March-2020-1.pdf (accessed 26 November 2021).

Cran, C. (2016). *The Art of Change Leadership.* Hoboken, NJ: Wiley.

Croson, R. and Gneezy, U. (2009). Gender differences in preferences. *Journal of Economic Literature* 47 (2): 448–474.

Cunningham, J. and Roberts, P. (2012). *Inside Her Pretty Little Head: A New Theory of Motivation and Why It Matters for Marketing.* London: Marshall Cavendish Business.

De Meuse, K.P. and Mlodzik, K.J. (2010). A second look at generational differences in the workforce: implications for HR and talent management. *People and Strategy* 33 (2): 50–58.

Deuskat, V.U. (1994). Gender and leadership style: transformational and transactional leadership in the Roman Catholic church. *Leadership Quarterly* 5 (2): 99–119.

Dimock, M. (2019). *Defining Generations: Where Millennials End and Generation Z Begins.* Pew Research Centre https://www.pewresearch.org/fact-tank/2019/01/17/where-millennials-end-and-generation-z-begins (accessed 23 November 2021).

Eagly, A.H. (2003). More women at the top: the impact of gender roles and leadership style. In: *Gender: From Costs to Benefits* (ed. U. Pasero), 151–169. Wiesbaden: Westdeutscher.

Eagly, A.H. and Carli, L.C. (2007). *Through the Labyrinth: The Truth About How Women Become Leaders.* Boston, MA: Harvard Business School Press.

Eagly, A.H. and Johannesen-Schmidt, M.C. (2001). The leadership styles of women and men. *Journal of Social Issues* 57 (4): 781–797.

Eagly, A.H. and Johnson, B.T. (1990). Gender and leadership style: a meta-analysis. *Psychological Bulletin* 108: 233–256.

Eckel, C.C. and Grossman, P.J. (2008). Men, women and risk aversion: experimental evidence. In: *Handbook of Experimental Economics Results,* vol. 1 (ed. C.R. Plott and V.L. Smith), 1061–1073. New York: Elsevier.

EgonZehnder (2021). Leaders & daughters global survey: Reversing the "She-cession": Retaining and Empowering Female Leaders, https://www.egonzehnder.com/reversing-the-she-cession (accessed 29/11/21).

Ely, R.J., Ibarra, H., and Kolb, D. (2011). Taking gender into account: theory and design for women's leadership development programs. *Insead Working Papers* 10 (3): 1–53.

Enticott, P., Johnston, P., Herring, S. et al. (2008). Mirror neuron activation is associated with facial emotion processing. *Neuropsychologia* 46: 2851–2854.

European Commission (2020). *Women in Economic Decision-Making in the EU: Progress Report*. Luxembourg: Publication Office of the European Union https://op.europa.eu/en/publication-detail/-/publication/8832ea16-e2e6-4095-b1eb-cc72a22e28df/language-en.

Evans, K.J. and Maley, J.F. (2021). Barriers to women in senior leadership: how unconscious bias is holding back Australia's economy. *Asia Pacific Journal of Human Resources* 59 (2): 204–226. http://doi.org/10.1111/1744-7941.12262.

Faizan, R., Nair, S.L.S., and Haque, A. (2018). The effectiveness of feminine and masculine leadership styles in relation to contrasting gender's performances. *Polish Journal of Management Studies* 17: https://doi.org/10.17512/pjms.2018.17.1.07.

Feldt, G. (2012). *No Excuses: Nine Ways Women Can Change How We Think About Power*. Berkeley, CA: Seal Press.

Forret, M.L. and Dougherty, T.W. (2004). Networking behaviours and career outcomes: differences for men and women. *Journal of Organizational Behaviour* 25 (3): 419–437.

Francis, T. and Hoefel, F. (2018). *True Gen': Generation Z and Its Implications for Companies*. McKinsey & Company https://www.mckinsey.com/industries/consumer-packaged-goods/our-insights/true-gen-generation-z-and-its-implications-for-companies (accessed 26 November 2021).

Franke, G. (1997). Gender differences in ethical perceptions of business practices: a social role theory perspective. *Journal of Applied Psychology* 82 (6): 920–934.

French, M.T., Mortensen, K., and Timming, A.R. (2021). 'A multivariate analysis of workplace mentoring and socializing in the wake of #MeToo. *Applied Economics* 53 (35): 4040–4058. http://doi.org/10.1080/00036846.2021.1896673.

Gardiner, M. and Tiggemann, M. (1999). Gender differences in leadership style, job stress and mental health in male- and female-dominated industries'. *Journal of Occupational and Organizational Psychology* 72: 301–315.

Griffiths, O., Roberts, L., and Price, J. (2019). 'Desirable leadership attributes are preferentially associated with women: a quantitative study of gender and leadership roles in the Australian workforce. *Australian Journal of Management* 44 (1): 32–49. http://doi.org/10.1177/0312896218781933.

Grossman, S. and Valiga, T.M. (2021). *The New Leadership Challenge: Creating the Future of Nursing*, 5e. Philadelphia, PA: FA Davis.

Grossman, M. and Wood, W. (1993). Sex difference in intensity of emotional experience: a social role interpretation. *Journal of Personality and Social Psychology* 65 (5): 1010–1022.

Guidice, R.B., Alder, C., and Phelan, S.E. (2009). Competitive bluffing: an examination of a common practice and its relationship with performance. *Journal of Business Ethics* 87: 535–553.

Gursory, D., Maier, T.A., and Chi, C.G. (2008). Generational differences: an examination of work values and generational gaps in the hospitality workforce. *International Journal of Hospitality Management* 27 (3): 448–458.

Hanna, J. (2012). Developing the global leader. Harvard Business School Working Knowledge (25 October) http://hbswk.hbs.edu/item/developing-the-global-leader (accessed 1 July 2016).

Harris, C., Jenkins, M., and Glaser, D. (2006). Gender differences in risk assessment: why do women take fewer risks than men? *Judgement and Decision Making* 1 (1): 48–63.

Hayes, B., Bonner, A., and Pryor, J. (2010). Factors contributing to nurse job satisfaction in the acute hospital setting: a review of recent literature. *Journal of Nursing Management* 18: 804–814.

Haynes, S. (2019). 'Now I Am Speaking to the Whole World.' How Teen Climate Activist Greta Thunberg Got Everyone to Listen. *Time*. https://time.com/collection/next-generation-leaders/5584902/greta-thunberg-next-generation-leaders (accessed 9/11/21).

Heilman, M.E. and Parks-Stamm, E.J. (2007). Gender stereotypes in the workplace: obstacles to women's career progress. In: *Social Psychology of Gender: Advances in Group Processes* (ed. S.J. Corell), 47–77. Greenwich, CT: JAI Press.

Hillstrom, L.C. (2018). *The# MeToo Movement*. ABC-CLIO.

Hoffman, H., Kessler, H., Eppel, T. et al. (2010). Expression intensity, gender and facial emotional recognition: women recognise only subtle facial emotions better than men. *Acta Psychologica* 135: 278–283.

Holm, H. (2005). Detection biases in bluffing: Theory and experiments. Working papers no. 30, pp. 1–45, Lund: Department of Economics, Lund University.

Huszczo, G. and Endres, M.L. (2017). 'Gender differences in the importance of personality traits in predicting leadership self-efficacy: gender differences in the importance of personality traits. *International Journal of Training and Development* vol. 21 (4): 304–317. http://doi.org/10.1111/ijtd.12113.

Kalaitzi, S., Czabanowska, K., Fowler-Davis, S., and Brand, H. (2017). 'Women leadership barriers in healthcare, academia and business. *Equality, Diversity and Inclusion: An International Journal* 36 (5): 457–474. http://doi.org/10.1108/EDI-03-2017-0058.

Kaufman, M.R., Dey, D., Crainiceanu, C., and Dredze, M. (2019). '#MeToo and Google inquiries into sexual violence: a hashtag campaign can sustain information seeking. *Journal of Interpersonal Violence* 36 (19–20): 9857–9867. http://doi.org/10.1177/0886260519868197.

Keepnews, D.M. and Shin, J.H. (2010). Generational differences among newly licensed registered nurses. *Nursing Outlook* 58 (3): 155–163.

Kogan, M. (2001). Human resource management: Bridging the gap. *Government Executive* (1 September) http://cdn.govexec.com/interstitial.html?v=2.1.1&rf=http%3A%2F%2Fwww.govexec.com%2Fmagazine%2Fmagazine-human-resources-management%2F2001%2F09%2Fbridging-the-gap%2F9752%2F (accessed 8 March 2016).

Lagace, M. (2003). Negotiating challenges for women leaders. Harvard Business School Working Knowledge (13 October) http://hbswk.hbs.edu/item/negotiating-challenges-for-women-leaders (accessed 8 March 2016).

Lerner, J.S. and Keltner, D. (2001). Fear, anger and risk. *Journal of Personality and Social Psychology* 81 (1): 146–159.

Lighthall, N.R., Sakaki, M., Vasunilashorn, S. et al. (2012). Gender differences in reward related decision processing under stress. *Scan* 7: 476–484.

Lyness, K.S. and Heilman, M.E. (2006). When fit is fundamental: performance evaluation and promotions of upper-level female and male managers. *Journal of Applied Psychology* 91: 777–785.

Madsen, S.R. and Andrade, M.S. (2018). 'Unconscious gender bias: implications for women's leadership development. *Journal of Leadership Studies* 12 (1): 62–67.

Marquis, B.L. and Huston, C.J. (2012). *Leadership Roles and Management Functions in Nursing: Theory and Application*, 7e. Philadelphia, PA: Lippincott, Williams & Wilkins.

Marshall, D.A. (2021). Changes Executives Need to Implement to Promote Women to Executive Positions. ProQuest Dissertations Publishing. https://www.proquest.com/openvie w/3225718d1ddae951640f7351d942abef/1?pq-origsite=gscholar&cbl=18750&diss=y (accessed 26/11/21).

McCrindle (2016). Gen Z and Gen Alpha infographic update. McCrindle Blog http:// mccrindle.com.au/the-mccrindle-blog/gen-z-and-gen-alpha-infographic-update (accessed 8 March 2016).

McCrindle (2021a). The generations defined. McCrindle Blog https://mccrindle.com.au/ insights/blog/the-generations-defined (accessed 22/11/21).

McCrindle (2021b). Understanding generation Alpha. McCrindle Blog https://mccrindle.com. au/insights/blog/gen-alpha-defined (accessed 22/11/21).

McCrindle (2021c) Four distinctives of generation Alpha. McCrindle Blog https://mccrindle. com.au/insights/blog/four-distinctives-of-generation-alpha (accessed 22/11/21).

McKinsey (2007). *Women Matter: Gender Diversity: A Corporate Performance Driver*. Paris: McKinsey & Co., Inc. www.raeng.org.uk/publications/other/women-matter-oct-2007 (accessed 1 July 2016).

McKinsey & Company (2021). Women in the workplace 2021. McKinsey & Co https://www. mckinsey.com/featured-insights/diversity-and-inclusion/women-in-the-workplace# (accessed 22/11/21).

Mercer (2020). Let's get real about equality: When Women Thrive global report. https://www. mercer.com/our-thinking/next-generation-global-research-when-women-thrive-2020. html#contactForm (accessed 23/11/21).

Moran, B. (1992). Gender differences in leadership. *Library Trends* 40 (5): 475–491.

Mousa, M., Boyle, J., Skouteris, H. et al. (2021). 'Advancing women in healthcare leadership: a systematic review and meta-synthesis of multi-sector evidence on organisational interventions. *eClinicalMedicine* 39: 101084. http://doi.org/10.1016/j.eclinm.2021.101084.

Nash, M., Davies, A., and Moore, R. (2017). 'What style of leadership do women in STEMM fields perform? Findings from an international survey. *PLoS One* 12 (10): e0185727. http:// dx.doi.org/10.1371/journal.pone.0185727.

Nelsey, L. and Brownie, S. (2012). Effective leadership, teamwork and mentoring: essential elements in promoting generational cohesion in the nursing workforce and retaining nurses. *Collegian* 19: 197–202.

Niederle, M. and Versterlund, L. (2007). Do women shy away from competition? Do men compete too much? *Quarterly Journal of Economics* 122 (3): 1067–1101.

Nielsen, S. and Huse, M. (2010). The contribution of women on boards of directors: going beyond the surface. *Corporate Governance* 18 (2): 136–148.

O'Hara, M.A., Burke, D., Ditomassi, M., and Palan Lopez, R. (2019). 'Assessment of millennial nurses' job satisfaction and professional practice environment. *The Journal of Nursing Administration* 49 (9): 411–417. http://dx.doi.org/10.1097/NNA.0000000000000777.

O'Reilly, N.D. (2015). *Leading Women: 20 Influential Women Share Their Secrets to Leadership, Business and Life*. Avon, MA: Adams Media.

Patel, G. (2013). *Gender Differences in Leadership Styles and the Impact within Corporate Boards*. London: Commonwealth Secretariat, Social Transformation Programmes Division.

Post, C., Lokshin, B. and Boone, C. (2021). Adding Women to the C-Suite Changes How Companies Think. Harvard Business Review. https://hbr.org/2021/04/research-adding-women-to-the-c-suite-changes-how-companies-think (accessed 26/11/21).

Rincón, V., González, M., and Barrero, K. (2017). 'Women and leadership: gender barriers to senior management positions. *Intangible Capital* 13 (2): 319–386. http://dx.doi.org/10.3926/ic.889.

Roberts, S. and Brown, D.K. (2019). 'How to manage gender bias from within: women in leadership. *The Journal of Business Diversity* 19 (2): 83–98.

Rose, A.S. (2021). 'Lessons from #MeToo: a critical reflective comment. *Journal of Marketing Management* 37 (3–4): 379–381. http://dx.doi.org/10.1080/0267257X.2020.1829320.

Rowe, M. (2009). *Find Yourself: The Mentoring You Need*. Cambridge, MA: MIT http://ombud.mit.edu/sites/default/files/documents/find_yourself_a_mentor.pdf (accessed 8 March 2016).

Sahoo, C.K. and Das, S. (2012). Women entrepreneurship and connective leadership: achieving success. *European Journal of Business and Management* 4 (3): 115–121.

Sandberg, S. (2015). *Lean In: Women, Work and the Will to Lead*. London: Penguin.

Sapienza, P., Zingales, L., and Maestripieri, D. (2009). Gender differences in financial risk aversion and career choices are affected by testosterone. *Proceedings of the National Academy of Sciences of the United States of America* 106 (36): 15268–15273.

Schumann, K. and Ross, M. (2010). Why women apologise more than men: gender differences in threshold for perceiving offensive behaviour. *Psychological Science* 21 (11): 1649–1655.

Seo, G., Huang, W., and Han, S.-H.C. (2017). 'Conceptual review of underrepresentation of women in senior leadership positions from a perspective of gendered social status in the workplace: implication for HRD research and practice. *Human Resource Development Review* 16 (1): 35–59.

Shen, W. and Joseph, D.L. (2021). 'Gender and leadership: a criterion-focused review and research agenda. *Human Resource Management Review* 31 (2): 100765. http://dx.doi.org/10.1016/j.hrmr.2020.100765.

Smith, J.E., von Rueden, C.R., van Vugt, M. et al. (2021). 'An evolutionary explanation for the female leadership paradox. *Frontiers in Ecology and Evolution* 9: 468. http://dx.doi.org/10.3389/fevo.2021.676805.

Stanley, D. (2010). Multigenerational workforce issues and their implications for leadership in nursing. *Journal of Nursing Management* 18: 846–852.

Stanley, D. (2011). *Clinical Leadership: Innovation into Action*. South Yarra, VIC: Palgrave Macmillan.

Stanley, D. (2014). Clinical leadership characteristics confirmed. *Journal of Research in Nursing* 19 (2): 118–128.

Stanley, D. (2019). *Values-Based Leadership in Healthcare: Congruent Leadership Explored*. London: Sage.

Stevanin, S., Voutilainen, A., Bressan, V. et al. (2020). Nurses' generational differences related to workplace and leadership in two European countries. *Western Journal of Nursing Research* 42 (1): 14–23. http://dx.doi.org/10.1177/0193945919838604.

Stevens, J. (2021). Tarana Burke - the woman behind the #MeToo movement [Television]. In *7.30 Report with Leigh Sales*. Australia: ABC.

Suk, J., Abhishek, A., Zhang, Y. et al. (2019). '#MeToo, networked acknowledgment, and connective action: how "Empowerment Through Empathy" launched a social movement. *Social Science Computer Review* 39 (2): 276–294. http://dx.doi.org/10.1177/0894439319864882.

Thunberg (2018) School strike for climate – save the world by changing the rules. https://www.youtube.com/watch?v=EAmmUIEsN9A&t=75s.

Tsui, L. (1998). The effects of gender, education and personal skills self-confidence on income in business management. *Sex Roles* 38 (5): 363–374.

Vinnicombe, S. (1999). The debate: do men and women have different leadership styles? *Management Focus* 12 (Summer): http://www.som.cranfield.ac.uk/som/dinamic-content/news/documents/p12_13.doc (accessed 1 July 2016).

Watts, J. (2019). Greta Thunberg, schoolgirl climate change warrior: 'Some people can let things go. I can't'; One day last summer, aged 15, she skipped school, sat down outside the Swedish parliament – and inadvertently kicked off a global movement. *The Guardian* (London). https://www.theguardian.com/world/2019/mar/11/greta-thunberg-schoolgirl-climate-change-warrior-some-people-can-let-things-go-i-cant (accessed 9/11/21).

Weber, E., Blais, A., and Betz, N. (2002). A domain-specific risk-attitude scale: measuring risk perceptions and risk behaviors. *Journal of Behavioural Decision Making* 15 (1): 263–290.

Weingarten, R.M. (2009). Four generations, one workplace: a Gen X-Y staff nurse's view of team building in the emergency department. *Journal of Emergency Nursing* 35 (1): 27–30.

Whiting, T. (2019). The Story of 16 Year Old Climate Activist Greta Thunberg. Medium https://tabitha-whiting.medium.com/greta-thunberg-i-promised-myself-i-was-going-to-do-everything-i-could-to-make-a-difference-cb6fade1904 (accessed 9/11/21).

Wilson, N. and Atlantar, A. (2009). *Director Characteristics, Gender Balance and Insolvency Risk: An Empirical Study*. Rochester, NY: Social Science Research Network http://papers.ssrn.com/sol3/papers.cfm?abstract_id=1414224 (accessed 8 March 2016).

World Bank (2021). *Labor Participation Rate, Female*, June 15. Washington, DC: World Bank https://data.worldbank.org/indicator/SL.TLF.CACT.FE.ZS (accessed 26 November 2021).

Zenger, J. and Folkman, J. (2012). *A Study of Leadership: Women Do It Better than Men*. Orem, UT: Zenger Folkman http://zengerfolkman.com/media/articles/ZFCo.WP.WomenBetterThanMen.033012.pdf (accessed 2 April 2016).

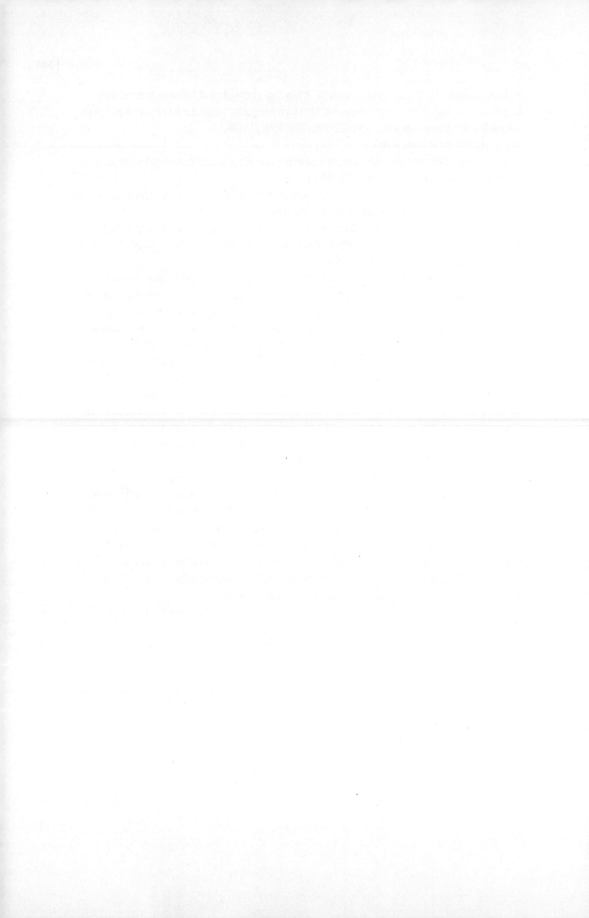

18

Power, Politics and Leadership
Alison H. James and Clare L. Bennett

That was a small lesson I learned on the journey. What is interesting and important happens mostly in secret, in places where there is no power. Nothing much of lasting value ever happens at the head table, held together by a familiar rhetoric. Those who already have power continue to glide along the familiar rut they have made for themselves.

Michael Ondaatje, 'The Cat's Table' p. 103 (Ondaatje (2012))

Introduction: Power and Politics

This chapter addresses the issues of power and politics as they relate to leadership for health professionals. Politics and power are central issues to health service delivery at every level of global healthcare, whether it is international influence on global healthcare agendas, national political policy or at local levels and contexts within organsiations. With such influence on our resources and direction in providing care, all healthcare professionals need to be aware and engaged in the relationship of power and politics on the outcomes of providing equity and effective care for patients.

The chapter outlines some definitions of power and politics and discusses what it means to exercise professional power as well as other types of power. It also considers the significance of a professional's capacity to influence, together with a number of types of influencing styles. Critical social theory is used to develop an argument for the role of professionals in relation to power and politics and our responsibility to provide equity and social justice. The chapter concludes with a discussion of politics and offers some practical approaches for how health professionals can deal with the media and become politically active, within the context of their professional responsibilities.

A Beginning

Like most phenomena in our lives, we begin to develop a sense of the characteristics of power and politics at an early age. Indeed, Howard and Gill (2000) suggest that children's interpretations are social constructions that cannot be independent of adult thought. Therefore, children assimilate information about power and politics through their contact with adults, or through cultural artefacts such as television, radio and the internet (Howard and Gill 2000). Recent studies have demonstrated that children at primary school level develop political views and understand basic perceptions (van Deth et al. 2011). So, it is clear the concepts of power and politics develop with a long history of pre-developed thoughts, ideas and expectations that shape our understanding of, and interaction with, all our social experiences.

Social experience suggests the involvement of people. As we all know, in the context of social relationships sometimes we have no power and sometimes we do; that is, according to social context, there are always differentials in power. The historical background of our nations, the relationships between governments and society, and relations within society itself often shape the overall policies and systems of health. Understanding this and where power sits and exercises that power can enlighten the overall picture of what is happening in healthcare in each of our nations, locally and globally. For example, the World Health Organization Commission on the Social Determinants of Health acknowledged health inequities exist due to 'a toxic combination of poor social policies and programmes, unfair economic arrangements, and bad politics' (CSDH 2008, p. 1), so it is important to consider the role of healthcare and social justice and the influences of power within.

Braynion (2004) asserts that power can be a vexed and difficult concept to define and that the definition will very much depend on the lens through which the phenomenon of power is considered. Roberts and Vasquez (2004, p. 197) cite *Merriam-Webster's* definition of power as 'the ability to act or produce an effect', and Huber (2000) believes that power can be perceived as the ability to exercise influence over others, either by coercion or persuasion. These views support the notion that power is exercised between people and is therefore specific to their relationship. People and relationships are central to healthcare, so it is important to consider these overarching influences within clinical practice.

Professional Power

Throughout this book you have been offered ideas and thoughts about the nature of clinical leadership, as well as the skills that allow for its operation in the practice setting. In this regard, you have been given opportunities to reflect on and analyse the meaning of clinical leadership for you as a health professional.

The operative word in the last sentence is 'professional'; that is, clinical leadership occurs in the context of professional practice. Therefore, it represents an activity carried out by professionals, where a profession is an occupational group that enjoys varying amounts of freedom and power, traditionally granted by governments (Wilding 1982). It is also acknowledged that the effectiveness of an interdisciplinary team is influenced by the balance of power within those relationships (McDonald et al. 2012); and to ensure the equal balance of team members feeling valued and being successful, it is often determined by effective leadership. If we acknowledge power balances exist in all our contexts of professional work, it is possible to recognise that power can have both positive and negative effects, and in being aware of this we can support decision-making for clinical leaders.

Professional leadership implies a capacity to communicate well, to remain visible and to act as a role model (particularly in a clinical context) for the values and beliefs relevant to the professional's role. Being aware of the shifting dynamics of power influences within these contexts can allow the development of a wider awareness and insight into the political potencies at work, whether that is from high levels or more local.

Power Base

Marquis and Houston (2012) and Bishop (2009) suggest that leadership cannot be effective without some measure of power to support it. French and Raven (1959), Bragg (1996), Braynion (2004), Bishop (2009) and Yoder-Wise (2015) propose that a number of sources exist for the exercise of power. They cite the following types of sources of power:

- **Reward power:** This is exercised by the ability to grant rewards or favours. It could include bonuses, special treats, time off or, indeed, anything of value.
- **Punishment, authoritarian or coercive power:** This type of power is derived from the capacity to generate fear. It may involve threats (real or implied) of transfer, work reassignment, lay-off, demotion or dismissal.
- **Legitimate power:** This is the power of authority and commonly accompanies titled positions. It implies feelings of obligation or responsibility, and its legitimacy arises from the authority associated with a job title.
- **Expert power:** This power comes from knowledge, expertise or experience that others value. It exemplifies the phrase 'knowledge is power'. It is often limited to a specialised area and usually fails to extend beyond this.
- **Referent or charismatic power:** This is power that is referred to a leader because others recognise or identify with that leader, or with what they symbolise. It can be paralleled with charismatic power and involves feelings of personal approval and acceptance, or it may be that the power comes from the reflective glow of being associated or connected with others in authority.
- **Resource power:** Controlling a variety of resources will imply a degree of power. This may be the control of budgets, staff promotion opportunities or the drug keys on a medical ward. It can be anything that has a relative value or that may be scarce.
- **Information or informational power:** This is derived from having access to selected or specialised information and knowledge or the means to control the sharing and directional information flow.

Reflection Point

If leadership cannot exist without some sort of power to support it, what sort of power do you feel you exercise in the course of your work duties? How does this manifest itself, and what examples can you think of where you have exercised this power? What were the effects on others as a consequence?

What sort of power do you think others hold within your team or department? Do you think others are aware of this power and its effects?

There are other types of power, such as connection power, where power is gained by having a connection with people perceived to be powerful. Marquis and Houston (2012) also identify self-power, where a person is able to gain power over their life so that with maturity, security and confidence they develop a degree of personal strength or resilience.

Recognising that there are different sources or types of power allows us to see that power in itself is not good or bad, positive or negative. Power is not about a balance between victory and loss. Instead, power is related to how it is used and to the purpose (good or evil) to which it is put (Marquis and Houston 2012). Foucault (1995) suggests power is not possessed, rather it is used, and that it is established within all contexts and interactions. So power does not belong to any one group or individual and therefore it is not an issue of taking sides or being in the powerful or less powerful group; rather, it lies in recognising that we all operate within a power structure and that the key is to understand the strategic elements of power (Foucault 1969).

Realising that power need not be positional – legitimate and related to a capacity to reward or punish – but is also related to expert power, knowledge, information and charisma means that influencing others through the appropriate use of power can enhance a health professional's personal and professional power base.

Powerlessness and Abuse

Brookes (2009, p. 241) describes powerlessness as 'a real or perceived state of having little or no power', which hints at the personal interpretation and emotion of this state. Within large organisations such as healthcare, many individuals may feel lacking in power and influence because they are not included in the decision-making process of wider policy and direction. However, in his distinction Brooks (2009) discerns between real powerlessness and that which is perceived. This clearly places perceived powerlessness within the realms of values and empowerment. If something is perceived, it may be possible to change, so with support and seeking out opportunities, it may be possible to change this state and change perception. Leaders who want teams and individuals to thrive will enable support and inclusion, seek out thoughts and opinions to demonstrate value and engagement, thereby strengthening commitment and suggesting degrees of power for all in decisions.

For some, power is an instrument of abuse and an enabler for negative outcomes for others. This can of course occur with determined consciousness or without realisation. Within healthcare, it is possible to consider historical examples of abuse of power through professions and hierarchy, and of course also through examples of when professional positions negatively manipulate patients. An extreme example of this in the UK was Harold Shipman, who used his power and position as a general practitioner to enable his crimes. However, day to day, less predetermined levels of power can be witnessed within teams and professions through cultures of behaviours and historical ritual which are not fully explored and questioned for rationale. For example, not so long ago, patients were expected to stay in bed and wash when the nurse enabled or authorised this as part of the daily routine. Strict rules of uniform colours and style often indicate levels of position and suggest levels of power over subordinates. In covert and abusive power, there is a potential for 'gaslighting', bullying and destabilisation, and it is in these contexts we must be transparent in our concern, as this most certainly devalues our professions and harms our patients.

Reflection Point

Sebring (2021) describes medical 'gaslighting' as 'the result of deeply embedded and largely unchallenged ideologies underpinning health-care services'.

What do you understand by the word 'power'? How is power derived and how is it maintained? In your opinion, is there a connection between power and leadership? How can negative use of power compromise patient care?

Influencing Styles

It is clear that power is related to influence (by what are called 'micropractices' by Gilson et al. (2014)). Exercising power often relies on a leader's capacity to use influence well. In turn, using influence well relies on a person's capacity to employ effective interpersonal and social skills to encourage others to change their attitudes, decisions or behaviours to comply with their requests (Bragg 1996). This often rests on the front-line leader's ability to manage power at a local level and to develop strategies to influence and 'empower' colleagues to support change, quality initiatives and impending innovations (Gilson et al. 2014). The following discussion on influencing styles provides one model for reflecting on some of the preferred influencing practices. Use of any influencing strategy is dependent on your own style or preference, the nature of your existing relationship with others and the personal style or preference of the individual you are attempting to influence.

As you reflect on your style, remember that if something is working, keep doing it; if it is not, try something different. If for any reason flexibility of style is an issue for you personally, think about how you operate on a day-to-day basis, intuitively shifting your style to achieve the desired effect. It is also important to recognise that while you may admire others for their style, this may not be effective or suitable for you, so simply emulating others is not always the best approach to take. Rather, consider what it is in those styles you feel is effective, and adapt this to suit your personal leadership approach.

Influencing styles include the following:

- **Assertive persuasion** – an attempt to influence someone through sheer weight of argument and counter-argument. This is a logical, calculated approach that attempts to overcome objections and resistance by appeals to sound reasoning. People will agree or disagree with your proposal because it is more or less effective, accurate, correct or true.
- **Reward and punishment** – an attempt to influence someone by using pressure or incentives to control their behaviour. Many negotiating and bargaining behaviours fit under this heading. Rewards may be offered for compliance; punishment or deprivation may be threatened for non-compliance. The use of power can be direct and aggressive (naked power) or more indirect, with veiled pressure from the use of status, prestige or formal authority. Whether people will agree or disagree is not the issue: the judgement of right or wrong is an evaluation based on a moral, social or arbitrary performance standard. The person making the evaluation sets themselves up as the judge.
- **Participation and trust** – an influencing style that increases people's commitment to the task by actively listening to them and involving them. It works best with the personal disclosure of one's own limitations; others are encouraged to be open and can more

easily see that their contribution is valued. People's ideas are encouraged and their commitment grows as more responsibility is delegated and communicated back to the participants. As this occurs, understanding and acceptance of their ideas are generated.

- **Common vision** – this influencing style tries to identify a common vision of the future for a group, and then group members have the vision strengthened so that through their collective or individual efforts the vision can become a reality. The power of this approach is in communicating the vision clearly, then in seeing the leader as trustworthy or dependable, and seeking others' ('followers'') commitment to working towards the vision.
- **Common values** – this form of influence can be overt or unconscious. It is closely aligned with congruent leadership and relates to the leader demonstrating their values and beliefs. Appeal is made to the values and emotions of the other(s), and images, metaphors and, more powerfully, actions are used to communicate enthusiasm and kindle excitement in a better future or a better way.

When attempting to influence others, it may be useful to follow a 'problem diagnosis' approach. By underpinning this to professional values, this will not only keep you focused on the desired outcomes, it can support your approach to the issues for others:

- **Step 1: Situation identification.** Begin by identifying a situation where it is important for you to increase your influence and power. Consider what values drive this need.
- **Step 2: Influence outcomes.** Now consider your desired outcome from this attempt at influence and how this links to your values. Consider what your objective is (e.g. to sell an idea, change an attitude, elicit certain behaviour). Describe your influence objective in specific behavioural terms (e.g. what you want the other person to do or say).
- **Step 3: Influence target.** Be specific about who you are trying to influence in the situation. If it is more than one person, identify the key individual whom it would be critical to influence, or most difficult for you to deal with effectively. In addition, describe the style of your influence target. How do they react to your influence attempts? What is it about the person that makes them difficult for you to influence?
- **Step 4: Situational factors.** Also consider any other characteristics of the situation that might affect your influence efforts (e.g. what the environment is like, what are the relationship dynamics).
- **Step 5: Description of past influence behaviour.** Consider any previous efforts to influence others. Do not evaluate your efforts; simply describe in detail how you tend to behave.
- **Step 6: Evaluation of past influence behaviour.** Now evaluate the effectiveness of your influencing attempts in this situation. What behaviour is effective or partially effective? Do you use influencing behaviour that is inappropriate? Do you use an appropriate style, but apply it poorly?
- **Step 7: Ideal influencing style.** Based on your analysis in Steps 1–6, describe what you believe to be the ideal influencing style or sequence of styles and behaviours to use. Do not be concerned at this time whether or not you can use the styles or behaviours that you identify. Describe what you believe would be the best strategy if you had an unlimited repertoire of influencing skills.

- **Step 8: Moderate your risk strategy.** Now decide on an influencing strategy – a combination or sequence of styles that takes your personal strengths into account. You may want to modify it somewhat to bring your risk down to a more acceptable level.
- **Step 9: Focus on the next contact.** What is the first step you plan to take with your influence target? Briefly describe the circumstances of this key meeting or contact. Then consider the single most important outcome you want from this crucial first step.

These steps are useful only if you understand strategies for increasing your influence. Some approaches to increasing your influence are outlined in Box 18.1.

The exercise of influence is how power is achieved. Power – any type of power, even positional power – is only potential until the user has mastered the ability to influence others and release the latent resource of that power (Bragg 1996). The key to releasing the potential resource of power is to unlock the process of influence. Some theoretical background may help, and this is addressed in the next section.

Box 18.1   Increasing Your Influence

Gain Greater Expertise
- Develop skills in new technologies
- Gain awareness of areas of knowledge you are lacking
- Gain more knowledge (general or specific)
- Attain knowledge that is of a specialised nature (but remember that specialisms come and go)
- Develop interpersonal skills that are of value (emotional intelligence)

Improve Personal Attraction
- Be pleasant at work
- Behave agreeably
- Be seen as trustworthy and likeable
- Avoid lengthy unresolved conflicts
- Dress (and smell!) to impress

Gain Legitimacy
- Can you articulate your values and beliefs?
- Are your values and beliefs consistent or compatible with those of the organisation or your colleagues?
- Are you seen to be demonstrating (living) your own or the organisation's values and beliefs?
- Can you articulate your vision?

Make an Effort
- Does what you do help or hinder your 'boss' or colleagues?
- What do you need to do to increase your departmental/organisational knowledge?
- Remember that effort equates to dedication and commitment.
- Contribute to organisational functions and be seen doing relevant and appropriate things.
- Arrive early, leave late – it all helps.

Critical Social Theory ·

Critical social theory is relevant to healthcare because it is centred on social justice and empowerment and the relationships among knowledge, ideology and power as core to learning and experience. While always relevant, in particular, the pandemic has highlighted that healthcare cannot be isolated from the impacts of social, economic and political positions that direct how it is funded, supported and distributed (James et al. 2021). All healthcare professions provide a service for society, within which lies a core responsibility to social justice. Developing knowledgeable clinical leadership with a renewed critical social consciousness is needed to attend realistically to our diverse populations and the issues which affect health globally, and to ensure nursing and all healthcare education includes global perspectives and inequities (James et al. 2021). Clinical leaders can apply critical social theory to challenge assumptions and stereotypes and reduce communication failures or misinformation and champion equity of healthcare for patients and communities.

Fundamentally, social justice and healthcare are intertwined, by the nature of the ethical and moral principles which are intrinsic to the professions. If this is accepted, then clinical leadership must also be centred on these purposes as knowledgeable authorities on matters of national health decision making, using power and influencing politics. As an example of current challenges, for this we can consider the pandemic, however, not as a new global phenomenon, as inequalities and pandemics are not contemporary problems as history tells us. Yet we are facing inequity in vaccine availability and distribution, and disbelief in science and misinformation. How clinical leaders apply power to politics is of great importance if patients are to receive equitable access and knowledgeable information.

Reflection Point

COVID-19 spread quickly spread around the world, and healthcare workers were called on to treat infected patients without knowing the full extent of spread, treatment or impact. As the spread increased in some countries quicker than others and while some approaches such as masking and physical distancing were advised, politicians took very different approaches to managing the effects and spread within society, from imposed 'lockdowns' to more lenient advisory approaches. Meanwhile, scientists rushed to develop vaccines. However, the availability of vaccines presented new ethical dilemmas for public health organsiations and politicians in allocating vaccinations and promoting the uptake.

What do you think the main dilemmas were in making decisions about distributing and vaccinating populations and groups?

Consider your own national response policy. Who made these decisions, what professional healthcare groups were involved and what do you know about the decision-making process?

What assumptions and stereotypes has this revealed, if any?

Power politics is sometimes not necessarily about mutuality or cooperation, but rather about achieving pre-determined end points. When professional groups engage, it is commonly through the application of countervailing power (Frankford 1997). In this way, power is subject centred; that is, it flows from one actor (a subject) towards another actor. Consequently, if this process is taken to be the traditional discourse of power, we can say the following about power:

- Power is a force applied by a 'wilful, rational, and autonomous subject' (Frankford 1997, p. 193).
- A second subject of power exists which, although equally wilful, rational and autonomous, is limited by its 'subjection' to the power of the first subject.
- Power can be created, transferred or possessed.
- The primary force of power lies in its ability to take hold of subjects' minds.
- Power is most effective when its action is invisible, and when it is invisible it minimises autonomy and freedom.
- The strongest antidote to this kind of power is transparency, as it helps to restore autonomy and freedom (Frankford 1997).

It is important to recognise that the term 'wilful' refers to an individual who is able to reflect and act on the basis of those reflections. However, to operate wilfully, an individual must be conscious (aware) of their social state. Therefore, in the traditional discourse of power, the application or use of (invisible) power would render the individual less able to be wilful.

Critical social theory evolved as a way of examining, or thinking about, the oppressive effects of society (Giroux 1983). It is not one discrete concept, but rather a conglomeration of theories (Fay 1987). A critical theory would want to explain a social order in such a way that the theory becomes a catalyst for transformation or shifts in power. Box 18.2 is a hypothetical example.

Box 18.2   Handmaidens in Healthcare

Imagine that the profession of medicine has a historical association with nursing, such that it is in the interests of medicine for nurses to carry out the orders of the doctors, that is, to support the practice of medicine (as I said, it is hypothetical).

Now, imagine that some nurses start to understand that the ways in which they care for individuals are limited by the subservient role they find themselves in towards medicine. Assume that this understanding develops, and as it develops it causes a great deal of suffering for those nurses who believe they could provide better care if they were not 'shackled' to medicine. These 'more aware' nurses are cognisant of their social state and believe that a crisis is looming, a crisis that could be resolved if only more nurses became aware of the need and potential for change.

However, these more enlightened nurses are unable to act because the majority of nurses remain ignorant of their 'handmaiden' state. Therefore, the suffering of the enlightened nurses is accentuated by the ignorance, or false consciousness, of some of their own group. Finally, assume that nursing represents the largest component of the healthcare workforce, and that if all nurses could have a different understanding of their social state, they would have the power to discard the shackles and alleviate their suffering by providing more effective (and autonomous) nursing care.

In explaining this situation, critical social theory would focus on the crisis and explain it as a function of the false consciousness of some of the group members. If explained in the right way, such a critique could lead to a change in consciousness and the transformation of nurses as a group; that is, by raising the consciousness of the oppressed, the critical theory enables the social group to achieve enlightenment. Enlightenment can be viewed as the ability of the group to see themselves in a different way. However, enlightenment is not enough; to achieve liberation, the social group must take action by becoming empowered. So, the aim of social action is emancipation.

Hence, the goal of critical social science is achieved through the instigation of a three-phase process: enlightenment, empowerment and emancipation (Fay 1987). According to Fay (1987), a fully formed critical theory would contain the following elements:

- **A theory of false consciousness:** This exemplifies how the self-understandings of a group (of people) are false. This is not to suggest that people are duped (although the earlier reference to power taking hold of subjects' minds implies this kind of process). Rather, false consciousness refers to a process whereby a group takes on the values and beliefs of a more dominant group and thus becomes oppressed (this effect is commonly witnessed following imperial colonisation).
- **A theory of crisis:** This examines the level of dissatisfaction within a group and the ways in which the crisis produced threatens the cohesion of society.
- **A theory of education:** This provides an account of the conditions necessary to achieve enlightenment.
- **A theory of transformative action:** This identifies the aspects of a society that require alteration in order to resolve the social crisis and provides a plan of action.

Thus, through enlightenment about their current position and their potential, the congruent leader can encourage the healthcare workforce to be empowered and to work towards reform.

Healthcare and Politics

Politics is defined as the 'process of human interaction within organisations' (Yoder-Wise 2015, p. 417) and can be seen working wherever people congregate (e.g. in families, in professional and interprofessional groups and in leisure activities). It is significant for clinical leaders to be aware of and consider, because politics is really about dealing with change (Missen 2009; Marquis and Houston 2012).

Advocacy and action are processes based on values and principles within healthcare, and professionals are predominantly ferocious when defending their patients' needs. Yet politics is often considered to be beyond the scope of a professional's responsibilities, and nurses in particular rarely take action into the socio-political platform As a result, the media, politicians, organised medicine and many healthcare executives or heads of departments of health have viewed nurses and nursing as powerless or irrelevant (Antrobus et al. 2009; Su et al. 2011; Yoder-Wise 2015). Recently, the pandemic has placed a further spotlight on the role of nurses and healthcare professionals which has emphasised the role of politics, health policy, and distribution of resources (Bennett et al. 2020). Within many countries, a historical lack of funding and focus on health and social care policy has resulted in the collapse and reduction of services and support to the public, as healthcare resources are focused towards managing the pandemic. However, this illumination of the importance of the health professions, the need for investment and overall widening interest in political leadership decision making could also emphsise the importance of involving nursing and other professions in policy direction. There may always be a dichotomy between political power and decision making to healthcare and its social justice values; however, how a government treats its people is often a marker of its own state of health.

Nurses have demonstrated influence on US health reforms, with nurses and professional nursing organisations across the United States mobilising to voice their needs and those of their patients to the Obama administration (Gardner 2009; Hahn 2009; Malloy 2009; Newland 2009; Tongue 2009). The same has been seen in the UK, where nurses and other professional groups spoke up to influence the outcome of the national election in mid-2010 (Dean 2010a, b; Staines 2010) and in the wake of the Francis Inquiry (Francis 2013). In Australia, health reforms are being influenced and orchestrated by powerful nursing lobby groups, such as nurse practitioners (NPs) and practice nurses, often with the support of professional organisations in an attempt to stimulate health reform and engage more actively in the politics of healthcare (Kearney 2010; Picton 2010; Thomas 2010). In reality, medicine as a whole has long had a powerful political voice, often out of all proportion to the size of its professional groups, and with carefully practised and well-directed comments it shows us the value of speaking up on 'political' issues.

Cohen et al. (1996) suggest that there are four stages to the political development of the profession of nursing, which also apply to other health professional disciplines:

- **Buy-in** – where the importance of activism is realised
- **Self-interest** – where the significance of politics is realised and political acumen is developed
- **Political sophistication** – where self-interest is eclipsed and there is a recognition that wider (public) benefit can be achieved with activism
- **Leading the way** – where genuine leadership is forthcoming on a range of healthcare platforms

Recent examples of healthcare being portrayed as both forces for good and manipulated by misinformation as conspirators of harm have been prevalent in particular regarding the promotion of vaccination, or supporters of mandatory vaccination for COVID-19, even though the majority within healthcare advocate for consent and personal choice (Wise 2021). This also serves as a warning about the delicate nature of politics and power and is a cautious reminder that the political landscape is often shaped by those seeking their own ends or serving their own agenda. Nothing gained will come easily, and, once an objective has been gained, vigilance is needed to monitor policy development and political backsliding or manipulation of the policies and the consequences.

If nurses and other health professionals are to engage in the politics of healthcare, clinical leaders may be best placed to bring clinical imperatives to the political debate and therefore must be cognizant with political agendas and policy (Yoder-Wise 2019; Bennett et al. 2020). Antrobus (2003) feels that political leadership occurs at the macro level and that the clinical leader's main aim is to deliver improved patient outcomes at the micro (clinical) or meso (strategic/executive) levels. However, if health professionals are genuinely going to have an impact on policymaking at local or national levels, there needs to be a strong clinical voice speaking for practitioners and patients at the political table (Antrobus et al. 2009; Missen 2009; Yoder-Wise 2015). Getting to the table requires clinical leaders to become politically astute, and to develop self-confidence and collaboration skills, as well as the capacity to work with a wide range of other professionals and people in healthcare (Kramer and Schmalenberg 2003). Clinical leaders also need to learn that change takes time and that the path to change can sometimes be convoluted (Jasper and Jumaa 2005; Marquis and Houston 2012). Finally, clinical leaders need to remain humble and congruent to their values, as staying at the table and engaging in politics require tact and focus.

Reflection Point

Consider the quote at the beginning of this chapter from 'The Cat's Table'.

Do you think you can influence what is regarded as 'macro' or wider level decisions in your profession? How do you think this could be best achieved?

Practical Politics

Dealing with the Media

Nursing and all health professionals have been forced into the media coverage as a consequence of the pandemic, and it is important to be aware of the intended and unintended consequences this brings. Social media has enormous potential for communication globally, and while this can be useful, the potential for negative influences is also acknowledged. This has been recognised by many of the professional regulatory bodies and guidance, such as that produced by the Nursing and Midwifery Council (NMC) in the UK, setting out the advantages and disadvantages while focusing professionals to maintain the values they align to while engaging in social media activities (NMC 2020). If nurses and health professionals are to distribute positive news about their contribution to the health system out into the wider society, the nursing profession needs to deal with the media effectively. Man (2010) put this simply in explaining Genghis Khan's leadership secret number one: controlling the message. In many ways, groups of nurses and key professional bodies have achieved this, but there is much that clinical leaders can do to harvest the bounty that media acumen can deliver.

Dealing with the media can be a minefield, so if you have had no specific training or if it is not an integral part of your role to liaise with the media, stick with a 'no comment' line. Most organisations have policies about dealing with the media, and these should be consulted before any contact or comment is offered.

It is worth noting that while the media are in the business of getting hold of news, it is possible through social media for every individual to 'be the media'. While this is effective, it is also fraught with dangers and risks. Most professional bodies have policies and guidelines for the use of social media, and for good reason. These guidelines should be considered and followed before the social media worlds of Twitter, Facebook and YouTube are used to 'spread the word'.

Becoming Politically Active

Becoming politically active does not mean handing out 'how to vote' leaflets on election day (although it could) or joining a political party (although that is an option). Here, it simply means gathering yourself to stand up for what you value and believe and joining in the discussion, debate or dialogue or taking action so that you gain a voice in your hospital, clinical environment, community, local area, city, state, country or even in the wider world. Becoming politically active does not mean becoming a 'radical' or 'extremist'. These approaches to politics often polarise debate and stifle collaboration, creativity and democratic discussion. Therefore, the following list offers information about how to become politically active in support of promoting the nurse's role and function without becoming a 'political radical'.

Becoming a politically active health professional can involve one of more of these strategies:

- Join a professional association (networking).
- Become involved in newsletter contributions (writing or distribution).
- Get involved in the committee structure and meetings of local or national professional associations.
- Recognise that if you are not looking to forward an opinion or view, someone else is. Someone is always listening – if it is not to you or your professional group, then they are hearing some other group's view.
- Write letters (not emails, as they are too easily deleted or ignored) to an individual member of parliament or local government official. Be clear and concise and explain the changes that you want to see. Keep your letter short and avoid blaming or being critical. Be positive and productive and provide your contact details so that they can reply; in fact, encourage a reply.
- Move issues from tactical to strategic by developing strategic objectives, identifying key stakeholders and constructing different messages for different stakeholders (Antrobus et al. 2009).
- Identify what you can do (in your clinical area, in your community, locally or nationally), not just what you would like to do.
- Engage with broader professional issues and gain a voice as a professional in the wider health arena and in health-related topics.
- Contribute to articles, publish in other ways and use the internet to express your views (there are a wide range of websites that seek to promote the cause of nursing and other professional groups).
- Support and sign petitions that matter to you.
- Become informed: use social media such as twitter, as they can be an excellent source of information. However, be cautious and critique, make sure the sources are robust and be professional if you are responding with a comment. Explore the internet and seek out conferences, join in, become involved. You *can* make a difference.

Reflection Point

Do you see yourself as politically active? Why and in what way? Are you a member of a union or a professional body? Are you a member of a club or sporting organisation? Do these organisations have a political agenda? What impact do these activities have on your political views and on the way you express yourself politically at work? Is politics something you feel you just do not do? Speak with your work colleagues about what they think about the nexus (union) of politics and your workplace or your professional discipline.

It's How You Use It!

This exploration of the concepts of power, politics and leadership has introduced some ideas and posed some questions aimed at prompting your thoughts. One of the ideas is that all nurses and other health professionals use power and are subjected to power and have the capacity to be political. What this suggests is the importance of being aware of the power dynamics operating in your practice area and in your own practice.

In the end, of course, the ways in which you use power, or support its use, will affect the care provided to individuals in your care. Therefore, it makes good sense to consider, and make rational choices about, the power relationships that you develop.

Case Study 18.1   Baroness Tanni Grey-Thompson DBE

Carys Davina Grey was born in 1969 in Cardiff, Wales and was soon known by the nickname her sister Sian gave her, evolving from 'Tiny' to Tanni.

Tanni was born with spina bifida and was a determined and independent child, keen to try a range of sports, and at age 13 years found that Wheelchair Racing was for her, winning the Junior National title for 100 m, and she was part of the British Wheelchair Racing Squad at age 17.

From her first Paralympic bronze medal in Seoul in 1988 for the 400 m, her achievements continued, including six victories in the London Wheelchair Marathon, four gold medals and a silver in the Barcelona Paralympics, where she also broke the 60-second barrier for 400 m. Winning a gold and three silver medals in Atlanta, four gold medals in the Sydney Paralympics and a gold in her final Games in Athens, Tanni had achieved 11 gold medals, World Championships and broke 30 world records across her athletics career.

Tanni has been recognised and received many honorary awards of recognition as she continued to be involved in sporting committees following her athletics career. She supported educational and campaign activities in the UK, using her experience and knowledge to promote Disability Rights and Welfare Reform, becoming a Dame Commander of the Order of the British Empire, and then Peer in the House of Lords in 2010.

(Continued)

Tanni gave birth to her daughter Carys in 2002, and she has also spoken about the challenges she faced from others while pregnant and her disagreement with the description of athletes with disabilities as 'inspirational': 'It is almost like you have to have had something dramatic or traumatic happen to you to justify your position as a disabled athlete'.

Tanni's Leadership

Tanni has demonstrated her personal style of leadership not only through her athletic achievements but how she elevated the issues within disability sport, voicing her opinions about the characterisation of athletes, the Paralympics and of the wider issues around disability rights. Being visible and knowledgeable in areas of influence, such as the House of Lords, and in the media, Tanni has demonstrated her ability to influence and appeal to the general public as well as long-established institutions.

Challenge: Tanni developed her enthusiasm and determination for her sport at a young age, and this meant she was very aware of the challenges within disabilities sport in the UK. What qualities of leadership do you think Tanni has demonstrated throughout her career? What have the challenges been for Tanni in making her voice heard, and how has she overcome this through her achievements and recognition?

What are the challenges and support systems for clinicians with disabilities to lead within our healthcare systems? Do we address issues such as prejudice, sexism and racism as leaders ourselves within healthcare? Reflect on any experiences you may have had of these.

Summary

- Politics and power are central issues in health service delivery, and health professionals should develop an awareness, interest and commitment to being politically engaged.
- Our social context influences our experience of power.
- Power is about the perceived ability to exercise influence over others.
- There are a number of different types of power: reward, punishment or coercive, legitimate, expert, charismatic, resource and informational power.
- Influence and power are related. There are different types of influence: assertive, reward and punishment, participation and trust, and common vision.
- Power, even professional power, is exercised within the context of the social 'theatre' in which the actors (subjects) operate. Critical social theory is used to explore catalysts for transformation or power shifts.
- Health professionals, and nurses in particular, are beginning to engage more effectively in the political side of healthcare. Clinical leaders may be best placed to bring clinical imperatives to the political debate.
- Dealing with the media can be difficult, and great care and appropriate preparation are required.
- Becoming politically engaged is advisable in the modern healthcare environment, and there are a number of options for doing this. It is about finding your 'professional voice' and taking a stand for your values and beliefs.

Mind Press-Ups

Exercise 18.1

Consider two types of leadership: transformational leadership and congruent leadership. What sources of power would you identify as being associated with the theories behind them, and why?

Exercise 18.2

What positive outcomes might be achieved for your future colleagues if, in the course of your work, you use your power and authority constructively?

Exercise 18.3

Consider your professional role in social justice. How can you apply these principles to current challenges in healthcare?

References

Antrobus, S. (2003). What is political leadership? *Nursing Standard* 17 (4): 40–44.

Antrobus, S., Macleod, A., and Masterson, A. (2009). *Developing political leaders in nursing*. In: *Leadership for Nursing and Allied Health Care Professions, Maidenhead* (ed. V. Bishop). Berkshire: McGraw-Hill.

Bennett, C., James, A., and Kelly, D. (2020). 'Beyond tropes: towards a new image of nursing in the wake of COVID-19. *Journal of Clinical Nursing* http://dx.doi.org/10.1111/jocn.15346.

Bishop, V. (ed.) (2009). *Leadership for Nursing and Allied Health Care Professions*. Maidenhead: McGraw-Hill.

Bragg, M. (1996). *Reinventing Influence: How to Get Things Done in a World without Authority*. London: Pitman.

Braynion, P. (2004). Power and leadership. *Journal of Health, Organisation and Management* 18 (6): 447–462.

Brooks, I. (2009). *Organisational Behaviour: Individuals, Groups and Organisation*, 4e. Financial Times: Prentice Hall.

Cohen, S.S., Mason, D.J., Kovner, C. et al. (1996). Stages of nursing political development: where we've been and where we ought to go. *Nursing Outlook* 44: 259–266.

Commission of Social Determinants of Health (2008). Closing the Gap in a generation: health equity through action on the social determinants of health. World Health Organization (www.who.int).

Dean, E. (2010a). Pay attention. *Nursing Standard* 24 (28): 22.

Dean, E. (2010b). It's time to boost the key role of ward sisters. *Nursing Standard* 24 (35): 12.

Fay, B. (1987). *Critical Social Science: Liberation and Its Limits*. Cambridge: Polity Press.

Foucault, M. (1969). *The Archaeology of Knowledge (L'Archéologie du savoir)* (trans. A. M. Sheridan-Smith). New York: Harper & Row.

Foucault, M. (1995). *Discipline and Punish: The Birth of the Prison*. New York: Vantage.

Francis, R. (2013). *Report of the Mid Staffordshire NHS Foundation Trust Public Inquiry*. London: HM Stationery Office.

Frankford, D.D.M. (1997). The normative constitution of professional power. *Journal of Health Politics, Policy and Law* 22 (1): 185–221.

French, J. and Raven, B. (1959). The basis of social power. In: *Understanding Organisational, Political and Personal Power: Leadership Roles and Management Functions in Nursing, Theory and Application*, 7e (ed. B.L. Marquis and C.J. Huston). Philadelphia, PA: Lippincott, Williams & Wilkins.

Gardner, D. (2009). The evolving voice of nursing in health care reform. *Nursing Economics* 24 (7): 255–259.

Gilson, L., Schneider, H., and Orgill, M. (2014). Practice and power: a review and interpretive synthesis focused on the exercise of discretionary power in policy implementation by front line providers and managers. *Health Policy and Planning* 29: iii51–iii69.

Giroux, H.A. (1983). *Theory and Resistance in Education*. London: Heinemann Education.

Hahn, J. (2009). Power dynamics, health policy and politics. *MEDSURG Nursing* 18 (3): 197–199.

Howard, S. and Gill, J. (2000). The pebble in the pond: Children's constructions of power, politics and democratic citizenship. *Cambridge Journal of Education* 30 (3): 357–358.

Huber, D. (2000). *Power and Conflict: Leadership and Nursing Care Management*. Philadelphia, PA: WB Saunders.

James, A.H., Carrier, J., and Watkins, D. (2021). 'Nursing must respond for social justice in this "perfect storm". Editorial. *Journal of Advanced Nursing* 77 (11): e36–e37. http://dx.doi.org/10.1111/jan.14957.

Jasper, M. and Jumaa, M. (2005). *Effective Healthcare Leadership*. Oxford: Blackwell.

Kearney, G. (2010). Nurses need to be political. *Australian Nurses Journal* 17 (11): 7.

Kramer, M. and Schmalenberg, C. (2003). Securing "good" nurse physician relationships. *Nursing Management* 34 (7): 34–38.

Malloy, D. (2009). AGH nurses meet with Obama to talk health care. *Tribune Business News* (September 11).

Man, J. (2010). *The Leadership Secrets of Genghis Khan*. London: Bantam.

Marquis, B.L. and Houston, C.J. (2012). *Leadership Roles and Management Functions in Nursing*, 7e. Philadelphia, PA: Lippincott, Williams & Wilkins.

McDonald, J., Jayasuriya, R., and Harris, M.F. (2012). 'The influence of power dynamics and trust on multidisciplinary collaboration: a qualitative case study of type 2 diabetes mellitus. *BMC Health Services Research* 12 (1): 63. https://doi.org/10.1186/1472-6963-12-63.

Missen, B. (2009). Mixing nursing and politics for the good of our health. *The Canadian Nurse* 105 (1): 34–35.

Newland, J. (2009). A call for active participation. *Nurse Practitioner* 34 (9): 5.

Nursing and Midwifery Council (2020). Social media Guidance. Social media guidance - The Nursing and Midwifery Council http://nmc.org.uk (accessed 15 September 2021).

Ondaatje, M. (2012). *The Cat's Table*. New York: Vintage ISBN-10: 9780099554424.

Picton, C. (2010). Time to engage with politics'. In: *Emergency Nurse*, vol. 18, no. 3, 3.

Roberts, D.W., and Vasquez, E. (2004). Power: an application to the nursing image and advanced practice. *AACN Clinical Issues: Advanced Practice in Acute and Critical Care* 15 (2): 196–204.

Sebring, J.C.H. (2021). Towards a sociological understanding of medical gaslighting in western health care. *Sociology of Health & Illness* 43: 1–14. http://dx.doi.org/10.1111/146 7-9566.13367.

Staines, R. (2010). Nurses join the campaign trail. *Nursing Standard* 24 (34): 62.

Su, S.F., Jenkins, M., and Liu, P.E. (2011). Nurses' perception of leadership style in hospitals: a grounded theory study. *Journal of Clinical Leadership* 21 (1–2): 722–780.

Thomas, L. (2010). Lee. *Australian Nursing Journal* 18 (3): 19.

Tongue, S. (2009). Obama's vision. *Nursing Standard* 24 (2): 64.

Van Deth, J.W., Abendschön, S., and Volmar, M. (2011). Children and politics: an empirical reassessment of early political socialization. *Political Psychology* 32 (1): http://dx.doi. org/10.1111/j.1467-9221.2010.00798.x.

Wilding, P. (1982). *Professional Power and Social Welfare*. London: Routledge & Kegan Paul.

Wise, J. (2021). COVID-19: France and Greece make vaccination mandatory for healthcare workers. *BMJ* 374: 1797. http://dx.doi.org/10.1136/bmj.n1797.

Yoder-Wise, P.S. (2015). *Leading and Managing in Nursing*, 6e. London: Mosby.

Yoder-Wise, P.S. (2019). A framework for planned policy change. *Nursing Forum* 55: 45–53. http://dx.doi.org/10.1111/nuf.12381.

19

From Empowerment to Emancipation – Developing Self-Leadership

Alison H. James and Clare L. Bennett

> *I am impelled, not to squeak like a grateful and apologetic mouse, but to roar like a lion out of pride in my profession.*
>
> John Steinbeck (1962)

Introduction: Elevating Your Voice

Within this chapter, we consider the concepts of empowerment and emancipation within clinical leadership. As the age of leadership theory within healthcare shifts from authoritarian models to relationship and values-based approaches, the defining characteristic for clinical leadership has changed to, 'listening to staff and arriving at a shared understanding of the challenges they face, empathising with and supporting them, rather than always imposing decisions from the top down' (The King's Fund 2020), so empowering and enabling has become a core role for leaders. However, while this shift to leadership approaches applies to all professions within healthcare, there remain historical professional silos and cultural influences, which mean the achievement of emancipation is challenging, for both leaders and followers.

Many authors feel that nurses display the characteristics of an oppressed group, showing signs that they lack self-esteem, autonomy, accountability or power (Friedson 1970; Greenleaf 1978; LeRoux 1978; Roberts 1983, 2000; Stein et al. 1990; Fulton 1997; Freshwater 2000). There is evidence to support the need to elevate and promote nursing leadership within healthcare delivery and ensure it is embedded and valued within nurse education (Kelly et al. 2016; James 2020). Indeed, the recognition to shift the stance of nursing from its angelic oppressed, and suppressed status to one of influencing professional and political decision making continued to gain pace during the pandemic, and is discussed further in Chapter 18 (Bennett et al. 2020). So, whether we consider leading within healthcare as a personal skill, a strategic concept, at local or global levels, across all healthcare professions it is worth considering what empowerment means and whether

Clinical Leadership in Nursing and Healthcare, Third Edition.
Edited by David Stanley, Clare L. Bennett and Alison H. James.
© 2023 John Wiley & Sons Ltd. Published 2023 by John Wiley & Sons Ltd.

emancipation can be enabled or whether it can only be achieved by the individual who seeks it.

To provide an effective and safe healthcare service, a multi-professional approach is needed; however, it has been suggested that to lead within these complex systems, creative leadership is required, shifting away from authoritarian hierarchy and control to capture the organic natural strengths of its workforce (Plesk and Wilson 2001). Within healthcare organsiations, there are multiple layers of professional cultures and hierarchies. To ignore the essential role of leadership within these would be naive and, indeed, dangerous, as many serious health reviews of failing leadership have been reported in recent years in the UK (Francis 2013). Embracing the interconnectedness of our professions and values can be empowering in itself and encourages a collaborative culture, nurtures trust and belonging and supports positive emancipation and self-efficacy of individuals within a workforce.

For a 'caring profession', nurses can be quite hostile towards each other at times, and bullying within the profession has been acknowledged as a continuing influence and to be a culturally disempowering obstacle, both within clinical areas and academia (Meissner 1986; Meissner 1999; Birks et al. 2017; Derbyshire and Thompson 2021). Recent research conducted by one of the authors demonstrated the emotional impact of experiencing negative examples of leadership (James 2020). This professional maleficence and purposeful self-destruction are counterintuitive to values-centred nursing, yet it must be acknowledged and addressed as disempowering if it is to be confronted. Perhaps clinical leaders could be the empowering force, breaking the oppressive bonds associated with a traditional view of hierarchy in nursing and healthcare. By seeking the clinical nurse leader's 'voice within' and by exploring the experience of clinical leaders, an understanding can be gained of their place in relation to oppression, empowerment, disempowerment and leadership. Then genuine opportunities for change, improvements in patient care and clinical developments may be achieved.

This chapter explores empowerment and considers how it may be conceptualised and viewed within the context of leadership for health professionals. It also explores the issues of disempowerment and oppression in relation to health professionals and considers how caring professionals can establish empowering behaviours to counteract these issues.

To begin exploring this area and its importance for clinical leadership, it is perhaps useful to attempt a definition of what we mean by both empowerment and emancipation within this context.

Defining Empowerment

Jones and Bennett (2018, p. 66) define empowerment as 'a process which enhances feelings of personal ability in individuals through positive feedback, as well as the identification and removal of the organsiational factors that lead to the feeling of powerlessness'. This definition accepts the influence of both the leader enabling and also being aware of the wider constraints which may inhibit empowerment. Simmonds (1998) indicates that empowerment is associated with helping people develop a critical awareness of their situation and enabling or facilitating them to master their environment to achieve self-determination. Rogers (1979) also sees empowerment as developing from personal growth and the exercise of personal power. Taken in its positive sense, empowerment can be viewed as liberating and allowing innovative and creative development.

However, here we also consider the contradictions. Empowerment is inextricably linked to context. Within organisations where policies and structures are contradictory or inhibiting, the opposite to empowerment can be inevitable, disempowering the individuals who work within. An example of this can be considered in the National Health Service (NHS) in the UK, where collaborative and compassionate leadership is now advocated, yet the traditional structures and institutionalisation of the professions continue to constrain empowerment and self-expression (Fisher and Kiernan 2019). So we know empowerment can be manipulated to advance the organisational needs or individual needs of the leader. The very notion of empowerment can suggest that the leader holds the power, paternalistically allowing individuals to reach for self-empowerment (Western 2019). It is important to consider both perspectives as we explore further these concepts within healthcare.

Clinically focused health professionals and clinical leaders, it may be speculated, represent the empowered few who are able to motivate and inspire others and excel in clinical care. Yet two significantly different perspectives can be presented: as a tool or as the result of personal choice. The decision to apply one or the other will reflect both the clinical leader's perspective on empowerment and their ability genuinely to lead change and development.

Box 19.1 A Little Horror Story, Part 1

Once upon a time … a male student nurse, on his second placement, was taken aside by his assessor (the student's preceptor/mentor and a senior RN on the surgical ward) into the sluice room. This was the first day of this placement, and needless to say, the student nurse was very nervous. This RN took it upon herself to welcome him to the ward. Her 'welcome', however, consisted of telling him that she did not like male nurses, that in her view they were lazy and had no place in nursing. The student nurse was not welcome and she would make sure that he had a difficult placement and would fail. Then she just left him to it. No handover, no guidance, no orientation … no hope. After this, the student was always given the 'heavy' bays and the more 'difficult' patients, and the RN was consistently and persistently rude, snappy and curt. The student's colleagues and fellow students said she was 'just like that' and in fact she seemed to pick on everyone, but he found her negative attention particularly difficult and struggled to cope. (*To be continued*)

The First Perspective: Empowerment as a Tool

Yoder-Wise (2015, p. 420) defines empowerment as a tool, declaring that it is 'the process by which we facilitate the participation of others in decision-making and taking action within an environment where there is an equitable distribution of power'. Other authors take a similar line, with Kreitner and Kinicki (1998) indicating that empowerment is the decentralisation of power, while French and Raven (1959) consider that expert power is the ability to exert influence through the possession of knowledge or skills that are useful to others. How this is developed can be central to your future career and professional development and relates to 'self-mastery' or recognising and releasing your own potential to achieve your self-determined goals. Self -mastery can also be considered a significant step towards personal leadership and emancipation.

Esterhuizen and Kooyman (2001) and Jones et al. (2000) suggest that empowerment can be developed in others by external agents, almost as if empowerment can be bestowed on them. This view is supported by comments made by well-meaning senior health professionals and managers, as they describe how they have 'empowered their staff', and ward managers who have hinted that through staff compliance with an appraisal process, they could 'make staff become more empowered'. To some extent, these views have grown from Kanter's (1977) theory of structural empowerment, where empowering workplace structures are described as those that support employees to accomplish their work in meaningful ways. Kanter (1977) sees employees as human capital needed to achieve organisational goals, with structural empowerment offered as an approach that influences employees' attitudes and behaviours to either increase or decrease organisational effectiveness. Laschinger et al. (2010) built on this work, linking empowerment to improving patient outcomes, and herein perhaps lies the key, ensuring when empowerment is proposed by clinical leaders, it is considered linked to the values of ensuring beneficence and improving patient care, and not as a tool or 'gift'.

The Second Perspective: Empower Walking

If clinical leaders are to be effective leaders, then core values should remain central to their vision, and they must also address the structural and cultural relationships within the workplace which encourage innovation, collaboration and trust. Empowerment in this context is not about one person bestowing a gift on another, as then it can be 'given' by someone in a position of power or authority, and can also be 'taken' by someone in a position of authority. Rather, it is about a leader creating the environment and the conditions within a context to enable the individual to develop self-mastery and create their own direction.

Building on this perspective is hinted at by Grossman and Valiga (2012, p. 195) when they define empowerment as 'a process in which individuals feel strengthened, in control, and in possession of some degree of power'. Within healthcare, we may sometimes consider our lack of power within an organisation; however, when it comes to patient care, there is potential for significant influence and direction based on expert knowledge and core values. Bishop (2009) proposes constructive facilitation of power to support both personal development and enhancing patient outcomes should be the focus of clinical leadership, and Rogers (1979) suggests that personal growth leads to personal power and so to empowerment. This perspective views empowerment as an action that an individual can take, rather than a tool used to impose empowerment on others. The second perspective can only be sustained if the first is rejected.

The book *Long Walk to Freedom* (Mandela 1994) about the life of Nelson Mandela can be used as an example of how empowerment is about personal growth, personal action and personal choice. Mandela's autobiography is a stark example of the life of a person who faced considerable personal obstacles and yet rose above the difficulties of living under an oppressive regime and imprisonment to lead his country. Even the title – where the word 'walk' is used in preference to 'road' or 'journey' – implies that the act of empowerment is about an individual's activity, choice and actions, and it is not a passive, not a 'given'.

The novel *The Power of One* by Bryce Courtenay (1989), about a young English boy growing up in South Africa, also deals with the theme of empowerment. Peekay is not a big person, but he grows up to become a boxer. Early in his life he is taught the maxim that 'little beat big when little smart, first with the head then with the heart'. Peekay faced considerable difficulties as he grew up, isolated and an outsider. This fictional story and Mandela's real-life biography both imply that empowerment is something that comes from within, something that emerges from the individual and something that relies on the individual's choice. In both these examples, empowerment was not dependent on a suitable environment, the person's authority, the beneficence of a senior colleague or favourable conditions.

The second perspective sees empowerment not as something that can be 'done' to others, but as something that remains in the domain of the individual and is reliant on the individual's ability to choose self-mastery. If clinical leaders demonstrate this approach, they will recognise that empowerment cannot be bestowed, given or imposed by them, or indeed be bestowed, given or imposed on them by others. The origin of the power to choose or to act is within the individual and can only be achieved by conscious choice or direct action by the individual concerned. As such, the power to choose or act rests squarely with the individual practitioner, client or person, aligning itself with the concept of accountability.

Bower (2000, p. 2) calls this 'knowing self' and also advocates self-inspection and self-knowledge as a way to developing leadership skills and personal empowerment (linked here to reflection and emotional intelligence). Nevertheless, the process of self-discovery, vital to empowerment, is not an easy one, as Rinpoche (1992, p. 31) states in this Buddhist extract:

> Yet how hard it can be to turn our attention within! How easily we allow our old habits and set patterns to dominate us! Even though they bring us suffering, we accept them with almost fatalistic resignation, for we are so used to giving in to them. We may idealise freedom, but when it comes to our habits, we are completely enslaved.

Viewed from the first perspective, empowerment comes from someone with the power or authority to give it, implying that such empowerment will be limited and transitory. When viewed from the second perspective, empowerment becomes a liberating, self-directing and personally uplifting prospect.

Unfortunately, much of the health service and management literature focuses on empowerment established from the first perspective. In a health service steeped in traditional, hierarchical structures, power – both personal and organisational – is held in place by position and authority. Clinical leaders (who may come from any level within the organisational structure) need to focus on empowerment from within and work on addressing the barriers that inhibit both themselves and others in their search for empowerment. Clinical leaders who employ congruent leadership (Stanley 2006a, b, 2008, 2011, 2014, 2019) engender a collaborative work approach that sees others following their lead as they live out their values and beliefs. These clinical leaders can demonstrate their professional traits or act out their core professional values in practice. Many have been able to engage in a choice to be empowered and are in a position to foster greater confidence among their colleagues and clients. These health professionals also benefit from improvements in healthcare environments, so they are more effectively supported in their progress and learning and are encouraged to promote greater staff participation and client choice. In this way barriers to empowerment are reduced, so that individual and professional empowerment can be achieved, although such barrier-busting interventions are not in themselves empowering.

Ultimately, the choice to engage with a supportive work environment or genuinely to participate in continuous professional development or any other liberating, stimulating or role-enhancing activity rests with the individual. Recognising that the individual has the power to choose, to engage with the organisation or with the client, is equally important as accepting that seeing empowerment as a tool will provide a diminished return. Teaching, encouraging, facilitating and directing are doing exactly what those words suggest – in a sense, showing a path to empowerment, but not actually empowering, because even if the barriers are down and even if the environment is the best it can be, it is still up to the individual to take that first step forward. If they do not choose self-empowerment, they will not cross the threshold.

Empowerment isn't the path, it's the walk and the choice about which path to take. Taking that risk, taking a chance, going out on a limb or to the edge requires empowerment from within and will happen independently of the state of the environment, professional position and leadership approach. If perfect conditions were the prerequisite for empowerment, nothing would ever get done.

Because power comes from within, you can facilitate it in others, but you cannot make it happen. Nelson Mandela was empowered and his will to act was a choice. He was not empowered by others: his countrymen, the government, his fellow prisoners or activists. His empowerment was not bestowed by others, and the obstacles and barriers he had to overcome and resist were immense. Yet accepting that empowerment comes from within is in itself liberating, because it allows individuals to focus on their own empowerment and to recognise the part they can play in taking down barriers for others. This is supported by Regan et al. (2016), who identified that linking values-focused leadership and empowerment led to the possibility of improving interprofessional collaboration, as health professionals developed more confidence and greater trust between themselves.

There is an ongoing challenge globally of retaining nurses and other healthcare professionals, and the recent pandemic has increased this as the demands and emotional feeling of powerlessness pervades our healthcare systems. Enabling empowerment is pivotal to the success of the clinical leader and to the effective accomplishment of their responsibilities. Indeed, it can create a legacy of meaningful support for others if applied with thought and consideration of its impact. It is even more vital to influence positive job satisfaction and staff retention, as these have been found to be interrelated and linked to autonomy, empowerment and agency (Gottileb et al. 2021). Beginning with self-reflection and awareness, clinical leaders should tap into the centre of their being, reflect on their practice and ask questions of their own self-mastery. They should also talk to, engage with, challenge and react to their colleagues, clients and managers. They should read about other ways of working or doing work, and engage with, initiate and become open to research, reflection, best practice and evidence-based practice. In this time of crisis and potential for feeling lack of having influence, leaders should embrace the new ways of working an innovation which was driven by necessity and see forward in a new light. They should explore their values and beliefs, look at their motives and explore the forces that drive them. Empowerment will not come to them and it will not be given to them, but from these steps they should be able to empower themselves and thus facilitate the journey of others.

Reflection Point

Che Guevara said, 'The revolution is made by man, but man must forge his revolutionary spirit day to day. Keeping the revolutionary spirit alive takes commitment and passion, belief and faith' (Knowles 2001, p. 354). What helps empower you? What are you committed to or passionate about? What do you believe in and what sustains your faith to keep going, day after day?

Box 19.2 A Little Horror Story, Part 2

The student was struggling. The clinical work and adjusting to the pace and drama of surgical nursing were difficult enough, but the senior RN's sniping and criticism, ridicule and miscommunication were really affecting his confidence and ability to function. The student took a few 'sickies' to avoid having to work with her and even made an appointment with an educator to discuss the problem discreetly. The educator knew about the RN's behaviour but declared that she was 'just like that' and other students had raised this problem in the past. What could she do? It was not an educational issue and the student was advised to discuss the matter with the hospital manager, the RN's boss, or to deal with it himself. The educator suggested that the student work harder and give the RN no reason to criticise or ridicule him.

The student did not want to go to the hospital manager, who by all accounts was a friend of the RN. So he reasoned he was just going to have to cope by rising above the matter. If the RN thought that male nurses were lazy, he would show her that they were not; in fact, she would see that this male nurse worked very hard. So the student began turning up a few minutes before work and leaving a few minutes later. He started helping other nurses with their patients and tried always to be one step ahead. If the RN came and said 'Have you taken out a wound drain?' or 'Have you done that set of obs?', he was more and more able to say 'Yes, done that', so giving her fewer faults to find and making her re-evaluate her stance. Other staff were also getting behind him and being supportive and were grateful for the help and effort he was making. Their support started to make the RN's ridicule and criticism seem petty or unfair and in time the sniping, nasty comments and ridicule began to subside.   (*To be continued*)

Oppression: Bridging the Power Divide

We contend that clinical leaders need to act as catalysts to lead change, empowering themselves and others, motivating, inspiring and leading nursing and the health service forward.

However, there is a raft of literature that claims that health professionals need to change because they may be disempowered and need inspiring, motivating and leading. This view is not new. Roberts (1983, 2000) – who is supported by Cleland (1971), Torres (1981), Clifford (1992), Oughtibridge (1998), Freshwater (2000), Watson and Shields (2009) and others – indicates that experts on nursing leadership have argued that the lack of nursing leaders is due to a lack of people with initiative, self-esteem and assertiveness in the nursing profession. They add that the style of leadership within nursing has evolved because nurses, like other groups throughout history, are oppressed. There is also debate on the anti-intellectualization of nurse education and the ongoing effects of this which are attributed to a number of contextual issues, including to leadership within nursing (Holmes and Lindsay 2018; Thompson and Clark 2018; Derbyshire et al. 2019; Racine and Vendenburg 2020).

Nursing has traditionally been oppressed because of being predominantly a female dominant in a patriarchal society and having evolved within a context dominated by the powerful hierarchical (male-dominated) medical profession. It may be that this perspective can be applied to other health professional groups. Bennett et al. (2020) discussed the tensions which emerged during the pandemic within images and language portrayed in the press and how this contributed to depicting nurses as heroes, or victims, rather than leading the vision for contributing to prevailing over the pandemic through knowledge and expertise. This oppressive state appears not to be waning, despite calls from the World Health Organisation (2020) for nursing to step up and lead globally. Nurses also display some of the characteristics of other oppressed groups, a lack of self-esteem and show passive aggression that extends into behaviours such as the 'horizontal violence' already mentioned (McNamara 2012;; Riskin et al. 2015; Wing et al. 2015). Freshwater (2000) sees such behaviour as the unexpressed or repressed expression of conflict within an oppressed group. Indeed, conflict within the oppressed group that is directed towards other members of the oppressed group is a further characteristic of oppression. Powerless groups, who are unable to act against their oppressors or feel unable to change their circumstances, frequently vent their frustrations on the least powerful within their own group. Horizontal violence appears to be an expression of this characteristic.

Characteristics of oppressed groups can be summed up as follows:

- They look and act differently from the dominant group (who set the norms) and their actions and looks are valued negatively. The looks and actions of the dominant group are associated with power and control; oppressors have a non-uniform dress and they make the rules.
- Assimilation – they try to look like the oppressor, which can lead to marginalisation and to further self-hatred and low self-esteem.
- Portrayed as victims or weaker versions of the dominant group.
- Dissociation from their own culture if it is perceived to be subordinate and attempts to emulate or 'fit in'.
- Passive aggression in the face of being powerless against the oppressor. This can lead to self- destructive behaviour and aggression as oppressed people turn on their own group.

- Horizontal violence – the oppressed cannot attack the oppressor so they turn on themselves or their own kind.
- They are often viewed as inherently violent or uncooperative, rather than this being seen as a result of oppression.
- Submission to authority.
- Fear of authority.
- Fear of change, even though change in the oppressive circumstances is required.
- Lack of faith in their own ability to take responsibility.
- Lack of confidence in their ability to change the status quo.

When studying oppression within Brazilian society, Freire (1971) found that oppressed groups learnt to hate themselves or their attributes (e.g. skin colour, language, clothing) because the dominant group set the norms for what was valued. Therefore, members of the oppressed group who attempted to succeed and escape their oppression could only do so by attempting to act and look as much as possible like the members of the dominant group – in effect, denying their own characteristics. This led to what Lewin (1948) called marginalisation and resulted when members of the oppressed group tried to escape but remained non-authentic members of the dominant group. This sort of behaviour often resulted in self-hatred, disapproval (from within their own group), frustration and conflict. Freire (1971) concluded that members of the oppressed group were then unable to unite against the dominant group and instead developed a passive-aggressive approach to dealing with the oppressor. Freire (1971) also proposed that the maintenance of oppression was supported by the educational system and by rewarding those in the oppressed group who supported the dominant views and values. Jobs, financial support and privileges were awarded to such people in the oppressed group, who worked to maintain the position of the dominant group and to subdue any potential revolt that might begin. As such, the subordinate group failed to establish any power base because its leadership was marginalised and it fostered, rather than diminished, conflict and frustration. As Freire (1971, p. 29) commented, 'it is the rare peasant who, if promoted to landowner, does not become the tyrant of the peasant'.

The position of nurse leaders has been evident in the UK during the pandemic as the visibility of nurse leaders has been significantly less than medical experts and politicians in the discussions portrayed to the public. There is also a need for nursing to be aware of the self-imposed and other-imposed self-fulfilling prophecy of nursing and leadership being misaligned, meaning our expectations and beliefs as leaders are not fully realised, and therefore we continue to conform to the oppressed underachievement expected. Leaders are commonly rewarded for maintaining the status, and furthermore, bullying can have a repetitive domino effect which reduces the profession and its status. The effects of the abuse of power and abuse in this context result in a devalued and oppressed workforce with risks to patient safety (Shorey and Wong 2021). Rather than contributing to the oppression, clinical leaders' professions should address the insidious undertones by:

- Clearly demonstrating professional values by addressing the negative cultures and inherited acceptance of bullying
- Demonstrating that a compassionate and values-based profession leads by example, pervading its philosophy throughout delivering care and services to patients, and to its workforce

- Demonstrating transparency in both how bullying is dealt with and how the positive effects of being free of negative cultures can elevate both self-value and improve workforce effectiveness

Liberated Leaders or Co-Oppressors?

It is prudent to ask whether nurses and other health professionals are in fact marginalised in the health service. It is also true to say that many nurses are from marginalised groups within Western society (indigenous/racially marginalised groups), and many more are from countries where women are still treated with less respect than men. With the progress of moving nursing in the UK to a degree level qualification, the aim was to elevate the profession, promoting the importance of research-based care and deserving of a place in decision making and expertise in patient care. However, the entry standard and educational level of nurses are still generally lower than those of medical and some allied health professionals. It could also be suggested that traditional medical values remain dominant within the health service, and that while today few nurses are viewed as 'handmaidens', the nursing characteristics of warmth, care, empathy, self-sacrifice and sensitivity are commonly viewed negatively within the target-driven, outcome-focused, financially constrained health service. Furthermore, having come so far in promoting the need for degree education in nursing, there are concerns of an increasing trend of anti-intellectualism, a focus on quantity rather than quality in nurse education and the corporate drivers of universities where nursing programmes are seen as money generators (Derbyshire et al. 2019; Racine and Vandenberg 2020).

It is also worth asking whether nursing and all health professionals have a positive public voice, or if the public perception of health professionals remains positive. Certainly, this has changed globally during the pandemic, with a rise of violence, stigmatisation and harassment reported (Devi 2020), and the volume of misinformation about the virus, vaccinations and conspiracy theories of the role of healthcare workers has been expedited by social media. The wider role of political leaders and communication has not sufficiently addressed this, and there are always alternative agendas at play. What is needed is considered and collaborative approaches to ensuring healthcare workers are not only seen to be valued by our political leaders and agendas to but also as professions with shared values, we ensure we lead the way in telling truth to power and evidence-based healthcare is amplified.

There are perhaps two ways for health professionals to move forward. The first rests on viewing empowerment as an act from within, as a conscious choice made by free will, in spite of oppression, disempowerment, institutional structures, gender bias and horizontal violence and current pandemic-induced challenges. This approach offers all health professionals an opportunity to write their own script, find their own voice and forge ahead. Secondly, clinical leaders represent the empowered few who have overcome the odds in spite of the structures that surround them. They can therefore be the few to whom other professionals look to lead their professional discipline out of the oppressive, semi-professional mire in which some professional disciplines appear to be stuck. To lead with values clearly displayed through actions and ensure the perceptions of healthcare workers shift from victims, angles and helpers, to leaders and influencers with expertise and knowledge which are needed, especially at this time.

It is vital to identify who the clinical leaders are, because if they are identified as the health professionals that foster (even unwittingly) the pattern of other nursing leaders, with the same characteristics as leaders of oppressed groups, then no progress is likely. Legacy is important in this context. If clinical leaders have broken free of oppression by accepting financial incentives, improved job status (e.g. nurse consultants, nurse practitioners or physician's assistants) and special privileges (prescribing rights/diagnostic privileges), simply to maintain the status quo or foster their own status and financial security, have they in fact merely become deluded, co-oppressors and highly paid frustrated conspirators? Have they instead moved into the marshland between their professional group and the oppressive, powerful manager and medical group, where they are now marginalised fringe-dwellers, no longer part of one group and still not accepted as part of the other? Leaders must create their own story, and while recalling how the profession was in years gone by, acknowledge that the provision of healthcare provided is far removed, patient needs have undeniably changed and our environments and contexts for delivery have also significantly shifted. Therefore, leaders within our professions must also do so, or be consigned to subservience.

Recalling that empowerment needs to be developed from within, simply inventing new titles or establishing new leadership positions will not foster empowerment. In fact, the introduction of consultant practitioners or nurse practitioners with potentially different values and agendas from the vast majority of nurses or professionals within the same discipline may have a negative impact on the dynamics of the oppressed group.

Clinical leaders are in a position to demonstrate that they have eclipsed their oppressed state and to offer a guiding light for all health professionals. Leaders can thrive at any level, as long as the core values underpinning their practice and professionalism stay strong, and as long as they keep patient care central to their aims.

Box 19.3   A Little Horror Story, Part 3

It would be delightful if I could support the theoretical perspectives offered in this chapter with a clear example of the power of the individual to rise above the oppressor and become truly empowered. However, this is a true story, and while this student nurse had achieved that to some extent, he was still dependent on the RN's assessment of competence to 'pass' the placement.

Things had improved. The student had started to write his own script. He was less threatened and able actually to enjoy elements of his time on the ward. Mostly, though, this was when the senior RN was not there. When she was, she continued to pick on the student whenever she could (often when there was no one about), and although the student was doing well and knew that the RN would really have to be creative if she wanted to find a reason to fail him, he was still worried that she would try to do just that.

Then serendipity played a hand. As the student walked into the sluice room one day, quite near the end of his placement, he found the senior RN vomiting into the open sluice. She was pregnant and had a serious bout of morning sickness. He offered to help, showed real and fitting sympathy, but she was so embarrassed that all she cared about was that he left her alone and did not tell anyone what had happened. He kept it secret for many years until he told me the story. After this incident, the now embarrassed RN never picked on the student again. She was not nice or polite, but she left him alone, and he passed the placement with flying colours.

> **Reflection Point**
>
> Reflect on this little horror story. Edmund Burke said, 'He that wrestles with us strengthens our nerves and sharpens our skill. Our antagonist is our helper' (Knowles 2001, p. 164). Have you ever had an antagonist that made you stronger? What made you strong and why?

How Can Oppressed Groups Liberate Themselves?

While clinical leaders may be held up as examples of the liberated few, it is also important that the majority of health professionals recognise approaches they can take to foster empowerment and escape from oppression. Exploring authentic and ethical leadership on psychological empowerment, Beiranvand et al. (2021) identified the impact on others, and combined with other recent evidence, it is possible to present a combination of characteristics, attitudes and styles which can both liberate the leader and the workforce using values-based leadership. These include:

- Transparency (Shirey et al. 2019)
- Self-awareness and self-efficacy (Alexander and Lopez 2018)
- Gaining trust and trusting others (Shirey et al. 2019)
- Respect and cooperation (Shirey et al. 2019; Beiranvand et al. 2021)
- Dignity and value in others' contributions (Lofti et al. 2018)
- Take a problem-solving approach by decision making and share the power balance (Beiranvand et al. 2021)

In order to stop, suppress or limit oppression, health professionals and nurses can act to give themselves more opportunity to find their 'voice within' and take steps towards becoming empowered. Remember, though, that no one will do it for you. Empowerment only comes from within, yet this is both a strength and a weakness in escaping oppression. However, here are a few activities and behaviours that can limit oppression and enhance empowerment:

- Become interconnected in your clinical area of work by discussing oppression as it relates to you. How do other professionals feel about oppression, their own professional constraints and identify common feelings of being undermined or oppressed? Talk about your oppression. If it is not recognised, described or acknowledged, then it cannot be changed, challenged or addressed. Recognise your strengths and that of others. Discuss what areas of work where you feel able to contribute, make decisions and are heard.
- Expose and destroy the myths associated with oppression. Oppressors would like you to think that being 'put down' and subservient is your natural state. It is not!
- Reject the negative images of your culture and replace them with pride and a sense of your ability to function autonomously. You will notice a number of famous women referred to throughout this book, and a number of historical issues that are discussed. As well as offering excellent examples of women with courage and drive, these are also examples of the use of the past to support and guide our journey into the future, so that we can avoid the mistakes and learn from the lessons of others.

- Autonomy must be acquired. Freedom is acquired by conquest, not by gift.
- Define yourself. Only you can do this. Reclaim your history and culture and create a sense of togetherness. What might your rallying cry be?
- Empowered leaders must come from within the group, not from the elite or from another group. This is a 'grassroots' approach. In this regard, recognising and celebrating your own view of clinical leadership is vital.
- Know what you want to achieve and what you believe. Set out your aims and objectives and be clear about your values.
- Be collegial, discuss a common area of healthcare you are interested in and form a multi-professional discussion group or journal review group. Share and be knowledgeable and confident in your locus of expertise.
- Be aware of what makes you feel good, what makes you feel positive and proud of your profession. Then, be vocal about this.
- Exercise your right to say 'no' if what you are being asked is not in your best interests, within your job responsibilities or will not enrich your own life or others' lives.
- Celebrate your accomplishments and the attainment of your dreams.
- Recognise and understand that nurses (and/or other health professional groups) are not inherently inferior.
- Develop leaders and leadership from the grassroots and avoid the elite leadership approaches of the past. Be clear what management and leadership are, how they overlap and how they are distinct.
- Foster personal and professional pride in your work and your achievements.
- Examine your 'voice within'. Develop a positive voice and eliminate the negative 'put down' voice.
- Rediscover the great cultural heritage of your professional discipline. What is nursing about, what is the history of physiotherapy, what is it that occupational therapists believe about their professional role and history? Share this in writing and with your colleagues.
- Take and make your own way, using your personal leadership style, clearly based in professional values.

Reflection Point

Considering the information given here on oppression, in your view, are nurses or other health professionals oppressed? Discuss this question with your colleagues. What are their views? Could it be that there are pecking orders within health? If so, how do you see them being structured? Has this changed during the pandemic?

Case Study 19.1   Jacinda Ardern

Jacinda Ardern was the world's youngest female head of state on her election at 37 years old. With a history of involvement in equality and justice, she became politically active at age 17. During her term, she has led the country following a terrorist attack and the natural disaster of Whakaari/White Island volcanic eruption. Her visibility and voice in the immediate aftermath manifested her style of leadership and

(Continued)

Case Study 19.1   (Continued)

established her on the world stage as a leader with both humility and ambition. Acting swiftly and ignoring calls for contemplation, she has made decisions which have had tangible outcomes, including the introduction of strict firearm regulations and decisive action to prevent the spread of COVID-19.

A champion for gender equality, she has stood her ground in the face of misogyny and made visible her support of working mothers by taking her own three-month-old daughter into the United Nations General Assembly. She further strengthened her commitment to the #MeToo movement and pledged to ensure equality as a global agenda and aim. In an act which aimed to emapathise with the communities, she took a 20% pay cut and has further demonstrated a refusal to engage in populist ideologies by standing with the disenfranchised in all areas of society.

Distinctive leadership approaches taken by Jacinda Ardern include the following:

- She uses 'we' not 'I' often to demonstrate inclusiveness and empathy.
- She demonstrates authenticity by acting on her decisions and rationalising.
- She has taken a modern and transparent approach to her leadership and is clearly visible as opposing traditional authoritarian styles amongst world leaders.
- She takes advice and makes decisions yet does not follow the popular choice always.
- In a crisis, she takes decisive action, is visible and takes responsibility for those actions.
- She demonstrates compassion and empathy, with strength in her convictions.
- She demonstrates humility and understanding of the population; for example, she held a press conference specifically aimed at children to enable their understanding of the pandemic and its implications.

Challenge: Jacinda Ardern has demonstrated a style of leadership which sets her apart from the majority of world leaders. It could be said she has empowered women in leadership roles by demonstrating empathy and compassion and being a leader who focuses on what is needed and follows this by taking action. How do you think she has enabled the discussion about women in leadership roles and the role of compassion and empathy in male-dominated power constructs? Do you think you could make your voice heard and that of others under pressure? She has also come across criticism for her style within the context of world politics. What are your views on this style, and are there contexts when this is not effective/ appropriate, or should she be praised for keeping her authenticity core to her approach?

Summary

- This chapter is about the relevance of empowerment and oppression to clinical leadership in healthcare.
- Empowerment is not the path, but the walk, and the choice about which path to take. This perspective of empowerment implies that nurses and other health professionals can liberate themselves and move forward in spite of the barriers and obstacles that may be acting against them.

- Empowerment can be defined as a tool, to be used to support or develop the empowerment of others, or as a choice, made by an individual to seize empowerment and take control over their life, both personal and professional.
- If nurses and other health professionals are able to access the power within themselves, then they will be able to empower themselves and set the conditions for empowerment in others.
- Clinical leaders may be the empowered few who have overcome some of the barriers in the health service to forge ahead and overturn the oppressive structures that impede their progress and success.
- Oppression remains an issue in the healthcare arena. Many nurses and other health professionals are still oppressed and display many of the signs of an oppressed group, and the pandemic has added to this.

Mind Press-Ups

Exercise 19.1

Do you think that nurses or other health professionals have inherited the values of the medical profession, and have they evolved? Discuss this question with your colleagues. What are their views?

Exercise 19.2

In your experience, have you ever encountered times when you have felt oppressed or been exposed to horizontal violence? Think about when this occurred and why it might have happened. How did you respond?

Exercise 19.3

Consider the characteristics of leaders of oppressed groups. Do any of these put you in mind of people you have worked for or with? In what way?

Exercise 19.4

How do historical stereotypes impinge on our profession's ability to influence the direction and quality of care and the health service?

Exercise 19.5

If nurses and some other clinically focused health professionals are oppressed, then taking steps to be liberated is vital. How can you take steps to liberate yourself (if you see the need) or to exercise your own empowerment?

References

Alexander, C. and Lopez, R.P. (2018). A thematic analysis of self-described authentic leadership behaviors among experienced nurse executives. *The Journal of Nursing Administration* 48 (1): 38–43.

Beiranvand, M.S., Beiranvand, S., Beiranvand, S., and Mohammadipour, F. (2021). 'Explaining the effect of authentic and ethical leadership on psychological empowerment of nurses. *Journal of Nursing Management* 1 (29): 1081–1090.

Bennett, C., James, A., and Kelly, D. (2020). 'Beyond tropes: towards a new image of nursing in the wake of COVID-19. *Journal of Clinical Nursing* https://doi.org/10.1111/jocn.15346.

Birks, M., Cant, R.P., Budden, L.M. et al. (2017). 'Uncovering degrees of workplace bullying: a comparison of baccalaureate nursing students' experiences during clinical placement in Australia and the UK. *Nurse Education in Practice* 25: 14–21. http://dx.doi.org/10.1016/j.nepr.2017.04.011.

Bower, F.L. (2000). *Nurses Taking the Lead*. Philadelphia, PA: WB Saunders.

Clifford, P.G. (1992). The myth of empowerment. *Nursing Administration* 16 (31): 1–5.

Courtenay, B. (1989). *The Power of One*. London: Penguin.

Derbyshire, P. and Thompson, R. (2021). 'Killing us softly with their wrongs: nursing academia's 'killer elite' continue unabated. *Journal of Nursing Management* 30 (1): 1–3. http://dx.doi.org/10.1111/jonm.13391.

Devi, S. (2020). 'COVID-19 exacerbates violence against health workers. *The Lancet* 396 (10252): 658.

Esterhuizen, P. and Kooyman, A. (2001). Empowering moral decision making in nurses. *Nurse Education Today* 21: 640–647.

Fisher, M. and Kiernan, M. (2019). Student nurses' lived experience of patient safety and raising concerns. *Nurse Education Today* 77: 1–5.

Francis, R. (2013). *The Report of the Mid Staffordshire NHS Foundation Trust Public Inquiry: Executive Summary*. London.: The Stationery Office.

Freire, P. (1971). *A Pedagogy of the Oppressed*. New York: Herder & Herder.

French, J. and Raven, B. (1959). The basis of social power. In: *Studies in Social Power* (ed. D. Cartwright), 150–167. Ann Arbor: Michigan Institute for Social Research.

Freshwater, D. (2000). Crosscurrent: against cultural narration in nursing. *Journal of Advanced Nursing* 32 (2): 481–484.

Friedson, E. (1970). *Profession of Medicine*. New York: Harper and Row.

Fulton, Y. (1997). Nurses' views on empowerment: a critical social theory perspective. *Journal of Advanced Nursing* 26 (3): 529–536.

Gottileb, L.N., Gottileb, B., and Bitzas, B. (2021). Creating empowering conditions for nurses with workplace autonomy and agency: how healthcare leaders could be guided by Strengths-Based Nursing and Healthcare Leadership (SBNH-L). *Journal of Healthcare Leadership* 3: 169–181.

Greenleaf, N. (1978). The politics of self-esteem. *Nursing Digest* 6: 1–7.

Grossman, S. and Valiga, T.M. (2012). *The New Leadership Challenge: Creating the Future of Nursing*, 4e. Philadelphia, PA: F. A. Davis.

Holmes, C. and Lindsay, D. (2018). "Do you want fries with that?": the McDonaldization of university education—some critical reflections on nursing higher education. *SAGE Open* 8 (3): 1–10. http://dx.doi.org/10.1177/2158244018787229.

James, A. H. (2020) *Perceptions and experiences of leadership. A Narrative Inquiry of leadership in undergraduate nurse education*. Thesis, Professional Doctorate in Advanced Healthcare Practice. Cardiff University, UK.

Jones, L. and Bennett, C.L. (2018). *Leadership, for Nursing, Health and Social Care Students*. Banbury: Lantern Publishing Ltd.

Jones, P.S., O'Toole, M.T., Hoa, N. et al. (2000). Empowerment of nursing as a socially significant profession in Vietnam. *Journal of International Scholarship* 32 (3): 317–321.

Kanter, R. (1977). *Men and Women of the Corporation*. New York: Basic Books.

Kelly, D., Lankshear, A., and Jones, A. (2016). 'Stress and resilience in a post-Francis world: a qualitative study of executive nurse directors. *Journal of Advanced Nursing* vol. 72: 3160–3168. http://dx.doi.org/10.1111/jan.13086.

Knowles, E. (ed.) (2001). *Oxford Dictionary of Quotations*, 5e. Oxford: Oxford University Press.

Kreitner, R. and Kinicki, A. (1998). *Organisational Behaviour*. New York: McGraw-Hill.

Laschinger, H.K.S., Gilbert, S., Smith, L.M., and Leslie, K. (2010). Towards a comprehensive theory of nurse/patient empowerment: applying Kanter's empowerment theory to patient care. *Journal of Nursing Management* 18: 4–18. http://dx.doi.org/10.1111/j.1365-2834.2009.01046.x.

LeRoux, R. (1978). Power, powerlessness and potential: nurses' role within the health care delivery system. *Image* 10: 75–83.

Lewin, K. (1948). *Resolving Social Conflicts: Selected Papers on Group Dynamics* (ed. G.W. Lewin). New York: Harper & Row.

Lofti, Z., Atashzadeh-Shoorideh, F., Mohtashami, J., and Nasiri, M. (2018). Relationship between ethical leadership and organisational commitment of nurses with perception of patient safety culture. *Journal of Nursing Management* 26 (6): 726–734.

Mandela, N. (1994). *Long Walk to Freedom*. London: Little, Brown.

McNamara, S.A. (2012). Incivility in nursing: unsafe nurse, unsafe patients. *ACORN Journal* 95 (4): 535–540. http://dx.doi.org/10.1016/j.aorn.2012.01.020.

Meissner, J.E. (1986). Nurses: are we eating our young? *Nursing* 89, 16 (3): 51–53.

Meissner, J.E. (1999). Nurses: are we eating our young? *Nursing* 99, 29: 2, 42–4.

Plesk, P.R. and Wilson, T. (2001). Complexity, leadership, and management in healthcare organisations. *British Medical Journal* 323: 746–749.

Racine, L. and Vandenberg, H. (2020). A philosophical analysis of anti-intellectualism in nursing: Newman's view of a university education. *Nursing Philosophy* 1: –22. http://dx.doi.org/10.1111/nup.12361.

Regan, S., Laschinger, H.K., and Wong, C.A. (2016). The influence of empowerment, authentic leadership, and professional practice environments on nurses' perceived interprofessional collaboration. *Journal of Nursing Management* 24: E54–E61.

Rinpoche, S. (1992). *The Tibetan Book of Living and Dying*. London: Rider.

Riskin, A., Eriz, A., Fouek, T. et al. (2015). The impact of rudeness on medical team performance: a randomized trial. *Pediatrics* 36 (3): 487–495. http://dx.doi.org/10.1542/peds.20shorey15-1385.

Rogers, C. (1979). *Carl Rogers on Personal Power*. New York: Delacorte.

Shirey, M.R., White-Williams, C., and Hites, L. (2019). Integration of authentic leadership lens for building high performing interprofessional collaborative practice teams. *Nursing Administration Quarterly* 43 (2): 101–112.

Shorey, S. and Wong, P.Z.E. (2021). A qualitative systematic review on nurses' experiences of workplace bullying and implications for nursing practice. *Journal of Advanced Nursing* 77: http://dx.doi.org/10.1111/jan.14912.

Simmonds, C.J. (1998). The rise of the supernurse is at the expense of others. *Nursing Times* 94 (37): 20.

Stanley, D. (2006a). Part 1: In command of care: clinical nurse leadership explored. *Journal of Research in Nursing* 2 (1): 20–39.

Stanley, D. (2006b). Part 2: In command of care: towards the theory of congruent leadership. *Journal of Research in Nursing* 2 (2): 132–144.

Stanley, D. (2008). Congruent leadership: values in action. *Journal of Nursing Management* 64: 84–95.

Stanley, D. (2011). *Clinical Leadership: Innovation into Action*. Melbourne, VIC: Palgrave Macmillan.

Stanley, D. (2014). Clinical leadership characteristics confirmed. *Journal of Research in Nursing* 19 (2): 118–128.

Stanley, D. (2019). *Values-Based Leadership in Healthcare. Congruent Leadership Explored*. London: Sage Publications.

Stein, L., Watts, D., and Howell, T. (1990). The doctor–nurse game revisited. *New England Journal of Medicine* 322: 546–549.

Steinbeck, J. (1962) Nobel Prize in Literature Banquet Speech. John Steinbeck – Banquet speech (http://nobelprize.org).

The King's Fund (2020). *NHS Leadership and Culture, Our Position*. NHS leadership and culture | The King's Fund (http://kingsfund.org.uk) Accessed September 2021.

Thompson, D.R. and Clark, A.M. (2018). Leading by gaslight? Nursing's academic leadership struggles. *Journal of Advanced Nursing* 74 (5): 995–997. http://dx.doi.org/10.1111/jan.13399.

Watson, R. and Shields, L. (2009). Cruel Britannia: a personal critique of nursing in the United Kingdom. *Contemporary Nurse* 32 (1–2): 42–54.

Western, S. (2019). *Leadership: A Critical Text*, 3e. London: Sage.

Wing, T., Regan, S., and Spence Lacchinger, H.K. (2015). The influence of empowerment and incivility on mental health of new graduate nurses. *Journal of Nursing Management* 23: 632–643.

World Health Organisation (2020). *The state of the world's nursing report*. https://www.who.int/publications/i/item/nursing-report-2020.

Yoder-Wise, P.S. (2015). *Leading and Management in Nursing*, 6e. St Louis: Mosby.

Bishop, V. (2009). *Leadership for Nursing and Allied Health Care Professions*. Maidenhead: Open University Press/McGraw-Hill Education.

Cleland, V. (1971). Sex discrimination: nursing's most pervasive problem. *American Journal of Nursing* 71: 1542–1547.

Derbyshire, P., Thompson, D.R., and Watson, R. (2019). 'Nursing's future? Eat young. Spit out. Repeat. Endlessly. *Journal of Nursing Management* 27: 1337–1340.

Oughtibridge, D. (1998). Under the thumb. *Nursing Management* 4 (8): 22–24.

Roberts, S.J. (1983). Oppressed group behaviour: implications for nursing. *Advances in Nursing Science* 5: 21–30.

Roberts, S.J. (2000). Development of a positive professional identity: liberating oneself from the oppressor within. *Advances in Nursing Science* 22 (4): 71–82.

Torres, G. (1981). The nursing education administrator: accountable, vulnerable, and oppressed. *Advances in Nursing Science* 3: 1–16.

20

Leading Through a Crisis

Alison H. James and Clare L. Bennett

> *. . . we cannot be content merely to experience but must seek to make sense of it, to know what is its cause and significance, to find the truth behind . . . the basic stimulus to the intelligence is doubt, a feeling that the meaning of an experience is not self-evident . . .*
>
> W. H. Auden (1907–1973) (2015, p. 44)

Introduction

This chapter explores how the recent experience of COVID-19 has placed challenges on leading healthcare systems globally. Clinical staff, clinical leaders, managers, health organisations and health services as a whole have encountered situations they were unprepared for and have had to become adaptable and quick-thinking, leading rapidly changing teams and situations, often with ineffective resources, ongoing uncertainty and community fear and confusion. While it is possible now to reflect on experiences of leadership during times of crisis, it is clear that there was little to draw from when this was first written about in the context of nurse leadership in 2020 (James and Bennett 2020). Pandemics are not new. The 1918 influenza pandemic killed an estimated 50 million people worldwide (CDC 2021) and remains the deadliest pandemic in recorded human history (Barry 2005; Arnold 2018). However, it is possible to consider some positives to have come from this most recent period of global upheaval, and it is important to learn from this experience, to try to make sense of decisions made and apply these for the future. This extraordinary challenge is a learning point for future healthcare leaders, and in particular, how to support teams and individuals through such times, when there is often ambiguity and confusion from political power and uncertainty of what further challenges lie ahead.

Clinical Leadership in Nursing and Healthcare, Third Edition.
Edited by David Stanley, Clare L. Bennett and Alison H. James.
© 2023 John Wiley & Sons Ltd. Published 2023 by John Wiley & Sons Ltd.

Defining Crisis

The word 'crisis' has become a woven thread of familiarity in daily conversation, in the media and within our places of work and home since the beginning of the pandemic. While the impact of COVID-19 has varied and fluctuated globally, all countries and healthcare systems have become familiar with its frequent inclusion in the wider contexts of global economies, travel and population well-being. The impacts will be far reaching and ongoing; however, let us consider its meaning and relevance going forward, as we are able to reflect on its usefulness for clinical leadership.

In understanding a term, it is often useful to explore synonyms, and the Merriam-Webster thesaurus (2021) associates 'boiling point', 'conjuncture', 'flash point' and 'crossroads' with the word *crisis*. These all suggest that a crisis is a point in time where decisions have to be made, where a situation reaches a place where there is no return and there is a need to drive forward and manage the drivers which forced the situation to this position. There have been considerable publications that have explored a host of regional and global pandemics and health catastrophes that have impacted on humans across the span of our history (the black death or plague, the 1918 influenza panademic and a host of others). However, Zhuravsky (2018) provides us with some insight to the earthquake disaster in Christchurch, New Zealand in 2011. While this was a contained crisis compared to COVID-19, the elements of the experience and response can provide learning from complex challenges, communication and coordination (see the Reflection point 1 in this chapter for background on this).

A crisis can be a short and immediate threat which requires quick decision making and actions, or a crisis can be an impactful and ongoing threat which requires quick decision making and action initially, with a need for ongoing and sustained collective planning. In both situations, it is known that no matter how prepared an organisation is, no matter how many policies are in place, the nature of a crisis means potentialities are unpredictable, and the endless hypothetical consequences and situations which may result are unconceivable.

Grint (2008) suggested distinguishing types of problems and correlating these with leadership, management, and command responses, which can be applied within a crisis situation. A 'tame problem', while complicated, involves low levels of uncertainty and may have happened previously. This therefore requires a management response. However, a 'wicked problem' consists of degrees of complexity, and the association between cause and effect is not fully evident and these problems are problematic and awkward (Grint 2008). This type of problem requires a leadership response, with collective positioning. Importantly, the leader's role within a complex wicked problem is to ask the right questions. Grint (2008) also suggests problems may be 'critical' or a 'crisis', demanding limited time for response, decision making and actions. In a crisis problem, there is need for command, when decisions are needed swiftly, answers provided and actions carried out. In such immediate crisis situations, for example, during the 7 July 2005 terrorist attack in London, this immediate and authoritative leadership is effective (James and Bennett 2020).

When considering what leadership knowledge and skills are needed during a crisis, James and Bennett (2020) assert these remain the same as any other time; however, the aptitude to modify and attune different aspects of leadership, according to the needs dictated by the various stages of a crisis, becomes imperative. For example, while collective and distributive approaches to leading are effective in usual circumstances, in immediate crisis situations, formal decision making through one channel of communication may be the most effective and valued approach. This was evident in the example provided in Chapter 10, of the San Jose mining disaster in Chile in 2010 where the rescue lasted 70 days, which required a longer-term approach of effective leadership and sustained teamworking, until the eventual desired outcome was reached with the rescue of all the trapped miners. Compare these examples with this current crisis, which spans across years and continents, continuing to take life and impacting the vulnerable.

James and Bennett (2020) suggest posing these questions during a crisis. Continuing to ask these of yourself as a leader can ensure you reframe and review the challenges and requirements, as they may often shift and change during the course of the crisis:

- What are the aims?
- What are the desired outcomes?
- How will I communicate these to the team?
- What approach should be applied to influence the team and ensure all team members work to their strengths?
- What resources are needed to support the team to achieve these outcomes?
- At what point will I review my approach and measure effectiveness?
- To what extent will my values anchor me to the application of ethically appropriate decisions and actions?

Reflection Point 1

Christchurch, New Zealand 2011

An earthquake with a magnitude of 6.3 struck, impacting the hospital and causing damage which compromised the hospital's functions, including water leaks, communications and electricity. Despite ongoing ground tremors of the building, which lasted for days, the staff continued to provide patient care, identifying risks and damage. With threat to life and delayed care a high possibility, the team adapted new approaches to provide solutions and ensure patient safety. Decisions were made to evacuate patients and close three medical wards, and within one week a new ward was created in a nearby hospital which did not usually have an acute facility or an emergency department. In the complexity of inadequate infrastructure and operational deficiencies, the team approached the crisis with creative and critical thinking, and infrastructure was installed, new operational procedures established and new models of care implemented. Despite a lack of experience in crisis events, the team responded rapidly and effectively (Ardagh et al. 2011; Dolan et al. 2011; Jacques et al. 2014; Zhuravsky 2018).

Consider the different characteristics of leadership that may be needed during a crisis and use the preceding examples to reflect on what approaches may be required, depending on the scale and urgency of the situation.

Deitchman (2013) developed a framework of 'formal' and 'informal' characteristics from the aviation, mining and nuclear power industries and the military, and these have been adapted by James and Bennett (2020) as outlined in the preceding section.

(Continued)

Case Study 14.1 (Continued)

Consider when these approaches could be effective and how you might apply them in your leadership approach to a crisis.

   Formal leadership characteristics

- Decisiveness
- Situational and emotional awareness
- Coordination of resources and workforce
- Communication
- Inspiring trust
- Calmness

   Informal leadership characteristics

- Motivation
- Autonomy
- Identifying personal strengths and values
- Emotional intelligence
- Sharing professional responsibility and burden
- Stepping up

Flexibility, Innovation and Resilience

While the immediate response of leading with a centralised, formal and hierarchical approach may be effective during the initial stages of a crisis event, the longer-term approach requires consideration of who has the best knowledge and experience of frontline issues. For longer term decision making, as we have seen in this pandemic, the professionals at the immediate coalface hold the expertise, which has been added to and built further from this experience. So, managers may need to release immediate control to allow clinical leaders to the return of autonomy, spontaneity and innovation based on this wide pool of expertise, even though that may well feel challenged. While allowing for innovation, maintaining a shared structure can ensure a balance exists between command and creativity (Lloyd-Smith 2020). A collective approach using a shared structure of agreed aims and decisions enables coordination and communication and embeds positive behaviours for ensuring effective care is provided (Faraj and Xiao 2006). This can result in a flexible yet stable organisation where the autonomy of teams can be highly creative and safe.

Within large and complex organisations, it is imperative that individuals and teams realise their interdependence in order to function effectively and safely. In a crisis situation, the status quo can be toppled, and individuals may focus on the issues in the immediate visual vicinity of the challenges, rather than thinking of the universal impacts of the wider organisation. Leaders can re-stabilise their organisation by sharing information to all areas and staff, in a timely and appropriate way, and ensure the implications of decisions made locally have been made with consideration of potential impact elsewhere in the system, thereby creating a collective response sensitive to the wider ramifications (Lloyd-Smith 2020).

While there has been a tendency in recent years for healthcare professionals to be told they must demonstrate resilience, there is perhaps now an emerging recognition that acknowledges that this discourse suggests individual failure if this is not achieved (Bodell 2020). As we work in a collective, it is perhaps more effective and beneficial to consider resilience to be a requirement of the organisation, rather than the individual. The responsibility then shifts to all, rather than focus on the individual. At the very least, there needs to be an understanding of the current pressures, signs of burnout and the 'inverse relationship' between burnout and resilience which has been explored previously by Guo et al. (2018). In their review of healthcare worker resilience during the pandemic, Baskin and Bartlett (2021) found that nurses recorded lower levels of resilience than other healthcare workers, and overall, even healthcare workers with moderate levels of resilience reported negative psychological effects. In times of crisis the chance of recovery may be more achievable if pressure is moved from individuals and professions to be resilient and instead placed on how the organisation responds as a whole. Conventional policies and planning become obsolete in times of crisis, and the need for improvisation is needed, as seen with the Christchurch earthquake example. However, it is also worth remembering improvisation can result in unpredictable outcomes, threatening the resilience of an organisation by creating unintended consequences of which some may well be negative, potentially causing further chaos. Leaders need to ensure the core values and aims of the organisation are maintained, which can provide some stability and ensure patient safety remains the priority (Crossan and Sorrenti 2001; Boin et al. 2010; Lloyd-Smith 2020).

Lessons Learnt for the Long Term

Reflecting so far on leadership during this crisis, it is evident that globally there have been many different approaches with varied outcomes in terms of maintaining services and safety for patients. If we view this crisis as an opportunity to learn for future challenges, we must have an open and honest debate as well as produce robust evidence to support improved approaches to leading our professions through such events. A crisis can provide many challenges to healthcare organisations and also to the staff who work within them, not least placing staff at risk by being the front-facing support to populations. Through this current turbulence, staff have faced great risk, emotional upheaval and now report rising threats and abuse from the people they aim to care for, as people vent frustrations of backlogs and delays on exhausted staff (Campbell 2021). Furthermore, staffing in many organisations was already an issue pre-pandemic. This has now been exacerbated through staff leaving, burnout and sickness (Andel et al. 2021). The emotional burden and moral distress cannot be underestimated, and in many areas there has been a rise in mental health issues and stress among healthcare workers who have struggled to cope with seeing suffering and death on an incredibly large scale over a sustained period, accompanied by the dilemma of knowing what they believe is the right action, while often not having the resources and support to fully implement it (Jameton 1984; Lake et al. 2020; Clark and Rogowski 2021; Andel et al. 2021; Freysteinson 2021). For clinical nursing managers, the impact has also been significant, with challenges of coordinating care and their workforce needs, expanding roles and responsibilities unsupported by preparation or training, and expectations of responding to the pandemic effects alongside routine service planning (Jackson and Nowell 2021). However, clinical leaders and managers have demonstrated strength and determination in maintaining quality care for patients and the workforce, while the strategic leadership response has often been to return from a shared distributive approach to transactional command approaches in order to mitigate the impact of the virus on other services (Rosser et al. 2020). The rapid increase in demands placed on health services has also meant a more public health and mass community approach to decision making, rather than person-centeredness. For practitioners, this is challenging and has caused moral distress as their usual approach to individual choice and care has been confounded (Rosser et al. 2020; de Campos and Daniels 2021). The changes to delivery of care, changing messages and information and varying support for staff have sometimes resulted in executive leaders being seen as remote and removed from reality (Ness et al. 2021). This lack of involvement in decision making by staff who previously felt engaged and listened to has resulted in increased disillusionment, which, in turn, may result in further impact on the workforce through staff leaving their professions. Thompson and Kusy (2021) agree with Frei and Morriss (2020) in comparing leadership approaches of teams who maintained cohesion and unity with those which fragmented; being honest and gaining trust was important for teams' morale and effectiveness, as well as authenticity, displaying competence and knowledge in decision making and being empathetic with staff.

Maintaining Compassion and Empathy in Leadership

With the pressure of trying to maintain professional values, support others and maintain high standards of care in times of crisis come far-reaching consequences, which accentuates the need for compassion and a value-based approach to care. In leadership, in organisational culture and in the delivery of care, a compassionate, collective and inclusive and values-driven or focused approach is needed. When faced with anger and frustration within society, this is undoubtedly difficult, yet all healthcare professions are grounded in compassion, care, courage, effective communication, a commitment to their clients and maintaining competence, so it is imperative that these remain the central approaches so that staff are enabled to thrive and survive in the face of the ongoing challenges. It is also important that society witness the strength this brings and how this can drive up quality patient care (De Zulueta 2016; West 2021). Klimecki et al. (2014) and Worline and Dutton (2017) suggests that compassion and empathy trigger neural networks associated with social connection and altruism, and that professional values are the motivating factor for healthcare professions, helping connect them and supporting a display of compassion and care that can improve engagement and unity.

Reflection Point 2

When we consider the benefits of taking a compassionate values-based approach to clinical leadership, it is possible to break down the concept, to see what and how this can be applied, and why it is perhaps so relevant during a crisis.

(Continued)

Read through this list of attributes, which are linked to compassion and a values-based approach to clinical leadership:

- Being present and aware of others' pain and suffering or challenges
- Having empathy with others' emotions and being aware also of one's own (applying emotional intelligence; see Chapter 15)
- Being motivated to find solutions and aim for improvements through thoughtful actions (see Chapter 13)
- Allowing reciprocity; being compassionate for others and for oneself
- Enabling the positive experience of compassion and a display of your own values to nurture compassion and reciprocal values in others
- Promoting small acts of kindness within the organisation and within your colleagues
- Praising acts of compassion and the application of appropriate values in others
- Viewing mistakes as learning and encourage transparency

Consider how you may apply these attributes in your clinical leadership approach. What might the challenges be in times of crisis? How might this approach benefit your own self- compassion and that of others?

Atkins and Parker (2012) suggest a compassionate leadership style requires four components:

- Attending
- Understanding
- Empathising
- Helping

Stanley (2017) suggest that a congruent leadership style requires the application of the leader's values and beliefs with their actions demonstrating a direct link between the leaders values and beliefs and what they do in real-world practice.

These approaches to clinical leadership provide support and links into the core values of the organisation, professional values and the values of the individual, providing legitimacy to the compassionate and values-based behaviours which in turn support others to respond with the same approach (Stanley 2017; West 2021). Bailey and West (2020) acknowledge that compassion also needs to be supported with the 'ABC of human needs at work':

Autonomy – During a crisis, there may be an overwhelming feeling of loss of control over circumstances, and staff may feel they have no say when being directed in stressful situations. Listening to staff and acknowledging their experience and knowledge as well as ensuring basic needs are met ensures a compassionate approach. Be honest and involve staff in decision making.

Belonging – Fear and uncertainty as well as worrying about what is ahead is more challenging if isolated. An inclusive, supportive environment supports staff through this time and encourages a collective multidisciplinary team approach to the challenges. This promotes flexibility and shared responsibility for each other and for patient care.

Competence – Staff shortages and high demand over a long period cannot be sustained. Time for sharing and discussion, to problem solve and be supported, is valuable and promotes feelings of being valued in staff. Promote your organisation as being learning focused, acknowledging the challenges and learning lessons by having a global perspective and acting on best practice and evidence.

Considering the Emotions of the Experience

> Without emotion our perception is inferior.
>
> Nayak (2016, p. 3)

In their study of nursing leaders during the pandemic, Freysteinson et al. (2021) found embodied leadership and heightened emotions were experienced. Intense emotions were also evidenced in studies by Cag et al. (2020) and Iheduru-Anderson (2020). Coping with the pressures of the pandemic have also removed time for contemplating ethical elements of decision making, placing increased stress on the emotions and risk to judgements (Markey et al. 2020). Prioritising with limited resources and in complex critical care situations has been termed as 'rationing care' (Schubert et al. 2013), and where decisions have to be made that contradict the values of the health professions, this causes moral distress and pressure. Failure to provide adequate care to vulnerable patients has also been raised as a concern (Faghanipour et al. 2020), and clinical leaders are essential anchors in ensuring values-driven approaches will thrive and remain prominent. The International Council of Nurses have recognised this in their revised 'Code of Ethics for Nurses' (2021), which aims to support nurses from lessons learnt in the pandemic and to equip them with guidance for the future. Complacency in ethical judgement should not be allowed to override decisions in a prolonged struggle, and health professionals must always concede that non-actions as well as actions have an effect, and how we 'see and not see' what we witness, and where our ethical values lie (Rest and Narvaez 1994, p. 23).

Acknowledging and relating the emotions of the pandemic experience is important for all, to give voice to what has been experienced and allow expression of the emotional impact. Emotions are an essential element of intelligence, linked to well-being and reasoning in humans (Nussbaum 2001). We must therefore place value on those and allow expression of these intelligent perceptions, to attempt to make sense, to analyse and move forward. O'Grady and Malloch (2018) view maintaining a moral compass through inner reflection and accepting of personal vulnerabilities as characteristics of authentic and values-based leadership. By encouraging this in teams, a clinical leader may acknowledge their own emotional position alongside staff, and gain respect through this transparency and open vulnerability, while also building trust. Courageous and successful leaders show their emotions to staff, recognise the impact this can have and reassure staff that what they are experiencing is difficult and normal (Thompson and Kusy 2021).

Leading for Self-Care and Well-being

Let us now consider what positive actions and strategies clinical leaders can take to support and encourage a return to some equilibrium for personal well-being. A range of approaches have been linked to current evidence, and while there are challenges in adopting new approaches when the pandemic still presents many areas with difficulties, they are presented here as a 'toolbox', for choice and appropriateness as directed by need and opportunity in the vast diversity our global healthcare settings present.

Clinical Leadership Strategies for Well-Being and Inclusion

- Provide opportunities for sharing stories of emotions and challenges in a safe place to avoid repressing emotions and building fear and frustration (Thompson and Kusy 2021)
- Mindfulness techniques have been found to decrease emotional tiredness and stress; explore ways of enabling staff to access these (Klatt et al. 2020)
- An environment of trust can support staff well-being; work to ensure trust is established in all areas of the workplace (Jena et al. 2018)
- Trust can produce engagement and innovation of staff; allow ideas to be offered and take actions forward to show these are valued contributions (-; Wah et al. 2018).
- Ensure less experienced staff have a buddy for support and mentorship. This is an effective and efficient approach for staff development (King's Fund 2021).
- Role model a positive, cohesive and compassionate approach so that staff will emulate positive leadership (King's Fund 2021).
- Focusing on effective fatigue strategies are associated with workforce recovery. Ensure staff know this is a priority (Whelehan et al. 2021).
- Provide clear and regular communication, especially when policies change rapidly. Consider daily communication briefings and opportunities for questions with timely responses based on clear rationale (Rosa et al. 2020; Lake et al. 2020).
- Involve staff in decision-making and planning to build staff morale and motivate an approach to challenges (Markey et al. 2020).
- Advocate for staff well-being and challenge resources for this if needed. Be visible to senior management and emphasise the need for well-being in your department (Markey et al. 2020).

Stories of the Crisis

> Nothing becomes real till it is experienced
>
> (Keats – 1795 1821) (1958).

While we can draw on theory to guide leadership approaches, the experiences of leadership in this pandemic, while hugely challenging, have provided a wealth of real-life stories. Personal stories and individual perceptions can make a significant contribution to the development of knowledge and thinking and provide unique perspectives on observations, emotions and sensory experiences (James et al. 2022). While stories may change and adapt as people recall aspects of their experience, they do have the power to connect people, often across countries and cultures. Within stories, there are often parallels in experiencing such events which enable a relationship to form, an association of emotions or experience, which can allow us to learn from each other. Sharing stories of leading through a crisis can provide others with learning and can reduce the isolation which leading in such situations can induce. It may be something you would want to consider doing with your teams in your clinical area, as it's also a way of valuing individuals' feelings and experiences. Many have found it has helped to write blogs, daily journals or to share wider, via social media.

A personal story This is a story of a unit manager in a nursing home during the pandemic. She narrates her experience here.

I started here in 2012, and I've loved nursing here. It's been a wonderful experience. The people here come from a wide and diverse background with all sorts of stories to tell. All who care for our residents are 'peoples' people, they enjoy being with each resident and they enjoy prioritising their care. It's important to have a sense of humour and our residents love that.

My mother was a nurse, and although at first, I didn't want to be a nurse, I found I became interested in nursing as a profession because I wanted to make some kind of difference, even if it was something small. It makes me get up in the morning, the fact that something I could do today would make a difference to someone else's life experience. I had a personal experience of how nurses can impact people's lives when a community nurse cared for a relative at home who was terminal. I was quite young, but the fact that she seemed to really direct and lead the care that was given inspired me. That nurse was empathetic, compassionate, yet strong and professional with an obvious real knowledge of her patient and what care was needed.

Being a nurse and leading a team has been a real challenge during this pandemic. We have all been afraid. You could feel the fear, not only in my residents but in my whole team. The worst feeling for me was not knowing what to expect. It was a struggle, as someone who is supposed to know what to do, how to enthuse and inspire, how to reassure people. I didn't know what to expect, and I didn't want to show them how worried I was. There were many sleepless nights for me. As the residents and the team became more aware of the numbers of deaths, because we all heard that on the TV every day, it was like a great wave was about to hit us and we were just waiting, not knowing what to do.

Some of the residents have been here a long time, and we have some great relationships built over that time. Families and relatives rely on us, they look to us for hope. That was hard in this pandemic. Especially when they were no longer allowed to visit their loved ones, looking in at us through windows, as if we were separate and isolated from the outside world.

The isolation, when it came, had a huge impact on us all. I had to ask my staff to stay at the home and not see their families. We all wondered if we would see our families again. It was like some surreal nightmare to begin with, and as the manager and leader, I was acutely aware of what I was asking my staff to do. That felt like a huge responsibility. I completely got it, if someone didn't want to stay, especially when we weren't sure about protective equipment supplies. It was emotionally breaking for me to see staff struggle with the dilemma. All I could do was be there, be determined and positive and be compassionate for all. Sometimes I did show them how much it meant to me,

---

(Continued)

and I certainly made sure I did everything my team were expected to do. I think that's important.

We worked together, that's for sure. We went out of the way to accommodate shift times, to be flexible and supportive of each other. There were no episodes of disagreement or niggling comments, which can sometimes happen in teams under pressure. They worked as one, all staff, together. They made time for each other as well. I noticed that. Even though the workload was intense, and the emotional strain was huge. There were some really dark times I won't go into. I noticed the staff in two's often, arms around each other. That made me feel so proud of what we were doing and how well we were doing it. I made sure they all knew that too. And every time there was an opportunity for music, for some light heartedness, for laughter, we made sure to make the most of it for us, and importantly for our residents.

Sometimes nursing homes have a bad reputation, and there have been some awful examples I know in the press. There are some excellent homes as well, and it's important this is reported too, isn't it? There was this campaign of clapping for healthcare workers. We all started off thinking, ok, that's nice. That soon wore thin with us as the pressure built, and frustration grew. A gesture was fine, but really, looking back now, and just thinking of the numbers of people who have passed, and still are. It's really something that makes me feels uncomfortable.

What did mean so much was the families and friends of the residents, and the families and friends of staff, who did so much to show their appreciation and support for us. We had so many lovely messages, and the food from the community as a whole. What really made me emotional were the comments from my team and the residents, when things finally began to ease. They appreciated my approach; one called me a 'guiding light'. That was a moment for me, when I thought, ok. I felt like I didn't know what to do most days, how to lead these people, but I must have done something right.

I have reflected on this time and wondered how, and if, this has changed me as a nurse, as a leader, how I think about healthcare, here and now. It certainly has taught me many lessons I never thought I would have to learn. Overall, I suppose it's the importance of being true to yourself, knowing your limits, knowing your strengths. Being compassionate, although you have to deal with the practicalities and the limitations placed on you as a manger and leader, if you remain compassionate, keep those values close and let others know that's who you are, they will come with you. All we can do is hope others learn, that we can see the end of this and that we are better individuals, by thinking of all those who are not here now.

Case Study 20.1 Julia Gillard

Julia Gillard was born in Barry, Wales in 1961, her family emigrated to Australian in 1966. She attended school in Adelaide and began her university studies at Adelaide University before transferring to Melbourne University and eventually graduating with a Bachelor of Law in 1986 and Bachelor of Art in 1989. In Melbourne, Julia worked with the Australian Union of Students and was secretary of the Socialist Forum. In 1985, Julia joined the Australian Labour party and was soon active in state politics in Victoria.

(Continued)

Case Study 20.1   (Continued)

Julia cited Welsh Labour politician Aueurin Bevan as one of her political heroes, and she was elected to the House of Representatives in 1998. She was a shadow minister (in opposition) between 2001 and 2007. Between 2007 and 2010, Julia became the deputy prime minister under Kevin Rudd. Julia held the portfolios of education, and Minister for Employment and Workplace Relations before she took on the Prime Minister's job after a leadership spill, replacing Kevin Rudd and becoming the 27th Australian Prime Minster and first woman in the role.

She stood for and won the next election to retain her place as Prime Minster, but held only a minority government and faced considerable opposition from the general public, some quarters of the media and the opposition, led by Tony Abbott, and some members of her own party. She faced the ongoing fall out of the 2007–2008 financial crisis, immigration challenges and the looming threat of climate change. As well on the domestic front, she dealt with issues in education, mental health and gambling policies.

In an August 2012 press conference regarding the AWU, Julia was critical of *The Australian* newspaper for writing about her connection to the affair and of what she called 'misogynist nut jobs on the internet'. Gillard said that she had been 'the subject of a very sexist smear campaign'. In early October, the opposition leader's wife, Margie Abbott, accused Julia's government of a deliberate campaign to smear Tony Abbott on gender issues.

Julia responded with her 'sexism and misogyny' speech, opposing a motion to remove her choice of Speaker of the House of Representatives, after revelations of inappropriate conduct on his part became public. The speech was widely reported around the world. In Laos soon after for an Asian-European leaders conference, Gillard described comments by many world leaders as complementing her on the speech. US President Barack Obama reportedly 'complimented' her on the speech in a private conversation following his re-election, and his Secretary of State Hillary Clinton praised the speech as 'very striking'.

Julia faced considerable pressure, mainly directed at her being a female and especially based on her stand for taking action on climate change. In the end, members of her own party conspired to generate a spill motion, and she was replaced in 2013 by Kevin Rudd. Julia congratulated him on his victory and then resigned from politics.

Julia expressed support for legal abortion in 2005 and again in 2012, saying 'Women must have the right to healthcare and women must have the right to choose'. Concerning euthanasia, Julia warned that it may, 'open the door to exploitation and perhaps callousness towards people in the end stage of life' and that she is not convinced that the policy of pro-euthanasia advocates contain 'sufficient safeguards', and she voted against a bill that would have legalised same-sex marriage 2011. She was a powerful advocate for addressing climate change and spoke out in favour of addressing inequality in politics. Julia Gillard faced many crises during her tenure as Australia's first female Prime Minister. Her speech based on her values about women's rights stands out as a high point in her political career, and her tenacity in addressing climate change points to her being a values-driven leader. Her is a small part of her speech:

(Continued)

I was also very offended on behalf of the women of Australia when in the course of this carbon pricing campaign, the Leader of the Opposition said, 'What the housewives of Australia need to understand as they do the ironing ...'. Thank you for that painting of women's roles in modern Australia.

And then of course, I was offended too by the sexism, by the misogyny of the Leader of the Opposition catcalling across this table at me as I sit here as Prime Minister, 'If the Prime Minister wants to, politically speaking, make an honest woman of herself ...', something that would never have been said to any man sitting in this chair. I was offended when the Leader of the Opposition went outside in the front of Parliament and stood next to a sign that said 'Ditch the witch'.

Challenge: It has been reported that women are better at leading in a crisis (Zenger and Folkman 2020). Do you agree, and why might this be? Julia Gillard faced considerable challenges from misogynistic and powerful men. How can we lead in a crisis if these other/external factors are impacting on the discussion/debate?

Summary

- This chapter is about leading during a crisis, reflecting on some of the lessons learnt from the COVID-19 pandemic and approaches to leading.
- Acknowledging the impact of the pandemic on staff is important, and exploring strategies to support well-being is an essential part of clinical leadership at this time.
- Maintaining compassion and a values-based focus in our teams and organisations is imperative, to demonstrate that core professional values and aims remain focused, so that we feel supported by our colleagues while also supporting them.
- Expressing experiences and emotions can be explored through telling our stories. Stories are a powerful way of expressing emotion and sharing to learn.

Mind Press-Ups

Exercise 20.1

Consider the case study and the emotions expressed.

Reflect on how you may have felt in this situation. Have you experienced something similar during the pandemic or in any other challenging situation? How do you think we can prepare our teams for these situations and the challenges faced?

Exercise 20.2

Do you think that nurses or other health professionals have experienced moral distress during the pandemic? Discuss this question with your colleagues. What are their views?

Exercise 20.3

In your experience, have you ever encountered times when you have felt unable to express your emotional reaction in a crisis? How did this impact your approach to your work environment?

Exercise 20.4

Consider the characteristics of leaders who demonstrate compassion or a values-based approach. Have you worked with a compassionate or values-focused leader? How did this make you feel?

Exercise 20.5

Do you think we look after our own and others' well-being at work? What can we do to improve this?

Exercise 20.6

How can we best learn from this crisis? How can we best share experiences of both positive and negative leadership during this time?

References

Andel, S.A., Tedone, A.M., Shen, W., and Arvan, M.L. (2021). Safety implications of different forms of understaffing among nurses during the COVID-19 pandemic. *Journal of Advanced Nursing* 00: 1–10. https://doi.org/10.1111/jan.14952.

Ardagh, M.W., Richardson, S.K., Robinson, V. et al. (2011). The initial health-system response to the earthquake in Christchurch, New Zealand, in February. *Lancet* 379: 2109–2115.

Arnold, C. (2018). *Pandemic 1918: The Story of the Deadliest Influenza in History*. New York: Penguin.

Atkins, P.W.B. and Parker, S.K. (2012). Understanding individual compassion in organizations: the role of appraisals and psychological flexibility. *Academy of Management Review* 37 (4): 524–546.

Auden, W.H. (2015). *The Complete Works of W.H. Auden*. Woodstock: Princeton University Press.

Bailey S. and West M. (2020). *Covid-19: why compassionate leadership matters in a crisis*. The King's Fund Covid-19: why compassionate leadership matters in a crisis. The King's Fund, (http://kingsfund.org.uk).

Barry, J.M. (2005). *The Great Influenza: The Story of the Deadliest Pandemic in History*. New York: Viking Press.

Baskin, R.G. and Bartlett, R. (2021). Healthcare worker resilience during the COVID-19 pandemic: an integrative review. *Journal of Nursing Management* 29 (8): 2329–2342. http://dx.doi.org/10.1111/jonm.13395.

Bodell, M. (2020). Calling for nurses to be resilient only implies failure when we struggle. Nursing Notes.

Boin, A., Hart, P., and Hart, P. (2010). Organising for effective emergency management: lessons from research. *Australian Journal of Public Administration* 69: 357–371.

Cag, Y., Erdem, H., Gormez, A. et al. (2020). Anxiety among frontline healthcare workers supporting patients with COVID-19: a global survey. *General Hospital Psychiatry* 68: 90–96. http://dx.doi.org/10.1016/j.genhosppsych.2020.12.010.

Campbell, D. (2021). *People are being very angry with us': A&E doctor on abuse of NHS staff.* 'People are being very angry with us': A&E doctor on abuse of NHS staff | NHS | The Guardian.

de Campos, A.P. and Daniels, S. (2021). Ethical implications of COVID-19: palliative care, public health, and long-term care facilities. *Journal of Hospice & Palliative Nursing* 23 (2): 120–127. http://dx.doi.org/10.1097/NJH.00000000000007.

Centers for Disease Control and Prevention (CDC) (2021). https://www.cdc.gov/flu/pandemic-resources/1918-commemoration/1918-pandemic-history.htm.

Clark, R.R.S. and Rogowski, J.A. (2021). Hospital nurses' moral distress and mental health during COVID-19. *Journal of Advanced Nursing* 00: 1–11.

Crossan, M. and Sorrenti, M. (2001). Making sense of improvisation. In: *Organizational Improvisation* (ed. K. Kamoche, M.P. Cunha and J.V. Cunha), 27–48. Abingdon, UK: Taylor & Francis Ltd.

De Zulueta, P.C. (2016). Developing compassionate leadership in health care: an integrative review. *Journal of Healthcare Leadership* 8: 1–10. http://dx.doi.org/10.2147/JHL.S93724.

Deitchman, S. (2013). Enhancing crisis leadership in public health emergencies. *Disaster Medicine and Public Health Preparedness* 7 (5): 534–540. https://doi.org/10.1017/dmp.2013.81.

Dolan, B., Esson, A., Grainger, P.P. et al. (2011). Earthquake disaster response in Christchurch, New Zealand. *Journal of Emergency Nursing* 37: 506–509.

Faghanipour, S., Monteverde, S., and Peter, E. (2020). COVID-19-related deaths in long-term care: the moral failure to care and prepare. *Nursing Ethics* 277 (5): 1171–1173. http://dx.doi.org/10.1177/09697.

Faraj, S. and Xiao, Y. (2006). Coordination in fast-response organizations. *Management Science* 52: 1155–1169.

Frei, F. and Morriss, A. (2020). Begin with trust: the first step in becoming a genuinely empowering leader. *Harvard Business Review* 98 (3): 112–121.

Freysteinson, W.M., Celia, T., Gilia, H., and Gonzalez, K. (2021). The experience of nursing leadership in a crisis: A hermeneutic phenomenological study. *Journal of Nursing Management* https://doi.org/10.1111/jonm.13310.

Grint, K. (2008). Wicked problems and clumsy solutions: the role of leadership. *Clinical Leader* 1 (2): 169–186.

Guo, Y., Luo, Y., Lam, L. et al. (2018). Burnout and its association with resilience in nurses: a cross-sectional study. *Journal of Clinical Nursing* 27 (1–2): 441–449. http://dx.doi.org/10.1111/jocn.13952.

Iheduru-Anderson, K. (2020). Reflections on the lived experience of working with limited personal protective equipment during the COVID-19 crisis. *Nursing Inquiry* 28 (1): https://doi.org/10.1111/nin.12382.

International Council of Nurses (2021). *Code of Ethics for Nurses. Revised.* ICN_Code-of-Ethics_EN_Web_0.pdf.

Jackson, J. and Nowell, L. (2021). The officer of disaster management' nurse managers' experiences during COVID-19: a qualitative interview study using thematic analysis. *Journal of Nursing Management* 29 (8): 2392–2400. http://dx.doi.org/10.1111/jonm.13422.

Jacques, C.C., McIntosh, J., Giovinazzi, S. et al. (2014). Resilience of the Canterbury hospital system to the 2011 Christchurch earthquake. *Earthquake Spectra* 30: 533–554.

James, A.H. and Bennett, C.L. (2020). Effective nurse leadership in times of crisis. *Nursing Management* 27: http://dx.doi.org/10.7748/nm.

James, A.H., Carrier, J., and Watkins, D. (2022). Perceptions and experiences of leadership in undergraduate nurse education: A narrative inquiry. *Nurse Education Today* https://doi.org/10.1016/j.nedt.2022.105313.

Jameton, A. (1984). *Nursing Practice: The Ethical Issues*. Englewood Cliffs, NJ: Prentice-Hall.

Jena, L.K., Pradhan, S., and Panigrahy, N.P. (2018). Pursuit of organizational trust: role of employee engagement, psychological well-being and transformational leadership. *Asia Pacific Management Review* 23: 227–234. https://doi.org/10.1016/j.apmrv.2017.11.001.

Keats, J. (1958). 'Letter to George and Georgiana Keats, 19 March 1819. In: *The Letters of John Keats*, vol. 2 (ed. H.E. Rollins). Harvard: Harvard University Press.

King's Fund (2021) Compassionate and inclusive leadership. The King's Fund (kingsfund.org.uk)

Klatt, M.D., Bawa, R., Gabram, O. et al. (2020). Embracing change: a mindful medical center meets COVID-19. *Global Advances in Health and Medicine* 9: 1–10. https://doi.org/10.1177/2164956120975369.

Klimecki, O.M., Leiberg, S., Ricard, M., and Singer, T. (2014). Differential pattern of functional brain plasticity after compassion and empathy training. *Social Cognitive and Affective Neuroscience* 9 (6): 873–879.

Lake, E.T., Narva, M.A., Holland, S. et al. (2020). Chronic hospital nurse understaffing meets COVID-19: an observational study. *BMJ Quality and Safety* https://doi.org/10.1136/bmjqs-2020-011512.

Lloyd-Smith, M. (2020). The COVID-19 pandemic: resilient organisational response to a low-chance, high-impact event. *BMJ Leader* 4: 109–112. https://doi.org/10.1136/leader-2020-000245.

Markey, K., Aparecida Arena Ventura, C., O'Donnell, C., and Doody, O. (2020). Cultivating ethical leadership in the recovery of COVID-19. *Journal of Nursing Management* 29: 351–355.

Merriam- Webster (2021). Crisis Synonyms | Merriam-Webster Thesaurus.

Nayak, A. (2016). Wisdom and the tragic question: moral learning and emotional perception in leadership and organisations. *Journal of Business Ethics* 137 (1): 1–13.

Ness, M.M., Saylor, J., DiFusco, L.A., and Evans, K. (2021). Leadership, professional quality of life and moral distress during COVID-19: a mixed-methods approach. *Journal of Nursing Management* 29 (8): 2412–2422. http://dx.doi.org/10.1111/jonm.13421.

Nussbaum, M.C. (2001). *The Fragility of Goodness*, 2e. Cambridge: Cambridge University Press.

Rest, J. R. & Narvaez, D. (1994) Moral Development in the Professions: Psychology and Applied Ethics, Hillsdale, NJ: Lawrence Erlbaum.

Rosa, W.E., Schlak, A.E., and Rushton, C.H. (2020). A blueprint for leadership during COVID-19. *Nursing Management* 51 (8): 28–34. http://dx.doi.org/10.1097/01. NUMA.0000688940.29231.6f.

Rosser, E., Westcott, L., Ali, P.A. et al. (2020). The need for visible nursing leadership during COVID-19. *Journal of Nursing Scholarship: An Official Publication of Sigma Theta Tau International Honor Society of Nursing* 52: https://doi.org/10.1111/jnu.12587.

Schubert, M., Ausserhofer, D., Desmedt, M. et al. (2013). Levels and correlates of implicit rationing of nursing care in Swiss acute care hospitals–a cross sectional study. *International Journal of Nursing Studies* 50 (2): 230–239. https://doi.org/10.1016/j.ijnurstu.2012.09.016.

Stanley, D. (2017). *Values Based Leadership in Healthcare: Congruent Leadership Explored.* London: Sage.

Thompson, R. and Kusy, M. (2021). Has the COVID pandemic strengthened or weakened health care teams? A field guide to healthy workforce best practices. *Nursing Administration Quarterly* 45 (2): 135–141.

Wah, N.C., Zawawi, D., Yusof, R.N.R. et al. (2018). The mediating effect of tacit knowledge sharing in predicting innovative behavior from trust'. *International Journal of Business and Society* 19 (3): 937–954. http://www.ijbs.unimas.my/images/repository/pdf/Vol19-no3-paper23.pdf.

West, M. A. (2021) Compassionate Leadership: Sustaining Wisdom, Humanity and Presence in Health and Social Care, London: The Swirling Leaf Press.

Whelehan, D.F., Algeo, N., and Brown, D.A. (2021). Leadership through crisis: fighting the fatigue pandemic in healthcare during COVID-19. *BMJ Leader* 5: 108–112. http://dx.doi. org/10.1136/leader-2020-000419.

Worline, M. and Dutton, J.E. (2017). *Awakening Compassion at Work: The Quiet Power.* Oakland, CA: Berrett-Koehler Publishers Inc.

Zenger, J. and Folkman, J. (2020). *Research: Women Are Better Leaders During a Crisis.* Harvard: Harvard Business Review https://hbr.org/2020/12/research-women-are-better-leaders-during-a-crisis.

Zhuravsky, L. (2018). 'When disaster strikes: sustained resilience performance in an acute clinical setting. In: *Delivering Resilient Health Care* (ed. E. Hollnagel, J. Braithwaite and R.L. Wears), 199–219. Milton: Routledge.

21

Clinical (Values-Based/Congruent) Leaders
David Stanley

> *He that would govern others, first should be the master of himself.*
> Philip Massinger, English dramatist, 1583–1640, in *The Bondman*, 1624

Introduction: Clinical Heroes

I see clinical leaders as practitioners who have gone to the edge and flown. Or perhaps they are the clinicians who have taken their strides clearly and decisively in the direction of their values and beliefs. Look about at those who have continued to turn up in the face of the devastation, hardship and risks and challenges (to their own and their family's health) during the COVID pandemic. They could not have done so if they didn't believe they were making a difference – acting under the influence of the better angels of their nature. Or those who have simply stood by those beliefs, working not because they wanted to change the world but because they knew that what they were doing was right and that their actions were making a difference – maybe not to the whole ward or unit, clinic, or hospital or world, but for the person they were with, at that moment. When acting out or role modelling their values and beliefs (even unconsciously), something was happening in their relationship with the client, patient or colleague that gave a clear signal about what they believed or what their values were.

Responding to these values and beliefs has seen others view clinicians as clinical leaders: not because of their creativity, or because they were visionaries, in powerful positions or wielded great authority, but because they are open and approachable, clinically knowledgeable and competent. They are visible in practice, role models for the practice they espouse and good communicators. They are supportive, empowered, can motivate others, inspire confidence, are honest, cope well with change and their actions are evident or match their values and beliefs.

These clinical leaders capture what it means to be a values-based or congruent leader, standing by their values in the execution and drive of their actions, putting their hands where their heart is, acting out and following through what they believe to be right. These

Clinical Leadership in Nursing and Healthcare, Third Edition.
Edited by David Stanley, Clare L. Bennett and Alison H. James.

leaders are not selling a vision or communicating a path for others to follow, they are living their vision and walking the path, role modelling with courage, commitment, conviction, care, compassion, and determination what they believe is the right thing to do. They are values-based or congruent leaders, but they are not the only people who have led this way.

Many Marys

The many Marys are offered as an example. Between 1854 and 1856, 229 nurses travelled officially to the Crimea and worked to care for wounded and dying soldiers in the military hospitals established near the war zone that were eventually managed by Florence Nightingale. Many other women travelled to the Crimea region unofficially. One such was Elizabeth Evans, the wife of Private Evans of the Fourth Regiment of Foot. She journeyed with him to the Crimean Peninsula and nursed the wounded men of his regiment. Clearly devoted, her dedication was acknowledged when she was awarded the Crimean Medal following the war.

However, it was Florence Nightingale who emerged from the war with iconic status, a legend even in her own time (Bostridge 2004). Henry Longfellow wrote a poem about her in 1857, 'Santa Filomena', which includes the lines (quoted in Brighton 2004, p. 308):

> A lady with a lamp shall stand
> In the great history of the land,
> A noble type of good,
> Heroic womanhood.

The 'lady with the lamp' has shone glorious and bright (and deservedly so). Her career was the result of her conviction, dedication and commitment to do something with her life, and in many ways Florence Nightingale can be seen as a values-based or congruent leader, standing by her values and beliefs and acting from the strength of her convictions, as did Elizabeth Evans.

I wonder, then, if Florence's lamp has blinded us to the many others who can rightly be called clinical heroes and values-based or congruent leaders? I believe there are indeed many, so here is some information on a few of the Marys, to remind us that there are many others who made their mark (Stanley 2007).

There were three nuns who travelled to the Crimea for whom Florence Nightingale had great respect. She was not always noted for her acceptance or patience with nurses from religious orders – she described some as being fit more for heaven than hospital (Woodham-Smith 1982). Nevertheless, she wrote generously and in complimentary tones about the care provided by Mary Clare Moore, Mary Stanislaus Jones and Mary Gonzaga Barry. The nuns worked without pay and under strict religious orders, and their desire to provide quality care often brought them into conflict with Florence, but their perseverance in the face of the conflict eventually won them her approval and admiration.

The other Mary that Florence was to encounter in the Crimea was Mary Seacole (see Chapter 4), a Jamaican Creole who travelled there unaided to care for the sick and wounded. She built a small hospital near the battlefront and successfully treated men suffering from diarrhoea, cholera, wounds and exhaustion (Brighton 2004). This Mary put herself in harm's way because she believed she could make a difference and contribute to the soldiers' welfare. I believe that she offers another fine example of a congruent leader.

Another Mary is Mary Jones, the superintendent of St John's House nursing sisterhood in London. According to Bostridge (2008, p. 427), Florence 'regularly consulted Mary Jones on all manner of nursing issues' and 'constantly deferred to the older woman's greater practical [clinical] experience'. Bostridge (2008) even suggests that the extent of her contribution to nursing matters (through Florence Nightingale) has meant that Mary Jones may have been overlooked as the real pioneer behind modern nursing. If this is the case, Mary may be an example of a congruent leader, leading from the wings with her values about collaboration and collegial support on show.

Not all the Marys that Florence Nightingale encountered survived their encounter intact. When the English Secretary of State at War Sidney Herbert suggested the establishment of a committee to recruit nurses to go the Crimean War, Florence Nightingale was accompanied by a number of other women. One of the prominent committee members was Mary Stanley, who worked with Florence to interview and prepare nurses for the trip to the Crimean Peninsula. Florence left with the first group of nurses, and Mary Stanley brought a second ship load over a few months later. By this time, Florence had established herself at Scutari Hospital and had firm control of the funds raised in England and was disinclined to share the soldiers fund or the glory or fame of the venture. Florence took some of Mary's newly arrived nurses, and after threatening to resign if Mary didn't leave, sent the other nurses and Mary away to a secondary hospital and deprived them of resources. Mary faced constant threats and snipes from Florence, and the two former friends fell out to the point that Mary had a breakdown and returned to England a few months later, leaving Florence to capture all the fame and manage the soldier's funds without oversight. When Queen Victoria decided to award a 'jewel' to the two women for their service during the war, Florence made it known (through letters to her sister) that if Mary was to get any reward or acknowledgement, she would refuse hers. Mary was never given the jewel and disappeared from the pages of history (Baylen 1974; Bostridge 2008).

This story reminds me that bullying, and conflict have never been far from the surface in the healthcare domain. One study by Lee et al. (2014) put the rate of bullying amongst nursing at 98%. While this is shocking, I am sure we have all thought, why is this so? *Graveyard Alive; A Zombie Nurse in Love* is a wonderful Canadian film that is based on a story about a shy nurse who is bullied and belittled and who gets her revenge when, as a zombie, she is able to manipulate, dominate and subsequently bully (and eat) her previous antagonists. Funny and bloody and sadly close to the mark in some places, however, zombification is not a strategy I recommend for dealing with bullies. The lesson from this film is that only by becoming a bully can we overcome bullies. And herein lies the issue embedded in the history of nursing and many others of the health professions.

Derbyshire et al.'s (2019) article, 'Nursing's Future? Eat Young. Spit out. Repeat. Endlessly' links bullying back 40-odd years when Meissner (1986) identified this theme and asked the question, 'Are we eating our young?' Although, looking at Florence Nightingale's treatment of Mary Stanley and other nurses during the Crimean War, I wonder if the link to our bullying past is more extensive?

Throughout the Crimean War, nurses fought over petty jealousies, leadership, access to resources and power, financial control, access to the soldier's souls and control of perceptions back in the UK. Letters and public information in the press carried great weight, and Florence Nightingale controlled much of this, but not all battles among her, other ladies, the nuns, the medical officers, the war department and the various aids and advisors to the Royal family and wider media were fought in destructive ways. Nursing grew from and thrived upon conflict, bitterness, jealousy and backstabbing, with one of the most bitter battles being fought between Florence Nightingale and Mary Stanley (Baylen 1974; Bostridge 2008).

Understanding how to manage and control conflict is vital if the leader's values are to be evident in their approach to leadership or if they are to be seen as values-based or congruent leaders. These are just a few of the Marys, but the reality is that there are thousands of front-line, clinical and client-focused health professionals in wards, clinics, units, operating theatres, ICUs, A&Es, community centres, rural and remote communities and surgeries, who make a difference to ordinary people by caring more than they think is wise, risking more than they think is safe, knowing more than is reasonably required, dreaming more than others think is practical, and giving more of themselves than might be considered prudent. These are values-based, values-focused or congruent leaders. They do not all carry lamps – and in reality, neither did Florence Nightingale (Stanley and Sherratt 2010) – but in my experience a lamp is not a prerequisite for excellent client care or for the recognition of a values-based congruent leader.

Clinical leaders are the genuine stars of the modern healthcare arena. Unfortunately, it is easy to lose sight of their efforts in the glare of government reform, competing political agendas, health service targets, audits, quality standard assessments, hospital and health department financial constraints or managerial burdens. Simply calling for a manager to be more compassionate will not change the foundational values the managers or leaders base their practice or leadership approach on. We need to be clear about what values are being sought and what values are vital for the delivery of quality, safe and compassionate care. However, the Marys are always there, in the shadows, in the wings, by the bedside, in the clinic, by the cot or on the road, and it is their effort, commitment, courage, teamwork, collaboration, conviction and dedication that shine brightly as a light for others to follow.

Values-Based or Congruent Leaders beyond the Ward

Throughout the book, there are clinical leaders' stories that offer examples to clarify values-based or congruent leadership from a health professional perspective and to support the theoretical foundation for why clinical leaders, who apply a values-based or congruent leadership approach, should be seen as effective leaders. Yet there are many others who can be identified as employing congruent leadership. I could have discussed the life and work of Mahatma (meaning 'great soul') Gandhi, Harriet Beecher Stowe, Nelson Mandela, Joan of Arc, Galileo Galilei, Edith Cavell, Mary Wollstonecraft, George Washington, Susan B. Anthony, Emmeline Pankhurst, Emily Murphy, Helen Keller, Odette Sansom, Oskar

Schindler, Franklin D. Roosevelt, Dian Fossey, Mairead Corrigan Maguire and Betty Williams, or many others.

I could also have discussed the actions of Rosa Parks, who refused to give up her seat to a white man on a bus in Montgomery, Alabama in 1955. A black woman, she was arrested under racially motivated laws and later, when asked to explain why she did not give up her seat, said simply, 'Our mistreatment was just not right, and I was tired of it'. Here was a congruent leader who stood (sat) for her values and beliefs, and by simply acting on those values and beliefs became a figurehead for the American civil rights movement.

Clinical leaders do no less when they refuse to continue with outdated practices when aware of evidence of better, more effective interventions, even if it means challenging traditional approaches to care or treatment. Clinical leaders do no less when they stand by a patient who voices a wish to be 'not for resuscitation' (NFR) in the face of physician or family opposition and reluctance. Clinical leaders do no less when they stand up for a student who feels bullied and ridiculed by a clinical teacher who has misunderstood, judged too early or not waited for all the relevant information when failing a student in practice. Clinical leaders do no less when they role model the value of vaccinations as a platform for stopping the spread of COVID-19 or any other pathogen. Clinical leaders do no less a hundred times a shift when they act out their values and beliefs about care and health practices as they fulfil their role in whatever clinical field or environment they are in.

Things often change when clinical leaders make a stand, but, like Rosa Parks, it is not always their intention to lead change as much as simply to make a stand. Rosa said that she was not angry, she just felt determined to take the opportunity to let it be known that she did not want to be treated this way anymore, and she had no idea how people would react to her arrest. What she did not know was that she was a leader and that she had followers. Clinical leaders often do not know this either. In the initial research study that supported the development of the theory of congruent leadership, half the clinical leaders who were identified did not recognise themselves as leaders. I suspect that the people who arrested Rosa Parks did not know they were dealing with a leader either. In the same way, I wonder if some managers, educators, organisations or departments of health recognise the leaders at work in the trenches, at the coalface or by the bedside.

However, I feel that it is vital that managers, educators, organisations, departments of health and other health practitioners do recognise the virtual army of clinical leaders who are there to drive, develop and support innovation and change, and bring about a quality health service. Organisational goals and patient-focused innovation can best be led by clinicians who are recognised and valued for the contribution they can bring to the organisation at every level, not just as facilitators of care or deliverers of treatments.

The First Step: Finding Your True Voice

Kouzes and Posner (2010) suggest that the first step on any leadership journey is to find your own true voice. What they are saying is that you have to choose your own values. The second step is to listen, observe and understand other people's values.

Personal values drive commitment. You can only commit to organisations, political action, personal ambition, professional progression or indeed anything else if there is a fit between what you are doing and what you value and believe. To lead effectively means being aware of what you believe, what your values are and where you stand. Clearly, belief alone is not enough. There must also be evidence, grown from research into clinical practice and experience. There must also be a commitment to breach the nexus of research, clinical practice and education, and a desire to be open and honest. Clinical leaders also need to act with dignity, respect and professionalism in communicating or proposing a change or innovation. They have to be resilient, courageous, compassionate, caring, calm and passionate, and have a robust sense of humour. Finally, a clinical leader should also be clinically competent, knowledgeable and visible, and act as a positive role model for the change or innovations being suggested or discussed. Once these features are established or clear, and progress is made towards their further development, it is possible to change a clinical practice standard, an in-service teaching module, a communication process, a clinical guideline, a ward routine, a departmental policy, an organisational strategy . . . the world.

Not convinced? Do some research of your own and read about Rosa Parks, Rosie Batty, Chai Jing, Alicia Garza, Patrisse Cullors and Opal Tometi and the leaders that were mentioned in the previous section, or the many others, congruent leaders all. Read on to consider the links between congruent leadership, innovation, change and quality.

Innovation, Change and Quality

Recognising the significance of values and beliefs and their impact on actions is vital, but in terms of influencing innovation, change and quality, it is also essential that clinical leaders understand the tools that can be used to facilitate change. Nurses and other health professionals in countries all over the world can be heard, sitting in tearooms or at the lunch table, discussing what is wrong with the health service, or how 'the recent changes in care delivery will have this or that impact' and 'if only they could do this or the other' or 'if only someone would listen to my view'. They complain, suggest, theorise and propose, but these ideas and opinions often go no further than that tearoom or lunch table. Sadly, what is left is a residue of disappointment, hopelessness, oppression or disenchantment with the clinical area, managers, colleagues, organisation, health service or government policy.

It could be that whining is the natural state of the hard-pressed health professional, but I do not believe that. Sometimes change or innovation is slow or resisted because health professionals have not learnt to listen to their 'true' or inner voice (Buresh and Gordon 2013) or do not understand their identity or culture (McAllister and Brien 2020) or simply have not learnt the skills associated with effectively managing or driving change and innovation, how to drive quality or the liberation of empowerment. It may also be that they are not clear about what leadership means, who can be leaders or who are recognised as leaders in clinical practice. So often, as I talk to clinically focused health professionals about leadership, the response I have had is, 'What, me? ... a leader, no . . . don't you want to talk to my manager?'

While managers might have the authority to support change, they might not have the practical or clinical insights to see what change is needed in practice or how quality can be improved. Thus, it is clinical leaders who are in an ideal position to see the change that is needed, and the value and impact that change and innovation can have for patient or client care. They may feel nevertheless that they lack the authority to take their ideas and suggestions further. Part of the proposition of this book is to point out that there are tools that clinical leaders can use to facilitate change, improve quality, and develop innovation without recourse to authority and power.

- The first lesson for clinical leaders is to know and understand the significance of their own values and beliefs.
- The second lesson is to recognise that they have followers, because followers recognise a match between the clinical leader's values and beliefs and their actions. People look to clinical leaders for clinical leadership even if the clinical leader is not aware of it.
- The third point is that change can occur and quality can be affected even without managerial power or formal authority, if clinical leaders can learn to use reflection and change management techniques, employ creativity, benefit from evidence-based approaches, network, delegate effectively, motivate others and minimise conflict. Then they can exercise considerable influence over clinical change and support substantial innovation and quality improvement.

Leadership in clinical practice need not be about vision, powerful authoritarian positions or budgetary control. Clinical leaders are the front-line, coalface, bedside doers (Stanley 2006a, 2006b, 2006c, 2008, 2009, 2010, 2011, 2012, 2014; Stanton et al. 2010; Stanley et al. 2012; Stanley et al. 2014; Scully 2015; Stanley et al. 2015; Stanley et al. 2017; Swanwick and McKimm 2017; Stanley and Stanley 2018; Stanley and Stanley 2019; Stanley 2019), and when they employ (or can learn to employ) collaborative strategies to limit conflict, approaches to motivating and influencing others and other change management and quality improvement techniques, they can be the force that will help deliver high-quality, more effective care and shape a better tomorrow for the health service (Stanley 2019).

Two Final Examples of Values-Based/Congruent Leaders

Mother Teresa

While she was not a health professional (initially), an outline of the life of Mother Teresa is offered here as another example of a congruent leader who was innovative and who changed the health and life outcomes for many people because she applied her values and beliefs to her actions.

When Agnes Gonxha Bojaxhiu (later known as Mother Teresa) set off for Darjeeling in 1929 to join the Sisters of Loreto, she was originally assigned the role of teacher at St Mary's High School, where she taught for 15 years. However, in 1946 she received what she described as 'a call from God' to give up her teaching role and 'follow Christ into the slums to serve him among the poorest of the poor'. She undertook some medical training and after many obstacles were overcome, she set up the Missionaries of Charity order, who took a fourth vow to give free help to the poorest people (the original three are poverty, chastity and obedience).

Her mission, in her words, was to 'care for the hungry, the naked, the homeless, the crippled, the blind, the lepers, all those who feel unwanted, unloved, uncared for throughout society, people that have become a burden to society and are shunned by everyone'. The first of the order's centres opened in Calcutta and from there others gradually spread across India. Mother Teresa was to be honoured with some of the world's greatest awards, but it remained her beliefs and values that centred her life. 'Love', she said, 'begins at home and it is not how much we do, but how much love we put in the action(s) that we do'. She is now acknowledged by the Catholic Church as a saint and I feel she is an example of a congruent leader. It could be argued that Mother Teresa is the very definition of a congruent leader, because her life was lived as a very testament to her values and beliefs.

Although I am not suggesting that congruent leadership is the same as religious devotion, I do believe that it is this type of leadership that clinically focused health professionals employ as they face the challenges of working in the ever-changing, increasingly difficult, financially constrained health service. Congruent leadership may not define a clinically focused leader's life, but the principles of congruent leadership do offer an explanation for how and why some health professionals do what they do and are followed in the way that they are.

Tank Man

My second example is not from a health professional perspective, but it demonstrates that congruent leadership theory can be applied across a range of areas.

On 5 June 1989, a single man dressed in a white shirt and black trousers stood defiantly before a long line of Red Army tanks as they attempted to leave Tiananmen Square in Beijing. When the tanks turned to avoid him, he stepped into their path. They turned back, again to avoid him, but again he stepped into their path. He stood his ground, until eventually the tanks' engines were turned off. The man then climbed up on the first tank and spoke to the commander. Although no one knows exactly what he said, it is reported that he chastised the tank commander for taking part in the brutal suppression (slaughter) of the protesters in Tiananmen Square.

His name is not known, nor is his fate, because at the end of the standoff he was grabbed by two men and he disappeared into the crowd that had gathered to watch. We will never know if these men were friends taking him to safety or goons taking him to a prison, or worse.

What is remarkable about this event is that although the student uprising that was a catalyst for his protest failed, the image of 'tank man' (captured on film and broadcast around the world), standing courageously before a line of lethal armaments, symbolises the raw heroism of an ordinary person and offers another example of congruent leadership.

Here was a man – not a great politician, not a military leader and not a person with assigned or titled leadership responsibility – literally standing for what he believed. He did not look on or shout his disapproval from the wings. He stood up, walked out and held his ground. He was not seeking to voice a vision or to take control and we do not even know his name. Yet *Time* magazine named him one of the 100 most influential people of the twentieth century. His influence, his leadership, came from the expression of his beliefs and values in action. He sought to defy the tanks and make a point about their inhumanity, but he did not seek to express a vision. Yet the image of him standing resolutely before the tanks in Tiananmen Square has been burnt into the global consciousness and influenced China's domestic and international policy in subtle yet significant ways. 'Tank man' is another example of a congruent leader.

Conclusion

Clinical leadership is evident in any clinical environment. It is practised by a clinical leader who is directly involved in providing nursing or other health professional care. Leaders who 'control' and manage from within offices or who fail to display values and beliefs that are in congruence with their actions are rarely seen as clinical leaders. Instead, clinical leaders are visible to their colleagues and considered to be clinically knowledgeable, skilled and competent clinicians (although not necessarily experts) who motivate and inspire others because their values, beliefs and guiding principles are on show and are recognised as such. These principles and values motivate and guide the clinical leader to act in ways that support patient/client rights and address issues of confidentiality, dignity, privacy and advocacy. When they address critical problems, face challenges and direct or provide care, it is the clinical leader's application of a values-based or congruent leadership style, based on values, beliefs and principles, that is evident.

Summary

- Clinical leaders are found in great numbers and across the spectrum of the health service.
- Clinical leaders display values-based or congruent leadership, matching their values and beliefs with their actions.
- Practitioners can be and often are congruent leaders who have gone to the edge and flown, stepped boldly in the direction of their values and beliefs or confidently stood by them.
- Conflict is evident in the healthcare area and needs to be subdued for values-based or congruent leadership to flourish.
- Values-based or congruent leaders can have a dramatic impact on the quality and initiatives that help make the health service better.
- Values-based or congruent leaders are not selling a vision or communicating a path for others to follow. They are living their vision and walking their path with conviction, commitment and determination and, whether they are aware of it or not, others see them as leaders and follow.

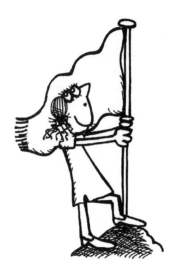

References

Baylen, J.O. (1974). The Florence nightingale/Mary Stanley controversy: some unpublished letters. *Medical History* 18 (5): 186–193.

Bostridge, M. (2004). The ladies with the lamps. *BBC History* (October), 18–19.

Bostridge, M. (2008). *Florence Nightingale: The Woman and Her Legend*. London: Penguin/Viking.

Brighton, T. (2004). *Hell Riders*. London: Viking.

Buresh, B. and Gordon, S. (2013). *From Silence to Voice: What Nurses Know and Must Communicate to the Public*, 3e. Ithaca, NY: IRL Press.

Derbyshire, P., Thompson, D.R., and Watson, R. (2019). Nursing's future? Eat young. Spit out. Repeat. Endlessly. *Journal of Nursing Management* 27: 1337–1340.

Kouzes, J.M. and Posner, B.Z. (2010). *The Truth about Leadership: The No-Fads, Heart of the Matter Facts you Need to Know*. San Francisco, CA: Jossey-Bass.

Lee, Y.J., Bernstein, K., Lee, M., and Nokes, K.M. (2014). Bullying in the nursing workplace: applying evidence using a conceptual framework. *Nursing Economics* 32 (5): 255–267.

McAllister, M. and Brien, D.L. (2020). *Paradoxes in Nurses' Identity, Culture, and Image. The Shadow Side of Nursing*. New York: Routledge.

Scully, N.J. (2015). Leadership in nursing: the importance of recognising inherent values and attributes to secure a positive future for the profession. *Collegian* 22 (4): 439–444.

Stanley, D. (2006a). Part 1: in command of care: clinical nurse leadership explored. *Journal of Research in Nursing* 2 (1): 20–39.

Stanley, D. (2006b). Part 2: in command of care: towards the theory of congruent leadership. *Journal of Research in Nursing* 2 (2): 132–144.

Stanley, D. (2006c). Recognising and defining clinical nurse leaders. *British Journal of Nursing* 15 (2): 108–111.

Stanley, D. (2007). Lights in the shadows. *Contemporary Nurse* 24 (1): 45–51.

Stanley, D. (2008). Congruent leadership: values in action. *Journal of Nursing Management* 64: 84–95.

Stanley, D. (2009). Leadership: behind the mask. *Australian College of Perioperative Nurses (ACORN)* 22 (1): 14–20.

Stanley, D. (2010). Clinical leadership and innovation. *Connections* 13 (4): 27–28.

Stanley, D. (2011). *Clinical Leadership: Innovation into Action*. Melbourne, VIC: Palgrave Macmillan.

Stanley, D. (2012). Clinical leadership and innovation. *Journal of Nursing Education and Practice* 2 (2): 119–126.

Stanley, D. (2014). Clinical leadership characteristics confirmed. *Journal of Research in Nursing* 19 (2): 118–128.

Stanley, D. (2019). *Values-Based Leadership in Healthcare: Congruent Leadership Explored*. London: Sage.

Stanley, D. and Sherratt, A. (2010). Lamp light on leadership: clinical leadership and Florence nightingale. *Journal of Nursing Management* 18: 115–121.

Stanley, D. and Stanley, K. (2018). Report: There where the "bullets can fly": Clinical Leadership in rural and remote north-western New South Wales. Research Report UNE Print ISBN: 978–64467–203-7.

Stanley, D. and Stanley, K. (2019). Clinical leadership and rural and remote practice: a qualitative study. *Journal of Nursing Management* 27 (6): 1314–1324.

Stanley, D., Cuthbertson, J., and Latimer, K. (2012). Perceptions of clinical leadership in the St. John ambulance service in WA. Paramedics Australasia. *Response* 39 (1): 31–37.

Stanley, D., Latimer, K., and Atkinson, J. (2014). Perceptions of clinical leadership in an aged care residential facility in Perth, Western Australia. *Health Care Current Reviews* 2, no. 2. http://www.esciencecentral.org/journals/perceptions-of-clinical-leadership-in-an-aged-care-residential-facility-in-perth-western-australia.hccr.1000122.php?aid=24341 (accessed 1 May 2016).

Stanley, D., Hutton, M. and McDonald, A. (2015). *Western Australian Allied Health Professionals' Perceptions of Clinical Leadership: A Research Report*, http://www.ochpo.health.wa.gov.au/docs/WA_Allied_Health_Prof_Perceptions_of_Clinical_Leadership_Research_Report.pdf (accessed 1 July 2016).

Stanley, D., Blanchard, D., Hohol, A. et al. (2017). Health professionals' perceptions of clinical leadership. A pilot study. *Cogent Medicine*. 4 (1).

Stanton, E., Lemer, C., and Mountford, J. (2010). *Clinical Leadership: Bridging the Divide*. London: Quay Books.

Swanwick, T. and McKimm, J. (2017). *ABC of Clinical Leadership*, 2e. Oxford: Wiley Blackwell.

Woodham-Smith, C. (1982). *The Reason Why*. Alexandria, VA: Time Life Books.

Index

Note: Tables are indicated by **bold** numbers. Figures are indicated by *italicized* page numbers